CHAPMAN AND NAKIELNY'S
GUIDE TO
RADIOLOGICAL
PROCEDURES

D1334239

This book is due for return on or before the last date shown below.

For Alexander and Olivia

For Elsevier
Content Strategist: Jeremy Bowes
Content Development Specialist: Helen Leng
Project Manager: Julie Taylor
Designer/Design Direction: Miles Hitchen
Illustration Manager: Jennifer Rose
Illustrator: David Gardner and Antbits Ltd

CHAPMAN AND NAKIELNY'S

GUIDE TO RADIOLOGICAL PROCEDURES

Edited by

Nick Watson MBChB MRCP FRCR
Consultant Radiologist,
University Hospital of North Staffordshire,
Stoke-on-Trent;
Senior Lecturer,
Keele University Medical School,
Keele, UK

SIXTH EDITION

SAUNDERS

ELSEVIER

Edinburgh • London • New York • Oxford • Philadelphia •
St Louis • Sydney • Toronto 2014

SAUNDERS
ELSEVIER

First edition 1981
Second edition 1986
Third edition 1993
Fourth edition 2001
Fifth edition 2009
Sixth edition 2014
  Reprinted 2015

ISBN 9780702051814
Ebook ISBN: 9780702054792

British Library Cataloguing in Publication Data
A catalogue record for this book is available from the British Library

Library of Congress Cataloging in Publication Data
A catalog record for this book is available from the Library of Congress

Notices
Knowledge and best practice in this field are constantly changing. As new research and experience broaden our understanding, changes in research methods, professional practices, or medical treatment may become necessary. Practitioners and researchers must always rely on their own experience and knowledge in evaluating and using any information, methods, compounds, or experiments described herein. In using such information or methods they should be mindful of their own safety and the safety of others, including parties for whom they have a professional responsibility. With respect to any drug or pharmaceutical products identified, readers are advised to check the most current information provided (i) on procedures featured or (ii) by the manufacturer of each product to be administered, to verify the recommended dose or formula, the method and duration of administration, and contraindications. It is the responsibility of practitioners, relying on their own experience and knowledge of their patients, to make diagnoses, to determine dosages and the best treatment for each individual patient, and to take all appropriate safety precautions.
    To the fullest extent of the law, neither the publisher nor the authors, contributors, or editors, assume any liability for any injury and/or damage to persons or property as a matter of products liability, negligence or otherwise, or from any use or operation of any methods, products, instructions, or ideas contained in the material herein.

ELSEVIER your source for books,
journals and multimedia
in the health sciences

www.elsevierhealth.com

  Working together
to grow libraries in
developing countries

The publisher's policy is to use **paper manufactured from sustainable forests**

www.elsevier.com • www.bookaid.org

Printed in China

Preface

Radiological techniques continue to evolve as the result of a combination of many factors; particularly the on-going advances in imaging hardware and software technology, and the continued refinement of the physicochemical properties of intravenous contrast media. Successive editions of this Guide have reflected this constant progress and the consequent continual evolution of our diagnostic and therapeutic armamentarium which is a central feature of our specialty. Even in the five years since the previous edition of this Guide, many routine day-to-day examinations have changed led, in particular, by advances in CT scanner technology. The barium enema, the IVP, V/Q isotope scanning and many invasive catheter angiographic examinations have now largely been replaced by their CT-based equivalents. Similar changes are seen reflecting advances in MR and ultrasound technology and radiologists continue to take on an ever-increasing role in therapeutic interventions previously the domain of the surgeon.

We set out to reflect these changes but retain the compact nature and accessible format and, therefore, the usefulness, of the Guide. All chapters have been thoroughly reviewed and, where appropriate, revised and rewritten to reflect current radiological practice, and a new chapter on patient consent has been added. As always, it is a difficult balance to ensure that current radiological practice is faithfully reflected but not to dismiss older techniques which may still be used in some centres or may continue to be required where there are contraindications to current preferred techniques such as MR imaging.

It has been a great privilege to be involved with this Guide; the 2nd edition of which rarely left my side as a junior radiologist. I hope the book continues to be a valued resource for the current generation of radiology trainees.

Nick Watson
2013

Acknowledgements

A number of new contributors have been involved in this latest edition to whom I am very grateful, but I would particularly like to acknowledge the work of previous contributors; J F C Oliff, F M Bryden, M S Moss and P C Thomas, whose chapters have been revised and updated.

I am also very grateful for the help given by colleagues, particularly; Dr John Oxtoby for reviewing the Nuclear Medicine elements of chapters 1, 7, 8 and 16; and senior radiographer colleagues Phil Andrews and Peter Sutton for their input into chapter 8.

I would like to acknowledge the great support I have had from Jeremy Bowes, Content Strategist, and Helen Leng, Content Development Specialist, at Elsevier.

Contents

Contents

Contents

List of contributors

Frances Aitchison MBChB FRCP FRCR
Consultant Radiologist, City Hospital, Birmingham; Senior
Clinical Lecturer, University of Birmingham, Birmingham, UK
Chapters 1 and 2

Victor Cassar-Pullicino FRCR
Consultant Radiologist, The Robert Jones and Agnes Hunt
Orthopaedic Hospital, Oswestry; Senior Clinical Lecturer,
University of Birmingham, Birmingham, UK
Chapters 12 and 14

Floriana Coccia MB ChB MRCPsych
Consultant Psychiatrist, Heartlands Hospital, Birmingham, UK
Chapter 20

Mark Cowling MRCP FRCR
Consultant Radiologist, University Hospital of North Staffordshire,
Stoke-on-Trent, UK
Chapters 9 and 10

Hilary Dobson FRCP FRCP
Consultant Radiologist, Clinical Director, West of Scotland Breast
Screening Service; Honorary Clinical Senior Lecturer, University of
Glasgow, Glasgow, UK
Chapter 17

Colm Forde MBBCh FRCR
Consultant Radiologist, Queen Elizabeth Hospital,
Birmingham, UK
Chapters 3 and 4

Jonathan Freedman MBChB MRCS FRCR
Consultant Radiologist, Heartlands Hospital, Birmingham, UK
Chapter 20

Peter Guest FRCP FRCR
Consultant Radiologist, Queen Elizabeth Hospital, Birmingham;
Senior Clinical Lecturer, University of Birmingham,
Birmingham, UK
Chapters 5 and 11

Amit Herwadkar MBBS FRCR
Consultant Neuroradiologist, Salford Royal Hospital, Salford, UK
Chapter 13

Arun Jacob FRCR
Consultant Radiologist, University Hospital of North Staffordshire,
Stoke-on-Trent, UK
Chapter 15

Zahid Khan MBBS DA FRCA FCCM FFICM
Consultant Anaesthesia and Critical Care, Queen Elizabeth
Hospital, Birmingham; Honorary Senior Clinical Lecturer,
University of Birmingham, Birmingham, UK
Chapters 18 and 19

Balashanmugam Rajashanker MRCP FRCR
Consultant Radiologist, Manchester Royal Infirmary and St Mary's
Hospital, Manchester, UK
Chapter 6

Polly Richards BA MBBS MRCP FRCR
Consultant Radiologist, St Bartholomew's Hospital, London, UK
Chapter 16

Nick Watson MRCP FRCR
University Hospital of North Staffordshire, Stoke-on-Trent;
Senior Lecturer, Keele University Medical School, Keele, UK
Chapters 7 and 8

General notes

RADIOLOGY

The procedures are laid out under a number of sub-headings, which follow a standard sequence. The general order is outlined below, together with certain points that have been omitted from the discussion of each procedure in order to avoid repetition. Minor deviations from this sequence will be found in the text where this is felt to be more appropriate.

Methods

A description of the technique for each procedure.

Indications

Appropriate clinical reasons for using each procedure.

Contraindications

All radiological procedures carry a risk. The risk incurred by undertaking the procedure must be balanced against the benefit to the patient as deduced from the information obtained. Contraindications may be relative (the majority) or absolute. Factors that increase the risk to the patient can be categorized under three headings: due to radiation; due to the contrast medium; due to the technique.

Risk due to radiation

Radiation effects on humans may be:

- hereditary, i.e. revealed in the offspring of the exposed individual, or
- somatic injuries, which fall into two groups: deterministic and stochastic.
  1. Deterministic effects result in loss of tissue function, e.g. skin erythema and cataracts. If the radiation dose is distributed over a period of time, cellular mechanisms allow tissue repair. There is then greater tolerance than if the dose had been administered

all at once. This implies a threshold dose above which the tissue will exhibit damage because the radiation dose exceeds the capabilities of cellular repair mechanisms.

2. Stochastic effects refer to random modifications to cell components, such as DNA mutations that can occur at any radiation dose; there is no threshold for stochastic effects.[1] Stochastic effects, such as malignancy, are 'all or none'. The cancer produced by a small dose is the same as the cancer produced by a large dose, but the frequency of occurrence is less with the smaller dose.

The current consensus held by international radiological protection organizations is that, for comparatively low doses, the risk of both radiation-induced cancer and hereditary disease is assumed to increase linearly with increasing radiation dose, with no threshold (the so-called linear no threshold model).[2] It is impossible to totally avoid staff and patient exposure to radiation. The adverse effects of radiation, therefore, cannot be completely eliminated but must be minimized. There is a small but significant excess of cancers following diagnostic levels of irradiation, e.g. during childhood[3] and to the female breast[4] and amongst those with occupational radiation exposure.[5] In the UK about 0.6% of the overall cumulative risk of cancer by the age of 75 years could be attributable to diagnostic X-rays. The most important factors which influence the risk of developing cancer after exposure to ionizing radiation are: (a) genetic considerations – specific gene mutations and family history; (b) age at exposure – children are, in general, more radiosensitive than adults; (c) sex – there is a slightly increased risk in females; (d) fractionation and protraction of exposure – higher dose and dose rate increase risk because of the influence of DNA damage.[6] (Typical average effective dose equivalents for some common examinations are given in Appendix I.)

There are legal regulations which guide the use of diagnostic radiation (see Appendices II and III). These are the two basic principles:

1. *Justification* that a proposed examination is of net benefit to the patient.
2. *ALARP* – doses should be kept *As Low As Reasonably Practicable*; economic and social factors being taken into account.[7]

Justification is particularly important when considering the irradiation of women of reproductive age, because of the risks to the developing fetus. The mammalian embryo and fetus are highly radiosensitive. The potential risks of in utero radiation exposure on a developing fetus include both teratogenic and carcinogenic effects. The risk of each effect depends on the gestational age at the time of the exposure and the absorbed radiation dose. The developing fetus is most vulnerable to radiation effects on the central nervous system between 8 and 15 weeks of gestational age and the risk of development of fatal childhood cancer may be greater if exposure occurs earlier in pregnancy.[8] The teratogenic risk of radiation is dose-dependent and exposure to ionizing radiation doses of less than 50 mGy has not been shown to be associated with different pregnancy outcomes compared with exposure to background radiation alone.[8] The carcinogenic risk of ionizing radiation is harder to calculate accurately. It is thought that the risk for the general population of developing childhood cancer is 1 in 500.[9] For a fetal radiation dose of 30 mGy the best estimate is of one excess cancer per 500 fetuses exposed,[10] resulting in a doubling of the natural rate. Most diagnostic radiation procedures will lead to a fetal absorbed dose of less than 1 mGy for imaging beyond the maternal abdomen/pelvis and less than 10 mGy for direct abdominal/pelvic or nuclear medicine imaging. There are important exceptions which result in higher doses, such as CT scanning of the maternal pelvis.

Almost always, if a diagnostic radiology examination is medically indicated, the risk to the mother of not doing the procedure is greater than the risk of potential harm to the fetus. However, whenever possible, alternative investigation techniques not involving ionizing radiation should be considered before a decision to use ionizing radiation in a female of reproductive age is taken. It is extremely important to have a robust process in place that prevents inappropriate or unnecessary ionizing radiation exposure to the fetus. Joint guidance from the Health Protection Agency, the College of Radiographers and the Royal College of Radiologists recommends the following:[9]

When a female of reproductive age presents for an examination in which the primary beam irradiates the pelvic area, or for a procedure involving radioactive isotopes, she should be asked whether she is or might be pregnant. If the patient cannot exclude the possibility of pregnancy, she should be asked if her menstrual period is overdue. Her answer should be recorded and, depending on the answer, the patient assigned to one of the following four groups:

1. **No possibility of pregnancy** – proceed with the examination.
2. **Patient definitely, or probably, pregnant** – review the justification for the proposed examination and decide whether to defer until after delivery, bearing in mind that delaying an essential procedure until later in pregnancy may present a greater risk to the fetus and a procedure of clinical benefit to the mother may also be of indirect benefit to her unborn child. If, after review, a procedure is still considered to be justified and is undertaken the fetal dose should be kept to the minimum consistent with the diagnostic purpose.

3. **Low-dose examination, pregnancy cannot be excluded** – a low-dose examination is defined as one in which the fetal dose is likely to be below 10 mGy. The vast majority of diagnostic examinations fall into this category. If pregnancy cannot be excluded but the patient's menstrual period is not overdue, proceed with the examination. If the period is overdue, the patient should be treated as probably pregnant and the advice in the section above followed.

4. **High-dose examination, pregnancy cannot be excluded** – a high-dose procedure is defined as any examination which results in a fetal dose greater than 10 mGy (e.g. CT of the maternal abdomen and pelvis). The evidence suggests that such procedures may double the natural risk of childhood cancer if carried out after the first 3–4 weeks of pregnancy and may still involve a small risk of cancer induction if carried out in the very early stages of an unrecognized pregnancy. Either of two courses can be adopted to minimize the likelihood of inadvertent exposure of an unrecognized pregnancy: (a) apply the rule that females of childbearing potential are always booked for these examinations during the first 10 days of their menstrual cycle when conception is unlikely to have occurred; or (b) female patients of childbearing potential are booked in the normal way but are not examined and are re-booked if, when they attend, they are in the second half of their menstrual cycle *and* are of childbearing potential *and* in whom pregnancy cannot be excluded.

If the examination is necessary, evaluation of the fetal dose and associated risks by a medial physicist should be arranged, if possible, and discussed with the parents. A technique that minimizes the number of views and the absorbed dose per examination should be utilized. However, the quality of the examination should not be reduced to the level where its diagnostic value is impaired. The risk to the patient of an incorrect diagnosis may be greater than the risk of irradiating the fetus. Radiography of areas that are remote from the pelvis and abdomen may be safely performed during pregnancy with good collimation and lead protection. Royal College of Radiologists guidelines indicate that legal responsibility for radiation protection lies with the employer, the extent to which this responsibility is delegated to the individual radiologist varies. Nonetheless, all clinical radiologists carry a responsibility for the protection from unnecessary radiation of:

- patients
- themselves
- other members of staff
- members of the public, including relatives and carers.[11]

Risk due to the contrast medium
The risks associated with administration of iodinated contrast media and magnetic resonance imaging (MRI) contrast are

discussed in detail in Chapter 2 and guidelines are given for prophylaxis of adverse reactions to intravascular contrast.

Contraindications to other contrast media, e.g. barium, water-soluble contrast media for the gastrointestinal tract and biliary contrast media, are given in the relevant sections.

Risks due to the technique

Skin sepsis can occur at the needle puncture site.

Specific contraindications to individual techniques are discussed with each procedure.

Contrast medium

Volumes given are for a 70-kg man.

Equipment

For many procedures this will also include a trolley with a sterile upper shelf and a non-sterile lower shelf. Emergency drugs and resuscitation equipment should be readily available (see Chapter 17).

See Chapter 9 for introductory notes on angiography catheters.

If only a simple radiography table and overcouch tube are required, then this information has been omitted from the text.

Patient preparation

1. Will admission to hospital be necessary?
2. If the patient is a woman of child-bearing age, the examination should be performed at a time when the risks to a possible fetus are minimal (see above). Any female presenting for radiography or a nuclear medicine examination at a time when her period is known to be overdue should be considered to be pregnant unless there is information indicating the absence of pregnancy. If her cycle is so irregular that it is difficult to know whether a period has been missed and it is not practicable to defer the examination until menstruation occurs, then a pregnancy test or pelvic ultrasound (US) examination may help to determine whether she is pregnant. Particular care should be taken to perform hysterosalpingography during the first 10 days of the menstrual cycle, so that the risks of mechanical trauma to an early pregnancy are reduced.
3. Except in emergencies, in circumstances when consent cannot be obtained, patient consent to treatment is a legal requirement for medical care.[12] Consent should be obtained in a suitable environment and only after appropriate and relevant information has been given to the patient.[13] Patient consent may be:
   (a) implied consent – for a very low-risk procedure, the patient's actions at the time of the examination will indicate whether they are content for the procedure to be performed
   (b) express consent – for a procedure of intermediate risk, such as barium enema, express consent should be given by the patient, either verbally or in writing

(c) written consent – must be obtained for any procedure that involves significant risk and/or side effects. The ability to consent depends more on a person's ability to understand and weigh up options than on age. At 16 a young person can be treated as an adult and can be presumed to have the capacity to understand the nature, purpose and possible consequences of the proposed investigation, as well as the consequences of non-investigation. Under the age of 16 years children may have the capacity to consent depending on their maturity and ability to understand what is involved. The radiologist must assess a child's capacity to decide whether to give consent for, or refuse an investigation. If the child lacks the capacity to consent, the parent's consent should be sought. It is usually sufficient to have consent from one parent. If the parents cannot agree, legal advice should be obtained.[14] When a competent child refuses treatment, a person with parental responsibility or the court may authorize investigations or treatment which is in the child's best interests. In Scotland the situation is different: parents cannot authorize procedures a competent child has refused. Legal advice may be helpful in dealing with these cases.

4. If an interventional procedure carries a risk of causing bleeding then the patient's blood clotting should be measured before proceeding. If a bleeding disorder is discovered, or if the patient is being treated with anticoagulant therapy, the appropriate steps should be taken to normalize clotting before performing the procedure.

5. Cleansing bowel preparation may be used prior to investigation of the gastrointestinal tract or when considerable fecal loading obscures other intra-abdominal organs. For other radiological investigations of abdominal organs, bowel preparation is not always necessary, and when given may result in excessive bowel gas. Bowel gas may be reduced if the patient is kept ambulant prior to the examination and those who routinely take laxatives should continue to do so.

6. Previous films and notes should be obtained.

7. Premedication will be necessary for painful procedures or where the patient is unlikely to cooperate for any other reason. Suggested premedication for adults and children is described in Chapter 18.

Preliminary images

The purpose of these films is:

1. to make any final adjustments in exposure factors, centring, collimation and patient position, for which purpose the film should

always be taken using the same equipment as will be used for the remainder of the procedure

2. to exclude prohibitive factors such as residual barium from a previous examination or excessive fecal loading
3. to demonstrate, identify and localize opacities which may be obscured by contrast medium
4. to elicit radiological physical signs.

Every radiographic view taken should have on it the patient's name, registration number, date and a side marker. The examination can only proceed if satisfactory preliminary films have been obtained.

Technique

1. For aseptic technique the skin is cleaned with chlorhexidine 0.5% in 70% industrial spirit or its equivalent.
2. The local anaesthetic used is lidocaine 1% without adrenaline (epinephrine).
3. Gonad protection is used whenever possible, unless it obscures the region of interest.

Images

When films are taken during the procedure rather than at the end of it, they have, for convenience, been described under 'Technique'.

Additional techniques *or* modifications of technique

Aftercare

May be considered as:

1. instructions to the patient
2. instructions to the ward.

Complications

Complications may be considered under the following three headings:

Due to the anaesthetic

1. General anaesthesia
2. Local anaesthesia:
   (a) allergic – unusual
   (b) toxic.

Anaesthetic lozenges contribute to the total dose. Symptoms of excessive dose are of paraesthesia and muscle twitching which may progress to convulsions, cardiac arrhythmias, respiratory depression and death due to cardiac arrest. Treatment is symptomatic and includes adequate oxygenation.

Due to the contrast medium

- Intravascular contrast media (see Chapter 2)
- Barium (see Chapter 3).

Due to the technique

Specific details are given with the individual procedures and may be conveniently classified as:

1. local
2. distant or generalized.

References

1. Tramblay E, Thérasse E, Thomassin-Nagarra E, et al. Quality initiatives: Guidelines for use of medical imaging during pregnancy and lactation. Radiographics 2012;32:897–911.
2. Wakeford R. Cancer risk modelling and radiological protection. J Radiol Prot 2012;32(1):N89–93.
3. Pearce MS, Salotti JA, Little MP, et al. Radiation exposure from CT scans in childhood and subsequent risk of leukaemia and brain tumours: a retrospective cohort study. Lancet 2012;380(9840):499–505.
4. Einstein AJ, Henzlova MJ, Rajagopalan S. Estimating risk of cancer associated with radiation exposure from 64-slice computed tomography coronary angiography. JAMA 2007;298(3):317–23.
5. Muirhead CR, O'Hagan JA, Haylock RGE, et al. Mortality and cancer incidence following occupational radiation exposure: third analysis of the National Registry for Radiation Workers. Br J Cancer 2009;100(1): 206–12.
6. Hricak HH, Brenner DJ, Adelstein SJ, et al. Managing radiation use in medical imaging: a multifaceted challenge. Radiology 2011;258:889–905.
7. International Commission on Radiological Protection. The optimization of radiological protection: broadening the process. ICRP publication 101. Ann ICRP 2006;36(3):69–104.
8. Wang PI, Chong ST, Kielar AZ, et al. Imaging of pregnant and lactating patients: Evidence-based review and recommendations, Parts 1 and 2. Am J Roentgenol 2012;198:778–92.
9. Advice from the Health Protection Agency, The Royal College of Radiologists and the College of Radiographers. Protection of Pregnant Patients during Diagnostic Medical Exposures to Ionising Radiation www.rcr.uk/docs/radiology/pdf/HPA_Diagnostic_Pregnancy.pdf; 2009.
10. International Commission on Radiological Protection. Pregnancy and medical radiation. Ann ICRP 2000;30(1):1–43.
11. Royal College of Radiologists. Good Practice Guide for Clinical Radiologists. 2nd ed. London, www.rcr.ac.uk/docs/radiology/pdf/BFCR(12)1_GoodPractice.pdf; 2012.
12. The Royal College of Radiologists. Standards for Patient Consent Particular to Radiology. London: The Royal College of Radiologists; 2005, BFCR(07)8.
13. General Medical Council. Consent: Patients and Doctors Making Decisions Together. London: General Medical Council; 2008.
14. General Medical Council. 0–18 years: Guidance for all Doctors. London: General Medical Council; 2007.

RADIONUCLIDE IMAGING

RADIOPHARMACEUTICALS

Radionuclides are shown in symbolic notation, the most frequently used in nuclear medicine being ^{99m}Tc, a 140-keV gamma-emitting radioisotope of the element technetium with $T_{1/2} = 6.0$ hours.

Radioactive injections

In the UK, the Administration of Radioactive Substances Advisory Committee (ARSAC) advises the health ministers on the Medicines (Administration of Radioactive Substances) Regulations 1978 (MARS). These require that radioactive materials may only be administered to humans by a doctor or dentist holding a current ARSAC certificate or by a person acting under their direction. Administration of radioactive substances can only be carried out by an individual who has received appropriate theoretical and practical training, as specified in the Ionising Radiation (Medical Exposure) Regulations 2000[1] (see Appendix III). These will place responsibilities on the referrer to provide medical data to justify the exposure, the practitioner (ARSAC licence holder) to justify individual exposure, and operators (persons who carry out practical aspects relating to the exposure).

Activity administered

The maximum activity values quoted in the text are those currently recommended as diagnostic reference levels in the ARSAC Guidance Notes.[2] The unit used is the SI unit, the megabecquerel (MBq). Millicuries (mCi) are still used in some countries, notably the US; 1 mCi = 37 MBq.

Radiation doses are quoted as the adult effective dose (ED) in millisieverts (mSv) from the ARSAC Guidance Notes.

The regulations require that doses to patients are kept as low as reasonably practicable (the ALARP principle) and that exposure follows accepted practice. Centres will frequently be able to administer activities below the maximum, depending upon the capabilities of their equipment and local protocols. Typical figures are given in the text where they differ from the diagnostic reference levels. In certain circumstances, the person clinically directing (ARSAC licence holder) may use activity higher than the recommended maximum for a named patient, for example for an obese patient where attenuation would otherwise degrade image quality.

ARSAC recommends that activities administered for paediatric investigations should be reduced according to body weight, but no longer in a linear relationship. The guidance notes include a table of suggested scaling factors based on producing comparable quality images to those expected for adults, with a minimum activity of 10% of the adult value for most purposes. However, organs develop at different rates (e.g. the brain achieves 95% of its adult size by age 5 years) and some radiopharmaceuticals behave differently in children, so the administered activity may need to be adjusted accordingly. It should be noted that when scaling activity according to the suggested factors, the radiation dose for a child may be higher than that for an adult.

Equipment

Gamma cameras usually have one or two imaging heads. Double-headed systems have the advantage of being able to image two sites simultaneously, which in many cases can roughly halve the imaging time. This can be a great advantage for SPECT (single-photon emission computed tomography) scans where minimizing patient movement can be critical.

Recent developments on double-headed systems include transmission line sources for measured attenuation correction, and coincidence imaging systems for PET (positron emission tomography). Hybrid systems are now available where multislice CT forms part of an integrated system as a single machine with either a double-headed gamma camera (SPECT-CT) or a PET scanner (PET-CT). Amongst a number of advantages is the better anatomical localization of abnormal areas of activity on co-registered or fused images.

All gamma cameras are now supplied with imaging computer systems, and the text assumes that all images are acquired by the computer for appropriate processing.

Technique

Patient positioning

The resolution of gamma camera images is critically dependent upon the distance of the collimator surface from the patient, falling off approximately linearly with distance. Every effort should, therefore, be made to position the camera as close to the patient as possible. For example, in posterior imaging with the patient supine, the thickness of the bed separates the patient from the camera, as well as interposing an attenuating medium. In this case, imaging with the patient sitting or standing directly against the camera is preferable.

Patient immobilization for the duration of image acquisition is very important. If a patient is uncomfortable or awkwardly positioned, they will have a tendency to move gradually and perhaps imperceptibly, which will have a blurring effect on the image. Point marker sources attached to the patient away from areas being examined can help to monitor and possibly permit correction for movement artefact.

Images

The image acquisition times quoted in the text should only be considered an approximate guide since the appropriate time will depend upon such factors as the sensitivity of the available equipment, the amount of activity injected and the size of the patient. An acceptable acquisition time will usually be a compromise between the time available, the counts required for a diagnostic image and the ability of the patient to remain motionless.

Aftercare

Radiation safety

Special instructions should be given to patients who are breastfeeding regarding expression of milk and interruption of feeding.[2] Precautions may have to be taken with patients leaving hospital or returning to wards, depending upon the radionuclide and activity administered. These precautions were reviewed following the introduction of the Ionising Radiation Regulations 1999 and the adoption of lower dose limits to members of the public, and appropriate guidance has been published.[3]

Complications

With few exceptions (noted in the text), the amount of biologically active substance injected with radionuclide investigations is at trace levels and very rarely causes any systemic reactions. Those that may occasionally cause problems are labelled blood products, antibodies and substances of a particulate nature.

References

1. The Ionising Radiation (Medical Exposure) Regulations. London: HMSO; 2000.
2. Administration of Radioactive Substances Advisory Committee. Notes for Guidance on the Clinical Administration of Radiopharmaceuticals and use of Sealed Radioactive Sources. Didcot: NRPB; 1998.
3. Working Party of the Radiation Protection Committee of the British Institute of Radiology. Patients leaving hospital after administration of radioactive substances. Br J Radiol 1999;72:121–5.

COMPUTED TOMOGRAPHY

Patient preparation

Many CT examinations require little physical preparation. An explanation of the procedure, the time it is likely to take, the necessity for immobility and the necessity for breath-holding whilst scanning chest and abdomen should be given. Waiting times should be kept to a minimum, as a long wait may increase anxiety. The patient should be as pain-free as is practical but too heavy sedation or analgesia may be counter-productive – patient cooperation is often required. Children under the age of 4 years will usually need sedation (see Chapter 18). Children should also have an intravenous (i.v.) cannula inserted at the time sedation is administered or local anaesthetic cream applied to two sites if i.v. contrast medium is needed. If these simple steps are taken, the number of aborted scans will be reduced and the resultant image quality improved.

Intravenous contrast medium

Many CT examinations will require i.v. contrast medium. Essential information should be obtained from the patient and appropriate guidelines followed (see Chapter 2). An explanation of the need for contrast enhancement should be given to the patient.

The dose of contrast (using 300 mg I ml^{-1}) will depend on the area examined: e.g. head – 50 ml; chest or abdomen – 100 ml, usually given at 2 ml s^{-1}. The chest is usually scanned at 20 s after the start of the contrast injection. For arterial phase images of the abdomen or pelvis the acquisition of the scan is usually begun 30 s after the start of the contrast injection and for portal venous phase images 60 s after the start of the contrast injection. For CT angiography, a technique of bolus tracking may be used where the density of contrast in the vessel is monitored directly during the injection to allow optimum acquisition timing. In children a maximum total iodinated contrast dose of 2 ml kg^{-1} body weight (300 mg I ml^{-1}) should be observed.

Oral contrast medium

For examinations of the abdomen, opacifying the bowel satisfactorily can be problematic. Plain water is recommended as a negative oral contrast medium for CT of the stomach and duodenum. Satisfactory opacification of the small and large bowel can be problematic. Water-soluble contrast medium (e.g. 20 ml Urografin 150 diluted in 1 l of orange squash to disguise the taste, preflavoured contrast such as 20 ml Gastromiro diluted in 1 l of water) or low-density barium suspensions (2% w/v) can be used. Timing of administration is given in Table 1.1. Doses of contrast media in children depend upon age.

Pelvic scanning

Rarely, it may be necessary to opacify the rectum using direct instillation of contrast medium or air via catheter. The concentration of contrast medium should be the same as for oral

Table 1.1 Timing and volume for oral contrast medium in CT

	Volume (ml)	Time before scan (min)
Adult		
Full abdomen and pelvis	1000	Gradually over 1 h before scanning
Upper abdomen, e.g. pancreas	500	Gradually over 0.5 h before scanning
Child		
Newborn	60–90	Full dose 1 h before scanning and a further half dose immediately prior to the scan
1 month–1 year	120–240	
1–5 years	240–360	
5–10 years	360–480	
Over 10 years	As for adult	

If the large bowel needs to be opacified then give the contrast medium the night before or 3–4 h before scanning

administration; 150 ml is adequate. Air contained within a vaginal tampon can be used to produce good negative contrast.

CT colonography

This requires thorough cleansing preparation of the large bowel and insufflation of air via a rectal catheter to adequately distend the colon during the examination.

MAGNETIC RESONANCE IMAGING

Patient preparation

As for CT scanning, a full description of the purpose and nature of the examination should be given to the patient and waiting times kept to a minimum. Some patients find the interior of the scanner a very disconcerting environment, and report claustrophobic and even acute anxiety symptoms. This may occur in as many as 10% of patients. Most of these patients are able to complete their examination, but approximately 1% of investigations may have to be curtailed as a result. To decrease the number of scans aborted, the counselling of, explanation to and reassurance of patients by well-trained staff should be routine. A small number of adult patients may require sedation before an MRI scan is undertaken. Sedation or general anaesthesia is often required for MRI scans in young children; details of suggested protocols are given in Chapter 18.

If i.v. contrast is required it is extremely helpful to insert the i.v. cannula before the examination begins. It is critically important that detailed preparation regarding patient safety is made for each MRI examination.

SAFETY IN MAGNETIC RESONANCE IMAGING

MRI has generally been a very safe process because of the care taken by equipment manufacturers and MRI staff. However, there are significant potential hazards to patients and staff due to:

1. electomagnetic fields:
   (a) static magnetic field
   (b) gradient magnetic field
   (c) radiofrequency field
2. the auditory effects of noise
3. inert gas quench
4. claustrophobia
5. i.v. contrast agents (see Chapter 2).

Effects due to magnetic fields

Static field
The strength of the static magnetic field used in MRI is measured in units of gauss or tesla (10 000 gauss = 1 tesla (T)). The earth's magnetic field is approximately 0.6 gauss.

Biological effects
Despite extensive research, no significant deleterious physiological effects have yet been proven.[1] There have been reports of temporary minor changes, such as alteration in electrocardiogram (T-wave elevation) presumed to be due to electrodynamic forces on moving ions in blood vessels which might result in a reduction of blood-flow velocity. Temporary and dose-correlated vertigo and nausea in patients exposed to static fields higher than 2 T have been found.[2] However, studies of volunteers exposed to 8 T static magnetic fields have shown no clinically significant effect on heart rate, respiratory rate, systolic and diastolic blood pressure, finger pulse oxygenation levels and core body temperature.[3] Teratogenesis in humans is thought unlikely at the field strengths used in clinical MRI.

Non-biological effects
There are two main areas of concern:

1. Ferromagnetic materials may undergo rotational or translational movement as a result of the field. Rotational movement occurs as a result of an elongated object trying to align with the field. This may result in displacement of the object, and applies to certain types of surgical clip. Not all materials implanted are ferromagnetic and many are only weakly so. Each type should be checked

1

individually for any such risk. In many cases, postoperative fibrosis (greater than 6 weeks) is strong enough to anchor the material so that no danger of displacement exists. Translational movement occurs when loose ferromagnetic objects are attracted to the field. Objects such as paperclips or hairgrips may reach considerable speeds and could potentially cause severe damage to patient or equipment, the so-called missile effect. In general, no object or equipment should be brought into the MRI environment unless it is proven to be:

- MRI safe (no known hazard in all MRI environments) or
- MRI conditional (no known hazard in a specified MRI environment with specified conditions of use).[4]

The safety of MRI conditional items must be verified with the specific scanner and MRI environment in which they are to be used.

2. Electrical devices such as cardiac pacemakers may be affected by static field strengths. Most modern pacemakers have a sensing mechanism that can be bypassed by a magnetically operated relay triggered by fields as low as 5 gauss. Relay closure can be expected in virtually all conventional cardiac pacemakers placed in the bore of the magnet and these patients must not enter the controlled MRI area. Recent engineering advances have produced the first generation of MRI conditional cardiac pacemaker devices but great care must still be taken.[5]

Gradient field

Biological effects

The rapidly switched magnetic gradients used in MRI can induce electric fields in a patient which may result in nerve or muscle stimulation, including cardiac muscle stimulation. The strength of these is dependent on the rate of change of the field and the size of the subject.[6] Studies have shown that the threshold for peripheral nerve stimulation is lower than that for cardiac or brain stimulation.[7] Although possible cardiac fibrillation or brain stimulation are major safety issues, peripheral nerve stimulation is a practical concern because, if sufficiently intense, it can be intolerable and result in termination of the examination. Recommendations for safety limits on gradient fields state that the system must not have a gradient output that exceeds the limit for peripheral nerve stimulation.[6] This will protect against cardiac fibrillation.

Non-biological effects

Rapidly varying fields can induce currents in conductors. Metal objects may heat up rapidly and cause tissue damage. Instances of partial- and full-thickness burns, arising when conducting loops (e.g. ECG electrodes or surface imaging coils) have come into contact with skin, are well recorded.

Radiofrequency field

Radiofrequency energy at frequencies above 10 MHz, deposited in the body during an MRI examination, will be converted to heat, which will be distributed by connective heat transfer through blood flow. Energy deposited in this way is calculated as the average energy dissipated in the body per unit of mass and time, the specific absorption rate (SAR). SAR values are dependent on the magnetic field strength and may be fourfold higher in a 3-T scanner than a 1.5-T scanner.[8] Guidelines on radiofrequency exposure are designed to limit the rise in temperature of the skin, body core and local tissue to levels below those where systemic heat overload or thermal-induced local tissue damage occur. The extent to which local temperature rises depends on the SAR and on the blood flow and vascularity of the tissue. Areas of particular concern include those most sensitive to heat such as the hypothalamus and poorly perfused regions such as the lens of the eye.

For whole-body exposures, no adverse health effects are expected if the increase in body core temperature does not exceed 1°C. In the case of infants and those with circulatory impairment, the temperature increase should not exceed 0.5°C. With regard to localized heating temperatures, measured temperature in focal regions of the head should be less than 38°C, of the trunk less than 39°C, and in the limbs less than 40°C.[6]

Noise

During imaging, noise arises from vibration in the gradient coils and other parts of the scanner due to the varying magnetic fields. The amplitude of this noise depends on the strength of the magnetic fields, pulse sequence and scanner design.

Noise levels may reach as much as 95 dB for long periods of time. This level is greater than agreed noise limits in industry. Temporary or even permanent hearing loss has been reported.

Where noise levels are excessive the use of earplugs or headphones is advised.

Inert gas quench

Where superconducting magnets are used the coolant gases, liquid helium or nitrogen, could vaporize should the temperature inadvertently rise. This could potentially lead to asphyxiation or exposure to extreme cold resulting in frostbite. To prevent this, a well-ventilated room with some form of oxygen monitor to raise an alarm should be installed.

Intravenous contrast medium

See Chapter 2.

Table 1.2 Questions which should be included in a screening questionnaire for magnetic resonance imaging patients and staff

Question to patient or staff member	Action
Do you have a pacemaker or have you had a heart operation?	Pacemaker – if present patient must not enter controlled area Heart operation – establish if any metal valve prosthesis, intravascular device or recent metallic surgical clip insertion and check MR compatibility
Could you possibly be pregnant?	See text
Have you ever had any penetrating injury, especially to the eyes, even if it was years ago?	Establish details. If necessary arrange X-ray of orbits or relevant area to determine if there is any metallic foreign body
Have you ever had any operations to your head, chest or neck?	Find out details. If any metallic aneurysm or haemostatic clips or metallic prosthesis/implant then check MR compatibility
Do you have any joint replacements or any other body implants?	Check details of surgery and MR compatibility of joint replacement or implant
Have you removed all metal objects and credit cards from your clothing and possessions?	This must be done before entering the controlled area

Recommendations for safety

Detailed MRI safety recommendations have been published by the American College of Radiology.[9] It is essential that all MRI units have clear MRI safety policies and protocols, including a detailed screening questionnaire for all patients and staff (Table 1.2).

Controlled and restricted access

Access to the scanning suite should be limited. Areas should be designated as restricted (5 gauss line) and, closer to the scanner, controlled (10 gauss line). No patient with a pacemaker should be allowed to enter the restricted area. Any person who enters this area should be made aware of the hazards; in particular the 'missile effect'. Any person entering the controlled area should remove all loose ferromagnetic materials, such as paperclips and pens, and it is advisable that wristwatches and any magnetic tape or credit cards do not come near the magnet. Other considerations include the use of specially adapted cleaning equipment, wheelchairs and trolleys. Fire extinguishers and all anaesthetic or monitoring equipment must be constructed from non-ferromagnetic materials.

Implants

As mentioned above, persons with pacemakers must not enter the restricted area. All other persons must be screened to ensure there is no danger from implanted ferromagnetic objects, such as aneurysm clips, prosthetic heart valves, intravascular devices or orthopaedic implants. Where an object is not known to be 'MRI safe' or 'MRI conditional', then the person should not be scanned. Lists of safe and unsafe implants are available[10] and should be consulted for each individual object.

Specific questioning is also advisable to assess the risk of shrapnel and intraocular foreign bodies.

Pregnancy

The developing fetus and embryo are susceptible to a variety of teratogens, including heat, being most sensitive during organogenesis. Increased static magnetic field strength, flip angle or number of radiofrequency pulses and decreased spacing between pulses will increase the SAR and therefore the radiofrequency energy deposited as heat on the fetus.[11] Although no conclusive evidence of teratogenesis exists in humans, scanning should be avoided, particularly during the first trimester, unless alternative diagnostic procedures would involve the exposure of the fetus to ionizing radiation. Before a pregnant patient is accepted for an MRI examination, a risk–benefit analysis of the request should be made. Pregnant staff members are advised to remain outside the controlled area (10 gauss line) and to avoid exposure to gradient or RF fields.

MRI contrast agents should only be used during pregnancy with extreme caution[11] (see Chapter 2).

Occupational exposure

The safety of MRI workers is regulated by the EU Medical Devices Directive (amend. Direct 93/42/EEC) and established safety standards have been set by the International Electrotechnical Commission (IEC/EN 60601-2-33, 2nd amendment 2007).

References

1. Hartwig V, Giovannetti G, Vanello N, et al. Biological effects and safety in magnetic resonance imaging: a review. Int J Res Public Health 2009;6(6):1778–98.
2. De Vocht F, Stevens T, van Wendel De Joode B, et al. Acute neurobehavioral effects of exposure to static magnetic fields: analysis of exposure–response relations. J Magn Reson Imaging 2006;23:291–7.

3. Chakeres DW, Kangarlu A, Boudoulas H, et al. Effect of static magnetic field exposure of up to 8T on sequential human vital sign measurements. J Mag Res Imaging 2003;18(3):346–52.

4. Shellock FG, Spinazzi A. MRI Safety Update 2008: Part 2, Screening Patients for MRI. Am J Roentgenol 2008;191(4):1140–9.

5. Shinbane JS, Colletti PM, Shellock FG. Magnetic resonance imaging in patients with cardiac pacemakers: era of "MR Conditional" designs. J Cardiovasc Magn Reson 2011;13(1):63.

6. The International Commission on Non-Ionizing Radiation Protection. Medical magnetic resonance (MR) procedures: protection of patients. Health Physics 2004;87(2):197–216.

7. Nyenhuis JA, Bourland JD, Kildishev AV, et al. Health effects and safety of intense gradient fields. In: Shellock FG, editors. Magnetic Resonance Procedures: Health Effects and Safety. New York: CRC Press; 2001. p. 31–53.

8. Chavhan GB, Babyn PS, Singh M, et al. MR imaging at 3.0T in children: technical differences, safety issues, and initial experience. RadioGraphics 2009;29(5):1451–66.

9. Kanal E, Barkovich AJ, Bell C, et al. ACR guidance document for safe MR practices. Am J Roentgenol 2007;188(6):1447–74.

10. Shellock FG. Reference Manual for Magnetic Resonance Safety, Implants, and devices. Los Angeles: Biomedical Research Publishing Company; or www.mrisafety.com; 2007.

11. Wang PI, Chong ST, Kielar AZ, et al. Imaging of pregnant and lactating patients: Part 1, Evidence-based review and recommendations Am J Roentgenol 2012;198(4):778–84.

Further Reading
Allisy-Roberts P, Williams J, editors. Magnetic resonance imaging. In: Farr's Physics for Medical Imaging. 2nd ed. Edinburgh, UK: Saunders; 2007.

ULTRASONOGRAPHY

Patient preparation

For many US examinations no preparation is required. This includes examination of tissues such as thyroid, breast, testes, musculoskeletal, vascular and cardiac. In certain situations simple preparatory measures are required.

Abdomen

For optimal examination of the gallbladder it should be dilated. This requires fasting for 6–8 h before scanning. If detailed assessment of the pancreas is required it can be helpful to have clear fluid filling the stomach, which can then act as a transonic 'window'.

Pelvis

To visualize the pelvic contents optimally, bowel gas must be displaced. This is easily accomplished by filling the urinary bladder to capacity. This then acts as a transonic 'window'. The patient should be instructed to drink 1–2 pints of water during the hour prior to scanning and to not empty their bladder. In practice, both abdominal and pelvic scanning are often performed at the same attendance. Oral intake of clear fluids will not provoke gallbladder emptying and so the two examinations can be combined. However, it should be noted that in normal subjects who drink a large volume of oral fluid prior to the scan to fill their bladder, the renal collecting systems may appear slightly dilated. If this is the case, the patient should be asked to empty their bladder and the kidneys rescanned. If the renal collecting system dilatation is significant it will persist after the bladder is emptied.

Endoscopic

Endoscopic examination of rectum or vagina requires no physical preparation but an explanation of the procedure in a sympathetic manner is needed.

Examination of the oesophagus or transoesophageal echocardiography requires preparation similar to upper gastrointestinal endoscopy. The patient should be starved for 4 h prior to the procedure to minimize the risk of vomiting, reflux and aspiration. Anaesthesia and sedation are partly a matter of personal preference of the operator. Local anaesthesia of the pharynx can be obtained using 10% lidocaine spray. Care to avoid overdose is essential as lidocaine is rapidly absorbed via this route. The maximum dose of lidocaine should not exceed 200 mg; the xylocaine spray metered dose applicator delivers 10 mg lidocaine per dose. Sedation using i.v. benzodiazepines such as Diazemuls 10 mg or midazolam 2–5 mg may also be necessary. If local anaesthetic has been used then the patient must be instructed to avoid hot food and drink until the effect has worn off (1–2 h).

Children

US examination in children can, in most cases, be performed with no preparation apart from explanation and reassurance to both child and parent. In some cases where the child is excessively frightened or where immobility is required, sedation may be necessary. With echocardiography in infants, sedation is essential to obtain optimal recordings. The sedation regimens described in Chapter 18 may be used.

2

Intravascular contrast media

HISTORICAL DEVELOPMENT OF RADIOGRAPHIC AGENTS

The first report of opacification of the urinary tract after intravenous (i.v.) injection of a contrast agent appeared in 1923 using an i.v. injection of 10% sodium iodide solution, which was at that time prescribed for treatment of syphilis and was excreted in the urine. In 1928 German researchers synthesized a compound with a number of pyridine rings containing iodine in an effort to detoxify the iodine. This mono-iodinated compound was developed further into di-iodinated compounds and subsequently in 1952 the first tri-iodinated compound, sodium acetrizoate (Urokon), was introduced into clinical radiology. Sodium acetrizoate was based on a 6-carbon ring structure, tri-iodo benzoic acid, and was the precursor of all modern water-soluble contrast media.

Until the early 1970s all contrast media were ionic compounds and were hypertonic with osmolalities of 1200–2000 mosmol kg^{-1} water, 4–7 × the osmolarity of blood. These are referred to as high osmolar contrast media (HOCM) and distinguished by differences at position 5 of the anion and by the cations sodium and/or meglumine. In 1969 Almén first postulated that many of the adverse effects of contrast media were the result of high osmolality and that by eliminating the cation, which does not contribute to diagnostic information but is responsible for up to 50% of the osmotic effect, it would be possible to reduce the toxicity of contrast media.

Conventional ionic contrast media had a ratio of three iodine atoms per molecule to two particles in solution, i.e. a ratio of $3:2$ or 1.5 (Table 2.1). In order to decrease the osmolality without changing the iodine concentration, the ratio between the number of iodine atoms and the number of dissolved particles must be increased.

Table 2.1 Schematic illustration of the development of contrast media

Description	Name	Chemical structure	Ratio of no. of iodine atoms/ions: no. of particles in solution	Osmolarity of a 280 mg I ml^{-1} solution	Osmolarity group
	Sodium iodide	Na$^+$ I$^-$	0.5		
	Diodone		1		
Ionic monomer	Diatrizoate (Urograffin, Hypaque) Metrizoate (Isopaque) Iothalamate (Conray)	 monomeric-monoacidic	1.5	1500	High
Ionic dimer	Ioxaglate (Hexabrix)	 dimeric-monoacidic	3	490	Low

2

Non-ionic monomer	Iopamidol (Niopam, Isovue) Iohexol (Omnipaque) Iomeprol (Iomeron) Ioversol (Optiray) Iopromide (Ultravist)	monomeric-non-ionic	3	470	Low
Non-ionic dimer	Iotrolan (Isovist) Iodixanol (Visipaque)	dimeric-non-ionic	6	300	Iso

Meg = meglumine; R = an unspecified side-chain.

Development to produce low osmolar contrast medium (LOCM) proceeded along two separate paths (Table 2.1). The first was to combine two tri-iodinated benzene rings to produce an ionic dimer with six iodine atoms per anion; ioxaglate (Hexabrix). The alternative, more successful, approach was to produce compounds that do not ionize in solution and so do not provide radiologically useless cations. Low osmolar contrast media of this type are referred to as non-ionic. These include the non-ionic monomers iopamidol (Niopam, Iopamiron, Isovue and Solutrast), iohexol (Omnipaque), iopromide (Ultravist), iomeprol (Iomeron) and ioversol (Optiray), which are now used widely.

For both types of LOCM the ratio of iodine atoms in the molecule to the number of particles in solution is 3:1 and osmolality is theoretically halved in comparison with high osmolar contrast material (HOCM). However, because of aggregation of molecules in solution the measured reduction is only approximately one-third (Fig. 2.1).

Further research led to the introduction of non-ionic dimers – iotrolan (Isovist) and iodixanol (Visipaque). These have a ratio of six iodine atoms for each molecule in solution with satisfactory iodine concentrations at iso-osmolality; they are, therefore, called iso-osmolar contrast media. The safety profile of the iso-osmolar

Figure 2.1 A plot of osmolality against iodine concentration for new and conventional contrast media. From Dawson et al.[1] (Reproduced by courtesy of the editor of *Clinical Radiology*.)

contrast agents is at least equivalent to LOCM, but any significant advantage of iso-osmolar contrast remains controversial.[2]

The low- and iso-osmolar contrast media are 5–10 times safer than the HOCM[3] and are used routinely in clinical practice. With development having reached the stage of iso-osmolality, further research is now targeted on decreasing the chemotoxicity and viscosity of iodinated contrast media.

References

1. Dawson P, Grainger RG, Pitfield J. The new low-osmolar contrast media: a simple guide. Clin Radiol 1983;34:221–6.
2. Morcos SK. Contrast-induced nephropathy: are there differences between low osmolar and iso-osmolar iodinated contrast media? Clin Radiol 2009;64:468–72.
3. The Royal College of Radiologists. Standards for Intravenous Iodinated Contrast Administration to Adult Patients, 2nd ed. BFCR(10)4. London: The Royal College of Radiologists; 2010.

ADVERSE EFFECTS OF INTRAVENOUS WATER-SOLUBLE CONTRAST MEDIA

The toxicity of contrast media is a function of osmolarity, ionic charge (ionic contrast agents only), chemical structure (chemotoxicity) and lipophilicity.

Adverse reactions after administration of non-ionic iodinated contrast media are rare, occuring in less than 1% of all patients.[1] Of these reactions, the vast majority are mild and self-limiting. The incidence of moderate or severe non-ionic contrast reactions is less than 0.001%.[2]

TOXIC EFFECTS ON SPECIFIC ORGANS

Vascular toxicity

Venous

1. Pain at the injection site – usually the result of a perivenous injection
2. Pain extending up the arm – due to stasis of contrast medium in the vein. May be relieved by abducting the arm
3. Delayed limb pain – due to thrombophlebitis as a result of the toxic effect on endothelium.

Arterial

Arterial endothelial damage and vasodilatation are mostly related to hyperosmolality. Contrast medium injected during peripheral arteriography may cause a sensation of heat or pain.

Soft-tissue toxicity

Pain, swelling, erythema and even sloughing of skin may occur from extravasated contrast medium. The risk is increased when pumps are used to inject large volumes of contrast medium during computed tomography (CT) examinations. Treatment should consist of the application of cold packs and elevation of the limb. Systemic steroids, non-steroidal anti-inflammatory drugs and antibiotics have all been shown to be useful.

Cardiovascular toxicity

1. Intracoronary injection of contrast media may cause significant disturbance of cardiac rhythm.
2. Increased vagal activity may result in depression of the sino-atrial and atrio-ventricular nodes, causing bradycardia or asystole.
3. Injection of hypertonic contrast medium causes significant fluid and ion shifts. Immediately after injection there is a significant increase in serum osmolality. This causes an influx of water from the interstitial space into the vascular compartment, an increase in blood volume, an increase in cardiac output and a brief increase of systemic blood pressure. Peripheral dilatation may cause a more prolonged fall of blood pressure. Injection into the right heart or pulmonary artery causes transitory pulmonary hypertension and systemic hypotension; injection into the left ventricle or aorta causes brief systemic hypertension followed by a more prolonged fall.

Haematological changes

1. In the presence of a high concentration of contrast medium, such as withdrawal of blood into a syringe of contrast medium, damage to red cell walls occurs and haemolysis follows. Haemolysis and haemoglobinuria have been reported following angiocardiography. It is advisable not to re-inject blood that has been mixed with contrast medium.
2. Red cell aggregation and coagulation may occur in the presence of a high concentration of contrast medium, e.g. 350 mg I ml^{-1}. However, disaggregation occurs easily and this is not likely to be of any clinical significance.
3. Contrast media may impair blood clotting and platelet aggregation. Low- and iso-osmolar contrast media have a minimal effect compared to HOCM.[3]
4. Contrast media have a potentiating effect on the action of heparin.
5. Thrombus formation occurs when blood is mixed with LOCM during injection. However, the role of the syringe is also significant; thrombus formation is maximal when blood is slowly withdrawn into a syringe so that it layers on top of the contrast medium, against the wall of the syringe, therefore this should be avoided.

Activation of coagulation by the tube material probably plays a significant role.

6. Contrast media have been shown to cause HbSS blood to sickle in vitro. Iso-osmolar contrast agents have a lesser effect and their use is indicated in this disease.[4] Beneficial diagnostic imaging with intravascular contrast can be performed without significant increased risk of serious complication in patients with sickle cell disease.[5]

7. When red blood cells are placed in a hypertonic contrast medium, water leaves the interior of the cells by osmosis and they become more rigid and less deformable. Iso-osmolar solutions also have an effect on red cell deformability, indicating that there may also be a chemical effect. Red cells that deform less easily are less able to pass through capillaries and may occlude them. This is the explanation for the transient rise in pulmonary arterial pressure during pulmonary arteriography and may also be a factor in contrast-induced nephropathy.

8. Transient eosinophilia may occur 24–72 h after administration of contrast medium.

Nephrotoxicity

Contrast-induced nephropathy (CIN) is one of the most serious adverse effects associated with the use of intravascular contrast media and is defined as an impairment of renal function (increase in serum creatinine >25% baseline value or 44 μmol l^{-1})[6] occurring within 3 days of contrast administration in the absence of an alternative aetiology. In those affected, the serum creatinine concentration starts to rise within the first 24 h, reaches a peak by 2–3 days and usually returns to baseline by 3–7 days. In rare cases patients may need temporary or permanent dialysis. The mechanisms of CIN are summarized below:[7]

1. Altered vascular haemodynamics:
   (a) adverse cardiotoxic effects
   (b) increased peripheral vasodilatation
   (c) renal vascular bed changes (increased blood flow followed by a more prolonged decrease)
   (d) increased rigidity of red cells.
2. Glomerular and tubular injury:
   (a) impaired perfusion
   (b) hyperosmolar effects
   (c) direct chemotoxic effects.
3. Interference with intratubular fluid volume and viscosity.

It was hoped that the iso-osmolar contrast agents might be less nephrotoxic than LOCM, however clinical trials have so far yielded conflicting results.[8] CIN has a complex aetiology and the

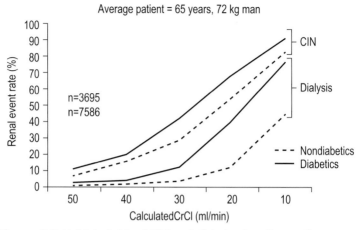

Figure 2.2 Validated risk of CIN and dialysis after diagnostic angiography and ad hoc angioplasty by creatinine clearance (CrCl) and diabetes. This assumes a mean contracts dose of 250 ml and a mean age of 65. (Adapted from Reference 9, with permission from Elsevier.)

positive benefit of reduction in osmolarity achieved with iso-osmolar contrast medium may be negated by the accompanying increase in viscosity.

There are a number of predisposing factors in CIN:

1. The single most important risk factor is pre-existing impairment of renal function; patients with normal renal function are at very low risk. A guide level of eGFR < 60 ml/min/1 is recommended to indicate renal impairment[3,9] (Fig. 2.2)
2. Diabetes mellitus
3. Dehydration
4. Sepsis
5. Age > 70 years
6. Use of very large doses of contrast medium
7. Multiple myeloma
8. Concomitant use of nephrotoxic drugs
9. Vascular disease.

A further hazard for patients who suffer impairment of renal function as a result of intravascular iodinated contrast is reduced renal clearance of other drugs, e.g. metformin, an oral hypoglycaemic drug which is exclusively excreted via the kidneys. The resultant accumulation of metformin may result in the development of the potentially fatal complication lactic acidosis.

See Table 2.2 for guidelines on prophylaxis of renal adverse reaction to iodinated contrast.

Table 2.2 Guidelines for prophylaxis of renal adverse reactions to iodinated contrast medium

Renal adverse reactions

Identification of patients at increased risk:

1. The referring clinician should identify patients with pre-existing renal impairment and inform the radiology department
2. eGFR (or serum creatinine) should be measured within 1 week before the administration of contrast in patients:
   a. **with previously known renal impairment**
   b. **who are diabetic and taking metformin**
   c. **who will undergo intra-arterial contrast injection**
   d. **with clinical history suggesting increased risk of renal impairment** (e.g. diabetes, renal surgery or administration of nephrotoxic drugs)

Precautions for patients with significant renal impairment (any patient with eGFR < 60 ml/min/1):

1. Consider an alternative imaging method, not using iodinated contrast media
2. In consultation with the referring clinic, 48 h before the procedure stop any treatment with metformin. This should be withheld for a further 48 h after the procedure and renal function re-assessed before restarting metformin treatment
3. 24 h before the procedure stop all nephrotoxic drugs, mannitol and loop diuretics
4. Start hydration either orally, or in the case of high dose or intra-arterial administration, intravenously. A suitable intravenous regimen is 1 ml/kg body weight per hour of normal saline for at least 6 hours before and after the procedure
5. Use the lowest dose of contrast consistent with a diagnostic result
6. Use low- or iso-osmolar contrast medium:
   - There is insufficient evidence to support the use of prophylactic administration of N-acetyl cysteine for patients at high risk of contrast nephropathy
   - There is no definite evidence that haemodialysis or peritoneal dialysis protect patients with impaired renal function from contrast-medium-induced nephrotoxicity
   - Patients with normal renal function (eGFR > 60 ml/min/l) receiving contrast can continue metformin treatment normally

Neurotoxicity

Contrast medium delivered to the brain via the arterial route during angiography or neurovascular intervention may rarely cross the blood–brain barrier with resultant cerebral oedema and altered neuronal excitability. Potential clinical effects include encephalopathy, seizures, cortical blindness and focal neurological deficits which are most often temporary but infrequently persistent.[10] Neurotoxicity is caused by both osmolality and chemotoxic effects.

Intravenous contrast medium may rarely provoke convulsions in patients with epilepsy or cerebral tumours.

Convulsions may also occur secondary to the cerebral hypoxia caused by hypotension ± cardiac arrest after severe contrast reaction.

Thyroid function

1. Iodinated contrast media may rarely cause thyroid dysfunction resulting in the development of either incident hyperthyroidism or incident overt hypothyroidism.[11] Iodide administration may result in the generation of intrathyroidal iodolactones or iodolipids which inhibit thyroid peroxidise activity and disrupt normal thyroid function. Patients with no known risk factors may be affected but those with goitre or proven detectable serum antibodies to thyroperoxidase are likely at increased risk, particularly in iodine-deficient geographic regions.
2. Contrast media may interfere with the accuracy of thyroid function tests.

IDIOSYNCRATIC REACTIONS

Adverse reactions can be classified in terms of severity as:

1. Mild: Nausea, vomiting, urticaria
2. Moderate: Mild bronchospasm, vasovagal reaction, tachycardia, diffuse erythema
3. Severe: Cardiovascular collapse, moderate or severe bronchospasm, laryngeal oedema, loss of consciousness or seizure.

Mild and moderate reactions are uncommon; major adverse reactions are very rare for both LOCM[12] and iso-osmolar iodinated contrast.[13] Adverse effects of low osmolar iodinated contrast are found in approximately 0.15% of all patients. In a large study of LOCM contrast doses[14] the adverse effects were categorized (Table 2.3).

The vast majority of adverse effects were managed with patient re-assurance or diphenydramine treatment and one death was presumed caused by LOCM (0.0003% of total patient group).

Fatal reactions

Deaths caused by iodinated contrast agents are very rare, occurring at a rate of 1.1–1.2 per million contrast media packages distributed. Most are attributed to renal failure, anaphylaxis or allergic reaction.[15]

Table 2.3 Categories of adverse effects of LOCM contrast doses[14]		
Category of adverse effect[14]	Proportion of adverse effect events ($n = 458$)	Proportion of total patient group ($n = 298\,000$)
Mild	81.6%	0.125%
Moderate	15.1%	0.02%
Severe	3.3%	0.005%

2

Almost every fatal reaction will occur in the minutes following injection and all patients must be under close observation during this time. The fatal event may be preceded by trivial events, such as nausea and vomiting, or may occur without warning. The majority of deaths occur in those over 50 years of age. Causes of death include cardiac arrest, pulmonary oedema, respiratory arrest, consumption coagulopathy, bronchospasm, laryngeal oedema and angioneurotic oedema.

Non-fatal reactions

1. Flushing, metallic taste in the mouth, nausea, sneezing, cough and tingling are common and related to dose and speed of injection.
2. Perineal burning, a desire to empty the bladder or rectum and an erroneous feeling of having been incontinent of urine are more common in women.
3. Urticaria.
4. Angioneurotic oedema. Most commonly affects the face. May persist for up to 3 days and its onset may be delayed.
5. Rigors.
6. Necrotizing skin lesions. Rare and mostly in patients with pre-existing renal failure (particularly those with systemic lupus erythematosus).
7. Bronchospasm. Predisposed to by a history of asthma and by therapy with ß-blockers. In most patients the bronchospasm is subclinical. Mechanisms include:
   (a) direct histamine release from mast cells and platelets
   (b) cholinesterase inhibition
   (c) vagal overtone
   (d) complement activation
   (e) direct effect of contrast media on bronchi.
8. Non-cardiogenic pulmonary oedema. During acute anaphylaxis or hypotensive collapse and possibly due to increased capillary permeability.

9. Arrhythmias.
10. Hypotension. Usually accompanied by tachycardia but in some patients there is vagal over-reaction with bradycardia. The latter is rapidly reversed by atropine 0.6–2 mg i.v. Hypotension is usually mild and is treatable by a change of posture. Rarely, it is severe and may be accompanied by pulmonary oedema.
11. Abdominal pain. May be a symptom in anaphylactic reactions or vagal overactivity. Should be differentiated from the loin pain that may be precipitated in patients with upper urinary tract obstruction.
12. Delayed-onset reactions – ($1\ h^{-1}$ week after injection) include nausea, vomiting, rashes, headaches, itching and parotid gland swelling. Late adverse reactions are commoner by a factor of three to four after iso-osmolar contrast medium injection. Risk factors for delayed reaction are previous contrast medium reaction, history of allergy and interleukin-2 treatment.[16]

MECHANISMS OF IDIOSYNCRATIC CONTRAST MEDIUM REACTIONS

Idiosyncratic contrast medium reactions are usually labelled anaphylactoid since they have all the features of anaphylaxis but are IgE-negative in over 90% of cases. However, patients who experience a severe anaphylactoid reaction to iodinated contrast should always be investigated for possible IgE-mediated allergy including skin testing and, if available, basophil activation testing.[17]

Possible mechanisms of non-IgE-mediated anaphylactoid reaction include those outlined below.

Histamine release

Histamine is the primary mediator of anaphylaxis/anaphylactoid reaction and contrast media cause the release of histamine from mast cells and basophils. This could provide a mechanism for the phenomena of flushing, urticaria, metallic taste, hypotension, collapse and angioneurotic oedema. While hyperosmolality is a factor, isosmolar concentrations of contrast media will also stimulate histamine release. Bronchospasm may be due to the effect of contrast medium on pulmonary-bed mast cells and dysrhythmias from the effect on cardiac mast cells.

Complement activation

Contrast medium may perhaps activate the complement system leading to the formation of anaphylatoxins which induce the release of histamine and other biological mediators from basophils and mast cells.[18]

Protein binding, enzyme inhibition and immune receptors

Contrast media are weakly protein-bound and the degree of protein binding correlates well with their ability to inhibit the enzyme acetyl cholinesterase. Contrast medium side effects such as vasodilatation, bradycardia, hypotension, bronchospasm and urticaria are all recognized cholinergic effects. It was previously thought that they might be related more to cholinesterase inhibition than osmolality; however, this has not been conclusively proven. It has also been postulated that weakly protein-bound drugs, such as iodinated contrast, may directly activate T cells which bear immune receptors. It is thought that these may interact with the drug and that contrast medium may have an effect on cytokine production by helper T cells to mediate the acute reaction.

Anxiety

Many years ago, Lalli[19] postulated that most contrast medium reactions are the result of the patient's fear and apprehension. The high autonomic nervous system activity in an anxious patient will be stimulated further when the patient experiences the administration of contrast medium. Furthermore, contrast medium crossing the blood–brain barrier can stimulate the limbic area and hypothalamus to produce further autonomic activity. This autonomic activity is responsible for contrast medium reactions by the sequence of events illustrated in Figure 2.3.

PROPHYLAXIS OF ADVERSE CONTRAST MEDIUM EFFECTS

Guidelines for prophylaxis of renal and non-renal adverse contrast media reaction are given in Tables 2.2 and 2.4. Sources used in these tables include documents of the Royal College of Radiologists,[3] Canadian Association of Radiologists[6] and the European Society of Urogenital Radiology[20] on contrast medium administration; the full text of these documents can be downloaded from the internet at www.rcr.ac.uk, www.car.ca and www.esur.org, respectively. General safety issues are:

- a doctor should be immediately available in the department to deal with any severe reaction
- facilities for treatment of acute adverse reaction should be readily available and regularly checked
- a patient must not be left alone or unsupervised for the first 5 min following injection of the contrast agent

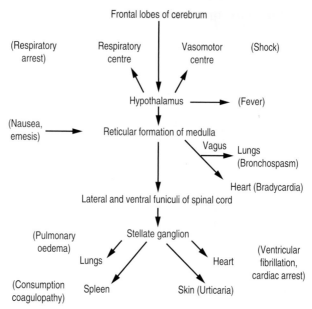

Figure 2.3 Central nervous system and contrast media reactions.

Table 2.4 Guidelines for prophylaxis of non-renal adverse reactions to iodinated contrast medium

Non-renal adverse reactions

Identification of patients at increased risk of anaphylactoid contrast reaction:

It is essential that before administration of iodinated contrast every patient must be specifically asked whether they have a history of:

1. **Previous contrast reaction** – associated with a sixfold increase in reactions to contrast medium.[18] Determine exact nature and specific agent used
2. **Asthma** – history of asthma associated with a six- to tenfold increase in risk of severe reaction.[21] Determine whether patient has true asthma or COPD and whether asthma is currently well controlled. If asthma not currently well controlled and examination is non-emergency, the patient should be referred back for appropriate medical therapy
3. **Previous allergic reaction requiring medical treatment** – determine the nature of the allergies and their sensitivity (there is no specific cross-reactivity with shellfish or topical iodine in acute reactions[22])

2

Table 2.4, Continued

Precautions for patients at increased risk of anaphylactoid contrast reaction:

1. Consider an alternative test not requiring iodinated contrast
2. If the injection is considered necessary:
   a. Use a non-ionic low or iso-osmolar contrast agent
   b. For previous reactors to iodinated contrast use a different non-ionic low- or iso-osmolar contrast to that used previously
   c. Maintain close supervision
   d. Leave the cannula in place and observe for 30 min
   e. Be ready to treat promptly any adverse reaction and ensure that emergency drugs and equipment are ready (see Chapter 19).

There are no conclusive data supporting the use of premedication with corticosteroids or antihistamines in the prevention of severe reactions to contrast media in patients at increased risk.[3,23] Pre-treatment with antihistamines is associated with an increased incidence of flushing.

Other situations:

Pregnancy – In exceptional circumstances, iodinated contrast may be given, see text

Lactation – No special precaution required

Treatment with ß-blockers – ß-blockers may impair the response to treatment of bronchospasm induced by contrast medium

Thyrotoxicosis – Intravascular contrast should not be given if the patient is hyperthyroid. Avoid thyroid radio-isotope tests and treatment for 2 months after iodinated contrast medium administration

Phaeochromocytoma – When diagnosis is made biochemically it is advised that α- and ß-adrenergic blockade with orally administered drugs is arranged before administration of iodinated contrast

Sickle cell anaemia – There is potential risk of precipitating a sickle cell crisis. Iso-osmolar contrast should be used[4]

Myelomatosis – Bence Jones protein may be precipitated in renal tubules. Risk is diminished by ensuring good hydration.

• the patient should remain in the department for at least 15 min after the contrast injection. In patients at increased risk of reaction this should be increased to 30 min.

Iodinated contrast in pregnancy and lactation

There is no evidence of mutagenic or teratogenic effects after intravenous administration of iodinated contrast to the mother during pregnancy but there is a potential impact on the neonatal thyroid gland. The fetal thyroid develops early in pregnancy and plays an important role in the development of the nervous system. It is recommended that iodinated contrast be used in pregnant women only when (a) no alternative test is available,

(b) information obtained from the study is useful to both mother and fetus during the pregnancy and (c) the referring physician considers it imprudent to delay the imaging study until after delivery.[24] A single in utero exposure to low osmolar iodinated contrast is unlikely to have any effect on thyroid function at birth,[25] however neonatal thyroid function should be checked during the first week of life.

Only small amounts of intravenous contrast medium reach the breast milk during lactation, approximately 0.5% of the dose received by the mother. It is considered safe for both mother and infant to continue breast feeding after iodinated contrast administration.[24]

References

1. Mortelé KJ, Oliva MR, Ondategui S, et al. Universal use of nonionic iodinated contrast medium for CT: evaluation of safety in a large urban teaching hospital. Am J Roentgenol 2005;184(1):31–4.

2. Hunt CH, Hartman RP, Hesley GK. Frequency and severity or adverse effects of iodinated and gadolinium contrast materials: retrospective review of 456,930 doses. Am J Roentgenol 2009;193:1124–7.

3. Aspelin P, Stacul F, Thomsen HS, et al. Effects of iodinated contrast media on blood and endothelium. Eur Radiol 2006;16(5):1041–9.

4. Losco P, Nash G, Stone P, et al. Comparison of the effects of radiographic contrast media on dehydration and filterability of red blood cells from donors homozygous for hemoglobin A or hemoglobin. S Am J Hematol 2001;68(3):149–58.

5. Campbell KL, Hud LM, Adams S, et al. Safety of iodinated intravenous contrast medium administration in sickle cell disease. Am J Med 2012;125(1):100e11–16.

6. Canadian Association of Radiologists. Consensus Guidelines for the Prevention of Contrast Induced Nephropathy, 2nd ed. Ottowa, Ontario: Canadian Association of Radiologists; 2011.

7. Seeliger E, Sendeski M, Rihal CS, et al. Contrast induced kidney injury: mechanisms, risk factors and prevention. Eur Heart J 2012;33(16): 2007–15.

8. Heinrich MC, Häberle L, Müller V, et al. Nephrotoxicity of iso-osmolar iodixanol compared with non-ionic low-osmolar contrast media: Meta-analysis of randomized controlled trials. Radiology 2009;250(1): 68–86.

9. McCullough PA, Soman SS. Contrast-induced neuropathy. Crit Care Clin 2005;21(2):261–80.

10. Leong S, Fanning NF. Persistent neurological deficit from iodinated contrast encephalopathy following intracranial aneurysm coiling. A case report and review of the literature. Interv Neuroradiol 2012;18(1):33–41.

11. Rhee CM, Bhan I, Alexander EK, et al. Association between iodinated contrast media exposure and incident hyperthyroidism and hypothyroidism. Arch Intern Med 2012;172(2):153–9.

12. Kopp AF, Mortele KJ, Cho YD, et al. Prevalence of acute reactions to iopramide: postmarketing surveillance study of 74,717 patients. Acta Radiol 2008;49(8):902–11.

13. Haussler MD. Safety and patient comfort with iodixanol: a postmarketing surveillance study in 9515 patients undergoing diagnostic CT examinations. Acta Radiol 2010;51(8):924–33.
14. Hunt CH, Hartman RP, Hesley GK. Frequency and severity of adverse effects of iodinated and gadolinium contrast materials: retrospective review of 456,930 doses. Am J Radiol 2009;193(4):1124–7.
15. Wysowski DK, Nourjah P. Deaths attributed to X-ray contrast media on U.S. death certificates. Am J Roentgenol 2006;186:613–15.
16. Bellin MF, Webb JA, Thomsen HS, et al. Late adverse reactions to intravascular iodine based contrast media: an update. Eur Radiol 2011;21(11):2305–10.
17. Trcka J, Schmidt C, Seitz CS, et al. Anaphylaxis to iodinated contrast material: nonallergic hypersensitivity or IgE-mediated allergy? Am J Radiol 2008;190(3):666–70.
18. Morcos SK. Acute serious and fatal reactions to contrast media: our current understanding. Br J Radiol 2005;78(932):686–93.
19. Lalli AF. Urographic contrast media reactions and anxiety. Radiology 1974;112(2):267–71.
20. European Society of Urogenital Radiology Contrast Media Safety Committee. ESUR Guidelines on Contrast Media, Version 7.0. www.esur.org, 2008.
21. Morcos SK, Thomsen HS. Adverse reactions to iodinated contrast media. Eur Radiol 2001;11(7):1267–75.
22. Schabelman E, Witting M. The relationship of radiocontrast, iodine and seafood allergies: a medical myth exposed. J Emerg Med 2010;39(5):701–7.
23. Davenport MS, Cohan RH, Caoili EM, et al. Repeat contrast medium reactions in premedicated patients: frequency and severity. Radiology 2009;253(2):372–9.
24. American College of Radiology. ACR Manual on Contrast Media. 7th ed. Reston, VA: American College of Radiology; 2010.
25. Bourjeily G, Chalhoub M, Phornphutkl C, et al. Neonatal thyroid function: effect of single exposure to iodinated contrast medium in utero. Radiology 2010;256(3):744–50.

CONTRAST AGENTS IN MAGNETIC RESONANCE IMAGING

HISTORICAL DEVELOPMENT

Shortly after the introduction of clinical MRI, the first contrast-enhanced human MRI studies were reported in 1981 using ferric chloride as a contrast agent in the gastrointestinal tract. In 1984, Carr et al. first demonstrated the use of a gadolinium compound as a diagnostic intravascular MRI contrast agent.[1] Currently, around one-quarter of all MRI examinations are performed with contrast agents.

MECHANISM OF ACTION

Whilst radiographic contrast agents use a direct alteration in tissue density to allow the visualization of structures, the MRI contrast agents act indirectly by altering the magnetic properties of hydrogen ions (protons) in water and lipid which form the basis of the image in MRI. To enhance the inherent contrast between tissues, MRI contrast agents must alter the rate of relaxation of protons within the tissues. The changes in relaxation vary and, therefore, different tissues produce differential enhancement of the signal (see Figs 2.4 and 2.5). These figures

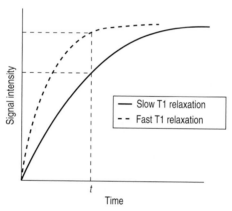

Figure 2.4 Signal intensity and T1 relaxation time.

Figure 2.5 Signal intensity and T2 relaxation time.

show that, for a given time t, if the T1 relaxation is more rapid then a larger signal is obtained (brighter images), but the opposite is true for T2 relaxation, where more rapid relaxation produces reduced signal intensity (darker images). There are different means by which these effects on protons can be produced using a range of MRI contrast agents.

MRI contrast agents must exert a large magnetic field density (a property imparted by their unpaired electrons) to interact with the magnetic moments of the protons in the tissues and so shorten their T1 relaxation time, which will produce an increase in signal intensity (see Fig. 2.4). The electron magnetic moments also cause local changes in the magnetic field, which promote more rapid proton dephasing and so shorten the T2 relaxation time. All contrast agents shorten both T1 and T2 relaxation times but some will predominantly affect T1 (longitudinal relaxation rate) and others predominantly T2 (transverse relaxation rate).

Agents with unpaired electron spins are potential contrast material for use in MRI. These may be classified under three headings:

1. *Ferromagnetic.* These retain magnetism even when the applied field is removed. This may cause particle aggregation and interfere with cell function, making them unsafe for clinical use as MRI contrast agents.
2. *Paramagnetic* – e.g. gadolinium contrast agents, which are by far the most widely used MRI contrast agents. Paramagnetic agents also include liver-specific manganese-based agents such as the manganese chelate Mn-DPDP (Telescan). These paramagnetic contrast agents have magnetic moments which align to the applied field, but once the gradient field is turned off, thermal energy within the tissue is enough to overcome the alignment. Their maximum effect is on protons in the water molecule, shortening the T1 relaxation time and hence producing increased signal intensity (white) on T1 images (Fig. 2.4).
3. *Superparamagnetic* – e.g. particles of iron oxide (Fe_3O_4). These cause abrupt changes in the local magnetic field which results in rapid proton dephasing and reduction in the T2 relaxation time, and hence producing decreased signal intensity (black) on T2 images (Fig. 2.5). Superparamagnetic compounds are available as large particles in a colloid suspension for oral ingestion as gastrointestinal contrast and also as small particles of iron oxide (SPIO) agents and ultrasmall particles of iron oxide (USPIO) agents. Both SPIO and USPIO agents have submicron global particle diameters and are small enough to form a stable solution which can be injected intravenously.

GADOLINIUM

Gadolinium compounds may be made soluble by chelation and can, therefore, either be injected intravenously or used as an oral preparation. In the chelation process large organic molecules form a stable complex around the gadolinium and reduce potential toxicity. The gadolinium (GD) chelates represent the largest group of MRI contrast media and are available in three forms:

1. Extracellular fluid (ECF) agents: by far the most commonly used form of gadolinium. Includes:
   (a) Gd-diethylenetriaminepenta-acetic acid (DTPA), Gadopentetate dimeglumine (Magnevist®)
   (b) Gd-DTPA-bismethylamide, Gadodiamide (Omniscan®)
   (c) Gd-DO3A, Gadoteridol (ProHance®).
   They all contain gadolinium, an 8-coordinate ligand binding to gadolinium and a single water molecule coordination site to gadolinium and all have a molecular weight similar to iodinated contrast agents. After intravenous injection they circulate within the vascular system and are excreted unchanged by the kidneys. The ECF agents do not cross the normal blood–brain barrier but do cross the abnormal blood–brain barrier. ECF agents are used for angiography but rapidly leak out of the vascular space into the interstitial space so are used only for dynamic arterial studies. There is a wide range of indications for ECF agents including improved detection rates and more accurate delineation and characterization of tumours.
2. Liver agents: the excretion pathway of the gadolinium chelates can be altered to produce compounds such as Gd-BOPTA, Gadobenate (Multihance®) and Gd-DTPA, Gadoxetate disodium (Primovist®) which are taken up by hepatocytes and cleared intact via the hepato-biliary system. These agents are used to improve detection of liver lesions which do not contain hepatocytes (therefore do not take up the contrast), such as liver metastases, and to characterize lesions which do take up the contrast, such as hepatocellular carcinoma. They can also be used to provide positive contrast (T1 weighted) of the hepato-biliary system.
3. Blood pool agents: these bind reversibly to human albumin resulting in higher relaxivity and longer persistence in the vascular space than ECF agents, allowing a wider range of vascular imaging, e.g. Gadofosveset trisodium (Vasovist®).

Dose

For ECF gadolinium agents, usually 0.1 mmol kg^{-1} body weight; up to 0.2 mmol kg^{-1} when used in low-field magnets.

Table 2.5 Acute adverse reaction rates for gadolinium contrast agents					
Study	Number of examinations	Mild	Moderate	Severe	Fatal
Morgan et al.[2]	28 078	0.63%	0.02%	0.014%	None
Abujudeh et al.[3]	32,659	0.13%	0.018%	0.006%	None
Dillman et al.[4]	78 353	0.05%	0.012%	0.005%	None
Hunt et al.[5]	158 439	0.03%	0.007%	0.0025%	None

Adverse reactions

Gadolinium contrast agents are very safe and well tolerated; they have a lower incidence of adverse reactions than iodinated contrast agents. Adverse reactions to gadolinium are mostly mild and self-limiting. These can be divided into acute and delayed reactions.

Acute adverse reactions
These are rare (Table 2.5) and are classified as:

1. **Mild**; e.g. nausea, vomiting, headache, dizziness, shaking, altered taste, itching, rash, facial swelling.
2. **Moderate**; e.g. tachycardia or bradycardia, hypertension, generalized erythema, dyspnoea, bronchospasm, wheezing, mild hypotension.
3. **Severe**; e.g. laryngeal oedema (severe or rapidly progressive), unresponsiveness, cardiopulmonary arrest, convulsions, clinically manifest cardiac arrhythmias.

Patients with a history of previous adverse reaction to gadolinium contrast agents have an increased likelihood of experiencing adverse reactions with a 30% recurrence rate of hypersensitivity reactions in those with previous reactions.[6] Those with asthma, documented allergies or previous adverse reaction to iodinated contrast are also at increased risk of adverse reaction.[7]

Delayed adverse reactions
1. Renal impairment – when used at the standard doses given above, gadolinium contrast agents do not cause significant impairment of renal function.

2. Nephrogenic systemic fibrosis (NSF) – this rare systemic disorder, first described in 2000, is characterized by increased deposition of collagen with thickening and hardening of the skin, contractures and, in some patients, clinical involvement of other tissues.[8] Most cases are mild but an estimated 5% have a progressive debilitating course.[9] NSF occurs in patients with renal disease and almost all patients with NSF have been exposed to gadolinium-based contrast agents within 2–3 months prior to the onset of the disease. The mechanism by which renal failure and gadolinium-based contrast agents trigger NSF is not known.

In 2009 the European Medicines Agency Committee for Medicinal Products for Human Use Scientific Advisory Group categorized gadolinium products according to risk of causing nephrogenic systemic fibrosis:

1. Low risk: macrocyclic chelates including gadoterate meglumine (Dotarem®), gadoteridol (Prohance®), gadobuterol (Gadovist®).
2. Medium risk: linear ionic chelates including gadoxetic acid (Primovist®), gadobenate dimeglumine (Multilane®).
3. High risk: linear non-ionic chelates including gadodiamide (Omniscan®) and linear ionic chelates including gadopentetate dimeglumine (Magnevist®) and made recommendations to minimize risk of NSF, which can be found at info@ema.europa.eu. Preventative guidelines have been shown to be extremely effective in protection of patients from NSF.[10]

Precautions for prevention of adverse reactions
Detailed guidelines are available from the American College of Radiology,[7] Royal College of Radiologists[11] and the European Society of Urogenital Radiology.[12] These form the basis for the following advice.

Acute adverse reactions
1. Identify patients at increased risk of reaction because of previous gadolinium reaction, asthma, allergies or previous adverse reaction to iodinated contrast.
2. For those at increased risk consider an alternative test not requiring a gadolinium agent.
3. If proceeding with i.v. gadolinium contrast:
    (a) patients who have previously reacted to one gadolinium-based contrast agent should be injected with a different agent if they are re-studied
    (b) although there is no clinical evidence of the effectiveness of premedication, it is suggested that consideration be given to the use of premedication such as oral prednisolone 30 mg orally 12 and 2 hours before contrast medium
    (c) those with an increased risk of adverse reaction should be monitored more closely after injection.

Delayed adverse reactions

1. Identify patients at risk of NSF; particularly patients with renal impairment, patients in the perioperative period after liver transplant, infants, neonates and the elderly.
2. For patients at increased risk consider an alternative test not requiring a gadolinium agent.
3. If proceeding with gadolinium contrast, the use of high-risk gadolinium contrast medium is contraindicated (see above). The lowest possible dose of low- or medium-risk gadolinium-based contrast agent should be used.

IRON-OXIDE MAGNETIC RESONANCE IMAGING CONTRAST AGENTS (SPIO AND USPIO)

After i.v. injection, the superparamagnetic SPIO contrast agents are taken up via the reticulo-endothelial system into the liver and spleen resulting in decreased signal intensity in normal liver and spleen on T2-weighted images. Malignant tumour tissue or other lesions which do not contain reticulo-endothelial cells will not take up the contrast and, therefore, retain their high MRI signal. Iron-oxide contrast agents are useful for detection of liver tumour, particularly hepatocellular carcinoma.[13]

The USPIO contrast agents have greater T1 shortening effects and a longer plasma circulation time than the SPIO agents. In addition, they have greater uptake in bone marrow and lymph nodes and are used for imaging bone marrow and lymph node metastases.[14]

GASTROINTESTINAL CONTRAST AGENTS

MR enteroclysis is increasingly widely used in the diagnosis of small bowel disease. During this examination, 1–3 litres of 0.5% methylcellulose solution in water, infused via a nasogastric tube (see Chapter 3) is used as the gastrointestinal tract contrast agent.

Other contrast materials can be used to distinguish bowel from adjacent soft-tissue masses. As with CT, all bowel contrast agents need to mix readily with the bowel contents to ensure even distribution. They must also be palatable. They can be divided into two groups:

Positive agents

These include fatty oils and gadolinium. They act by T1 shortening effects and appear white on T1 images.

Negative agents

These include ferrite and barium sulphate (60–70% w/w). These act by T2 shortening effects and appear black on T2 images.

MRI contrast agents in pregnancy and lactation

MRI contrast agents should not be routinely given to pregnant patients.[7] Although there are no reports of teratogenic or mutagenic effects in humans, there are no case-controlled prospective studies in large numbers of patients and the precise risk to the fetus is not known. Gadolinium chelates may accumulate in the amniotic fluid and remain there for an indefinite period of time with potential dissociation of toxic free gadolinium ion. The decision to administer an MRI contrast agent to a pregnant patient should be made on a case-by-case basis and accompanied by a thoughtful and well-documented risk–benefit analysis.

Only tiny amounts of gadolinium-based contrast medium given intravenously to a lactating mother reach the milk and a minute proportion entering the baby's gut is absorbed. The use of gadolinium contrast agents is considered safe during lactation.[15]

References

1. Carr DH, Brown J, Bydder GM, et al. Intravenous chelated gadolinium as a contrast agent in NMR imaging of cerebral tumours. Lancet 1984;1(8375):484–6.
2. Morgan DE, Spann JS, Lockhart ME, et al. Assessment of adverse reaction rates during gadoteridol-enhanced MRI imaging in 28,078 patients. Radiology 2011;259(1):109–16.
3. Abujudeh HH, Kosaraju VK, Kaewlai R. Acute adverse reactions to gadopentetate dimeglumine and gadobenate dimeglumine: experience with 32,659 injections. Am J Roentgenol 2010;194(2):430–4.
4. Dillman JR, Ellis JH, Ellis JH, et al. Frequency and severity of acute allergic-like reactions to gadolinium-containing i.v. contrast media in children and adults. Am J Roentgenol 2007;189(6):1533–8.
5. Hunt CH, Hartman RP, Hesley GK. Frequency and severity or adverse effects of iodinated and gadolinium contrast materials: retrospective review of 456,930 doses. Am J Roentgenol 2009;193:1124–7.
6. Jung JW, Kang HR, Kim MH, et al. Immediate hypersensitivity reaction to gadolinium based MR contrast media. Radiology 2012;264(2):414–22.
7. American College of Radiology. ACR Manual on Contrast Media. 7th ed. Reston, VA: American College of Radiology; 2010.
8. Cowper SE, Robin HS, Steinberg SM, et al. Scleromyxoedema-like cutaneous diseases in renal dialysis patients. Lancet 2000;356(9234):1000–1.
9. Reiter T, Ritter O, Prince MR, et al. Minimising risk of nephrogenic systemic fibrosis in cardiovascular magnetic resonance. J Cardiovasc Magn Reson 2012;14(1):31.
10. Wang Y, Alkasab TK, Narin O, et al. Incidence of nephrogenic systemic fibrosis after adoption of restrictive gadolinium based contrast guidelines. Radiology 2011;260(1):105–11.

11. The Royal College of Radiologists. Gadolinium-based Contrast Media and Nephrogenic Systemic Fibrosis. BFCR(07)14. London: The Royal College of Radiologists; 2007.
12. European Society of Urogenital Radiology Contrast Media Safety Committee. ESUR Guidelines on Contrast Media, Version 7.0. www.esur.org, 2008.
13. Gandhi SN, Brown MA, Wong JG, et al. MR contrast agents for liver imaging: what, when, how. Radiographics 2006;26(6):1621–36.
14. We L, Cao Y, Liao C, et al. Diagnostic performance of USPIO enhanced MRI for lymph node metastases in different body regions: a meta-analysis. Eur J Radiol 2011;80(2):582–9.
15. Tremblay E, Thérasse E, Thomassin-Naggara I, et al. Quality initiatives: guidelines for use of medical imaging during pregnancy and lactation. RadioGraphics 2012;32(3):897–911.

Further Reading

Edelman RR, Hesselink JR, Zlatkin MB, et al. Clinical Magnetic Resonance Imaging. 3rd ed. Philadelphia, PA: Saunders Elsevier; 2006.
Symposium on Nephrogenic Systemic Fibrosis. J Am Coll Radiol 2008;5(1):21– 56 [Special Issue].

CONTRAST AGENTS IN ULTRASONOGRAPHY

During the late 1960s, the first reported use of ultrasound (US) contrast was published describing the intracardiac injection of agents during echocardiography. Considerable progress has now been made in the development and clinical application of US contrast agents and these are now used more widely to assess vascularity and tissue perfusion. US contrast agents contain microbubbles of air, nitrogen or fluorocarbon gas coated with a thin shell of material such as albumin, galactose or lipid. The contrast is usually injected intravenously, but in order to cross the pulmonary filter and reach the arterial circulation the microbubbles must be 3–5 μm diameter, approximately the size of a red blood cell. Bubbles of this size only remain intact for a very short time in blood. The bubbles do not pass through the vascular endothelium therefore they provide pure intravascular contrast. The effect of a bolus injection is to increase the echo signal from blood by a factor of 500–1000. After about 5 minutes the gas from the bubbles had diffused into the blood and the very small mass of shell material is then metabolized.[1]

Clinical applications of US contrast agents include the following:[2,3]

1. Identification and characterization of solid lesions, particularly in the liver,[4] but also in the spleen, pancreas, kidney, prostate, ovary and breast.
2. To assist US-guided interventions such as biopsy.

3. Voiding urosonography can be used to detect vesico-ureteric reflux in children; here US contrast is administered directly into the bladder.

4. Assessment of fallopian tubal patency at hysterosonosalpinography.

5. Determination of disease activity in patients with inflammatory bowel disease.

There are a number of different microbubble contrast agents available. Levovist® is one of the most widely used; it consists of microbubbles of air enclosed by a thin layer of palmitic acid in a galactose solution and is stable in blood for 1–4 min. SonoVue®, another microbubble contrast agent, is an aqueous suspension of stabilized sulphur hexafluoride microbubbles.

The US agents in clinical use are well tolerated and serious adverse reactions are rarely observed. These agents are not nephrotoxic and may be used in patients with any level of renal function.[5] Allergy-like reactions occur rarely and adverse events are usually mild and self-resolving.[6]

References

1. Wilson S, Burns PN. Microbubble-enhanced US in body imaging: What role? Radiology 2010;257:24–39.
2. Quaia E. Microbubble ultrasound contrast agents: an update. Eur Radiol 2007;17(8):1995–2008.
3. Furlow B. Contrast-enhanced ultrasound. Radiol Technol 2009;80(6): 547–61.
4. Piscaglia F, Lencioni R, Sagrini E, et al. Characterization of focal liver lesions with contrast enhanced ultrasound. Ultrasound Med Biol 2010;36(4): 531–50.
5. Wilson S, Greenbaum L, Goldberg BB. Contrast enhanced ultrasound; what is the evidence and what are the obstacles? Am J Roentgen 2009;193(1):55–60.
6. Jakobsen JA, Oyen R, Thomsen HS, et al. Safety of ultrasound contrast agents. Eur Radiol 2005;15(5):941–5.

Further Reading

Burns PN, Wilson SR. Microbubble contrast for radiological imaging 1. Principles. Ultrasound Q 2006;22(1):5–13.

Wilson SR, Burns PN. Microbubble contrast for radiological imaging 2. Applications. Ultrasound Q 2006;22(1):15–18.

Gastrointestinal tract

Methods of imaging the gastrointestinal tract

1. Plain film
2. Barium swallow
3. Barium meal
4. Barium follow-through
5. Small bowel enema
6. Barium enema
7. Ultrasound (US):
   (a) Transabdominal
   (b) Endosonography
8. Computed tomography (CT)
9. Magnetic resonance imaging (MRI)
10. Angiography
11. Radionuclide imaging:
    (a) Inflammatory bowel disease
    (b) Gastro-oesophageal reflux
    (c) Gastric emptying
    (d) Bile reflux study
    (e) Meckel's scan
    (f) Gastrointestinal bleeding.

INTRODUCTION TO CONTRAST MEDIA

BARIUM

Barium suspension is made up from finely ground barium sulphate (the contaminant barium carbonate is poisonous). The particles of barium must be very small (in the range of 1 μm) to make them more stable in suspension. To prevent the particles clumping a non-ionic suspension medium is used. The resulting solution has a pH of 5.3 which makes it stable in gastric acid.

Table 3.1 Barium suspensions and dilutions with water to give a lower density

Proprietary name	Density (w/v) – use
Baritop 100	100% – all parts gastrointestinal tract
EPI-C	150% – large bowel
E-Z-Cat	1–2% – computed tomography of gastrointestinal tract
E-Z HD	250% – oesophagus, stomach and duodenum
E-Z Paque	100% – small intestine
Micropaque DC	100% – oesophagus, stomach and duodenum
Micropaque liquid	100% – small and large bowel
Micropaque powder	76% – small and large bowel
Polibar	115% – large bowel
Polibar rapid	100% – large bowel

There are many varieties of barium suspensions in use. Ingredients are designed to optimise mucosal coating and to make it palatable. In most situations the preparation will be diluted with water to give a lower density (Table 3.1) and must be shaken well immediately before use.

Examinations of different parts of the gastrointestinal tract require barium preparations with differing properties:

1. *Barium swallow*, e.g. Baritop® 100% w/v or E-Z HD® 200–250% 100 ml (or more, as required).
2. *Barium meal*, e.g. E-Z HD® 250% w/v. A high-density, low-viscosity barium is required for a double-contrast barium meal to give a good thin coating that is still sufficiently dense to give satisfactory opacification. It also contains simethicone (an anti-foaming and coating agent) and sorbitol (a coating agent).
3. *Barium follow-through*, e.g. E-Z Paque® 60–100% w/v 300 ml (150 ml if performed after a barium meal). This preparation contains sorbitol, which produces an osmotic hurrying and is partially resistant to flocculation.
4. *Small bowel enema*, e.g. either one 300 ml can of Baritop 100% w/v or two tubs of E-Z Paque made up to 1500 ml (60% w/v). N.B. As the transit time through the small bowel is relatively short in this investigation, there is a reduced chance of flocculation. This enables the use of barium preparations which are not flocculation-resistant. Gastrografin can be added to the mixture as this may help reduce the transit time still further.

5. *Barium enema*, e.g. Polibar 115% w/v 500 ml or more, as required. Reduced density between 20% and 40% w/v for single contrast examinations.

Advantages

1. The main advantage of barium over water-soluble contrast agents is that it results in better coating and thus better mucosal detail.
2. Low cost.

Disadvantages

1. Subsequent abdominal CT is rendered difficult (if not impossible) to interpret. Patients may need to wait for up to 2 weeks to allow satisfactory clearance of the barium. There may also be some reduction in US quality. It is advised that CT and/or US are performed before the barium study.
2. High morbidity associated with barium in the peritoneal cavity.

Complications

1. *Perforation.* The escape of barium into the peritoneal cavity is rare. If large amounts enter the peritoneal cavity it is extremely serious and will produce pain and severe hypovolaemic shock. Treatment should consist of aggressive intravenous fluid resuscitation, emergency surgery with copious washout and antibiotics. A 50% mortality rate is quoted and of those that survive, 30% will develop granulomata and peritoneal adhesions. Intramediastinal barium also has a significant mortality rate. It is imperative that a water-soluble contrast medium be the initial agent used for any investigation in which there is a risk or suspicion of perforation.
2. *Aspiration.* Aspirated barium is relatively harmless. Sequelae include pneumonitis and granuloma formation. Physiotherapy is the only treatment required (for both aspirated barium and low osmolar contrast material (LOCM)), and should be arranged before the patient leaves hospital.
3. *Intravasation.* This very rare complication may result in a barium pulmonary embolus, which carries a mortality of 80%.

   For further complications (e.g. constipation and impaction), see the specific procedure involved.

WATER-SOLUBLE CONTRAST AGENTS

There are numerous water-soluble contrast agents available. Two agents of particular note are Gastrografin® and Gastromiro®. Gastrografin is an aniseed-tasting, high osmolarity contrast agent (sodium amidotrizoate and meglumine amidotrizoate) containing a wetting agent for oral or rectal use. Although primarily used in diagnosis, its high osmolarity is exploited to help achieve bowel catharsis in CT colonography, to diagnose and treat meconium ileus and also in adhesive small bowel obstruction. Its use needs to be especially carefully monitored in the frail and the very young owing to potential profound fluid and electrolyte disturbance. It should be diluted 4–5-fold for rectal administration.

Low osmolar contrast agents may be given orally but taste unpleasant. Gastromiro, a low osmolarity contrast agent (containing iopamidol), is a more palatable orange-flavoured alternative.

Indications

1. Suspected perforation.
2. Meconium ileus.
3. To distinguish bowel from other structures on CT. A dilute (c. 3%) solution of water-soluble contrast medium (e.g. 30 ml of Gastrografin in 1 l of flavoured drink) is used so that minimal artefact 'shadow' is produced.
4. LOCM is used if aspiration is a possibility.

Complications

1. HOCM can precipitate pulmonary oedema if aspirated (not LOCM).
2. HOCM can cause hypovolaemia and electrolyte disturbance due to the hyperosmolality of the contrast media drawing fluid into the bowel (not LOCM).
3. May precipitate in hyperchlorhydric gastric acid (i.e. 0.1 M HCl) – not non-ionic.

GASES

1. Oesophagus, stomach and duodenum – Carbon dioxide and, less often, air are used in conjunction with barium to achieve a 'double contrast' effect. For the upper gastrointestinal tract, CO_2 is administered orally in the form of gas-producing granules/powder (sodium bicarbonate) which when mixed with fluid (citric acid) produces gas. The requirements of these agents are as follows:
   (a) Production of an adequate volume of gas – 200–400 ml
   (b) Non-interference with barium coating
   (c) No bubble production
   (d) Rapid dissolution, leaving no residue
   (e) Easily swallowed.
2. Large bowel – For the large bowel, room air is administered per rectum via a hand pump attached to the enema tube. Carbon dioxide can also be administered by hand pump and is said to be resorbed more quickly, cause less abdominal pain, but produce inferior bowel distension when compared to air.[1] CO_2 insufflating pumps are in common usage in CT colonography.

PHARMACOLOGICAL AGENTS

Hyoscine-N-butylbromide (Buscopan®)

This is an antimuscarinic agent thus inhibiting both intestinal motility and gastric secretion. It is not recommended in children.

Adult dose

20 mg i.v.

The advantages of hyoscine include its immediate onset of action, relatively short duration of action (approx. 5–10 min) and its relatively low cost. Disadvantages include short-lived antimuscarinic side effects which include blurring of vision, a dry mouth, transient bradycardia followed by tachycardia and rare side effects said to include urinary retention and acute gastric dilatation. A particular side effect is that hyoscine can precipitate acute-angle closure glaucoma (AACG) in those patients who are susceptible to this because it dilates the pupil. In the UK patients who have AACG are almost always treated surgically in both eyes to prevent any recurrence. Pupillary dilatation has no role to play in the most common sort of glaucoma, open angle glaucoma, which accounts for 90% cases. Denying patients hyoscine on the basis of previous history of glaucoma is now not thought justified. Instead the following precautions are thought sufficient for the administration of hyoscine.[1]

Do

- Ask clinicians to identify patients who have *unstable* cardiac disease
- Ask whether there is a history of allergy to hyoscine
- Warn patients to expect blurred vision and not to drive until this has worn off
- Patient information leaflets should include 'in the rare event that following the examination you develop painful, blurred vision in one or both eyes, you must attend hospital immediately for assessment.'

Don't

- Administer hyoscine if the patient has unstable cardiac disease
- Routinely enquire whether there is a history of glaucoma, prostatism, porphyria, or myasthenia gravis.

Glucagon

This polypeptide hormone produced by the alpha cells of the islets of Langerhans in the pancreas has a predominantly hyperglycaemic effect but also causes smooth muscle relaxation. It is used in USA as an alternative to hyoscine which is not licensed there.

Adult dose
- 0.2–0.5 mg i.v. (or 1 mg i.m.) for barium meal.
- 0.5–0.75 mg i.v. (1.0–2.0 mg i.m.) for barium enema.
- 1 mg i.m. for CT or MRI small bowel imaging.

Advantages
1. More potent smooth muscle relaxant than hyoscine. Arrests small bowel peristalsis more reliably and lasts longer compared with hyoscine.[2]
2. Short duration of action (approximately 15–20 min), similar in length to hyoscine.
3. It does not interfere with the small-bowel transit time.

Disadvantages
1. May cause nausea (common), vomiting (uncommon) and abdominal pain (rare).
2. May paradoxically cause hypoglycaemia, especially in those who have fasted.
3. Hypersensitivity reactions (rare).
4. Relatively long onset of action (1 min), similar to hyoscine.
5. Relatively high cost compared with hyoscine.

Contraindications
1. Phaeochromocytoma. Glucagon can cause the tumour to release catecholamines, resulting in sudden and marked hypertension (5–10 mg phentolamine mesilate may be administered i.v. in an attempt to control the blood pressure).
2. Caution is advised in the following conditions:
   - (a) Insulinoma: an initial increase in blood glucose may be followed by severe hypoglycaemia
   - (b) Glucagonoma.

Metoclopramide (Maxolon®)

This dopamine antagonist stimulates gastric emptying and small-intestinal transit.

Adult dose
10–20 mg oral OR 10 mg i.m. OR 10 mg by slow i.v. injection.

Advantages
1. Produces rapid gastric emptying and, therefore, increased jejunal peristalsis.
2. Anti-emetic.

Disadvantages
Dystonic side effects may occur if the dose exceeds 0.5 mg kg^{-1}. This is more likely to occur in children/young adults. Intramuscular administration of an anticholinergic drug (for example, biperiden 5 mg or procyclidine 5 mg)[3] is usually effective within 20 min.

General points

In all barium work a high-kV technique is used (90–110 kV).

As in all radiological procedures, the ALARP (*As Low As Reasonably Practicable*) principle should be adhered to.

As regards women of child-bearing age, the '10-day rule' is generally applied for both upper and lower gastrointestinal investigations.

Barium has superior contrast qualities and, unless there are specific contraindications, its use (rather than water-soluble agents) is preferred.

3

References

Gases

1. Holemans JA, Matson MB, Hughes JA, et al. A comparison of air, carbon dioxide and air/carbon dioxide mixture as insufflation agents for double contrast barium enema. European Radiology 1998;8:274–6.

Pharmacological agents

1. Dyde R, Chapman AH, Gale R, et al. Precautions to be taken by radiologists and radiographers when prescribing hyoscine-N-butylbromide. Clinical Radiology 2008;63:739–43.
2. Froehlich JM, Daenzer M, von Weymarn C, et al. A peristaltic effect of hyoscine N-butylbromide versus glucagon on the small bowel assessed by magnetic resonance imaging. European Radiology 2009;19:1387–93.
3. van Harten PN, Hoek HW, Kahn RS. Acute dystonia induced by drug treatment. British Medical Journal 1999;319:623–6.

Further Reading

Other

Karanikas ID, Kakoulidis DD, Gouvas ZT, et al. Barium peritonitis: a rare complication of upper gastrointestinal contrast investigation. Postgraduate Medical Journal 1997;73:297–8.

Useful summaries of product characteristics may be obtained at: www.medicines.org.uk.

CONTRAST SWALLOW

Indications – suspected oesophageal pathology

1. Dysphagia
2. Painful swallow
3. Anaemia (with a barium meal)
4. Assessment of tracheo-oesophageal fistulae
5. Assessment of the site of perforation.

Contraindications

None.

Contrast medium

1. E-Z HD 200–250% or Baritop 100% w/v, 100 ml (or more, as required)
2. Water-soluble contrast agent if perforation is suspected (e.g. Conray, Gastrografin)
3. LOCM (approx. 300 mg I ml^{-1}) is safest if there is a risk of aspiration.

N.B.

1. Gastrografin should **NOT** be used for the investigation of a tracheo-oesophageal fistula or when aspiration is a possibility. Use LOCM instead.
2. Barium should **NOT** be used initially if perforation is suspected. If perforation is not identified with a water-soluble contrast agent then a barium examination should be considered.

Equipment

Rapid fluoroscopy images, rapid exposures (6 frames s^{-1}) or video recording may be required for assessment of the laryngopharynx and upper oesophagus during deglutition.

Patient preparation

None (but as for barium meal if the stomach is also to be examined).

Technique

1. Start with the patient in the erect position, right anterior oblique (RAO) position to project the oesophagus clear of the spine. An ample mouthful of barium is swallowed and this bolus is observed under fluoroscopy for dynamic assessment to assess the function of the oesophagus. Then further mouthfuls with spot exposure(s) to include the whole oesophagus with dedicated AP views of the gastro-oesophageal junction.
2. Coned views of the hypopharynx should be obtained with a frame rate of 3–4 per second to include AP, lateral and oblique views whilst the patient swallows contrast.
3. The patient is placed semi-prone in a 'recovery position' in a left posterior oblique (LPO) position with their right arm by their side behind their back and the left arm used to support the cup containing contrast. One further swallow with a single bolus is observed under fluoroscopy to assess motility with the effect of gravity eliminated. A distended single-contrast view should be obtained as the patient rapidly sips and swallows contrast as this best identifies hernias, subtle mucosal rings and varices.

4. Modifications may be required depending on the clinical indication.

   (a) If dysmotility is suspected barium should be mixed with bread or marshmallow bolus and observed under fluoroscopy correlating symptoms with the passage of the bolus in the erect position.

   (b) If perforation is suspected a control film may be useful to identify pneumomediastinum and ideally the patient should be examined in four positions (prone/supine/left lateral/right lateral) with water-soluble contrast first, and if this is negative then with barium contrast.

   (c) To demonstrate a tracheo-oesophageal fistula in infants, a 'pull back' nasogastric tube oeosphagogram may be performed if the standard oesophagogram is negative.[1] This technique is particularly useful in patients known to aspirate or in ventilated patients. Suction and nursing support should be available should aspiration occur. The patient is positioned prone with the arms up and the table may be tilted slightly head down. A nasogastric tube is introduced into stomach and then withdrawn to the level of the lower oesophagus under lateral screening guidance. Ten to 20 ml of LOCM is syringed in to distend the oesophagus which will force the contrast medium through any small fistula which may be present. The process is repeated for the upper and mid oesophagus. It is important to watch for aspiration into the airway from overspill which can lead to diagnostic confusion.

Aftercare

Eat and drink as normal but with extra fluids.

Complications

1. Leakage of barium from an unsuspected perforation
2. Aspiration.

Reference

1. Hiorns MP. Gastrointestinal tract imaging in children: current techniques Pediatric Radiology 2011;41:42–54.

BARIUM MEAL

Methods

1. *Double contrast* – the method of choice to demonstrate mucosal pattern.
2. *Single contrast* – uses:

   (a) children – since it usually is not necessary to demonstrate mucosal pattern

   (b) to demonstrate gross pathology only, typically very frail patients unable to swallow gas granules.

Indications

1. Failed upper gastrointestinal endoscopy or patient unwilling to undergo endoscopy
2. Dyspepsia
3. Weight loss
4. Gastrointestinal haemorrhage (or unexplained iron-deficiency anaemia)
5. Partial obstruction
6. Assessment of site of perforation – it is essential that a water-soluble contrast medium, e.g. Gastrografin or LOCM, is used.

Contraindications

Complete large-bowel obstruction.

Contrast medium

1. E-Z HD 250% w/v 135 ml
2. Carbex granules (double contrast technique).

Patient preparation

1. Nil orally for 6 h prior to the examination
2. No contraindications to the pharmacological agents used.

Preliminary image

None.

Technique

The double contrast method (Fig. 3.1):

1. A gas-producing agent is swallowed.
2. The patient then drinks the barium while lying on the left side, supported by their elbow. This position prevents the barium from reaching the duodenum too quickly and so obscuring the greater curve of the stomach.
3. The patient then lies supine and slightly on the right side, to bring the barium up against the gastro-oesophageal junction. This manoeuvre is screened to check for reflux, which may be revealed by asking the patient to cough or to swallow water while in this position (the 'water siphon' test). The significance of reflux produced by tipping the patient's head down and simultaneously drinking water is debatable, as this is non-physiological – 24-hour pH probe monitoring is the best current investigation. If reflux is observed, images are taken to record the level to which it ascends.
4. An i.v. injection of a smooth muscle relaxant (Buscopan 20 mg or glucagon 0.3 mg) may be given to better distend the stomach and to slow down the emptying of contrast into duodenum. The

Figure 3.1 Barium meal sequence. Note in a, b, c and d, the patient position is depicted as if the operator were standing at the end of the screening table looking towards the patient's head.

administration of Buscopan has been shown not to affect the detection of gastro-oesophageal reflux or hiatus hernia.

5. The patient is asked to roll onto the right side and then quickly over in a complete circle, to finish in an RAO position. This roll is performed to coat the gastric mucosa with barium. Good coating has been achieved if the areae gastricae in the antrum are visible.

Images

There is a great variation in views recommended. One scheme is:

1. Spot exposures of the stomach (lying):
    (a) RAO – to demonstrate the antrum and greater curve
    (b) Supine – to demonstrate the antrum and body
    (c) LAO – to demonstrate the lesser curve en face
    (d) Left lateral tilted, head up 45°– to demonstrate the fundus.
        From the left lateral position the patient returns to a supine position and then rolls onto the left side and over into a prone position. This sequence of movements is required to avoid barium flooding into the duodenal loop, which would occur if the patient were to roll onto the right side to achieve a prone position.
2. Spot image of the duodenal loop (lying):
    (a) Prone – the patient lies on a compression pad to prevent barium from flooding into the duodenum.
        An additional view to demonstrate the anterior wall of the duodenal loop may be taken in an RAO position.
3. Spot images of the duodenal cap (lying):
    (a) Prone
    (b) RAO – the patient attains this position from the prone position by rolling first onto the left side, for the reasons mentioned above
    (c) Supine
    (d) LAO.
4. Additional views of the fundus in an erect position may be taken at this stage, if there is suspicion of a fundal lesion.
5. Spot images of the oesophagus are taken, while barium is being swallowed, to complete the examination.

Modification of technique for young children

The main indication will be to identify a cause for vomiting. The examination is modified to identify the three major causes of vomiting – gastro-oesophageal reflux, pyloric obstruction and malrotation, and it is essential that the position of the duodeno-jejunal flexure is demonstrated:

1. Single-contrast technique using 30% w/v barium sulphate and no paralytic agent.

2. A relatively small volume of barium – enough to just fill the fundus – is given to the infant in the supine position. An image of the distended oesophagus is exposed.

3. The child is turned semi-prone into a LPO or RAO position. An image is taken as barium passes through the pylorus. The pylorus is shown to even better advantage if 20–40° caudocranial angulation can be employed with an overhead screening unit. Gastric emptying is prolonged if the child is upset. A dummy coated with glycerine is a useful pacifier.

4. Once barium enters the duodenum, the infant is returned to the supine position, and with the child perfectly straight a second image is taken as barium passes around the duodenojejunal flexure. This image should just include the lower chest to verify that the child is straight.

5. Once malrotation has been diagnosed or excluded, a further volume of barium is administered until the stomach is reasonably full and barium lies against the gastro-oesophageal junction. The child is gently rotated through 180° in an attempt to elicit gastro-oesophageal reflux.

In newborn infants with upper intestinal obstruction, e.g. duodenal atresia, the diagnosis may be confirmed if 20 ml of air is injected down the nasogastric tube (which will almost certainly have already been introduced by the medical staff). If the diagnosis remains in doubt, it can be replaced by a positive contrast agent (dilute barium or LOCM if the risk of aspiration is high).

Aftercare

1. The patient must not drive until any blurring of vision produced by the Buscopan has resolved.

2. The patient should be warned that their bowel motions will be white for a few days after the examination and may be difficult to flush away.

3. The patient should be advised to eat and drink normally but with extra fluids to avoid barium impaction. Occasionally laxatives may also be required.

Complications

1. Leakage of barium from an unsuspected perforation
2. Aspiration
3. Conversion of a partial large bowel obstruction into a complete obstruction by the impaction of barium
4. Barium appendicitis, if barium impacts in the appendix (exceedingly rare)
5. Side effects of the pharmacological agents used.

N.B. It must be emphasized that there are many variations in technique, according to individual preference, and that the best way of becoming familiar with the sequence of positioning is actually to perform the procedure oneself.

SMALL BOWEL FOLLOW-THROUGH

Methods

1. Single contrast
2. With the addition of an effervescent agent
3. With the addition of a pneumocolon technique.

Indications

1. Pain
2. Diarrhoea
3. Anaemia/gastrointestinal bleeding unexplained by colonic or gastric investigation
4. To assess small bowel Crohn's disease status
5. Partial obstruction
6. Malabsorption.

Contraindications

1. Complete or high-grade obstruction. This is usually better evaluated by CT examination (without oral contrast) using the intraluminal fluid caused by the obstruction as a natural contrast agent.
2. Suspected perforation (unless a water-soluble contrast medium is used).

Contrast medium

E-Z Paque 100% w/v 300 ml usually given divided in 10–15-min increments, although some radiologists give the full 300 ml at once. The transit time through the small bowel has been shown to be reduced by the addition of 10 ml of Gastrografin to the barium. In children, 3–4 ml kg^{-1} is a suitable volume.

In general water-soluble small bowel contrast studies are avoided as contrast becomes diluted in small bowel fluid resulting in poor mucosal detail compared with barium. An exception is in adhesional small bowel obstruction where conservative investigation and 'treatment' with water-soluble contrast agents, frequently Gastrografin, may reduce the need for surgical intervention.[1] In this case limited images are usually acquired at 1, 4 and 24 h, stopping once contrast is seen in the colon.

Patient preparation

Metoclopramide 20 mg orally may be given before or during the examination.

Preliminary image

Plain abdominal film is used if high-grade small bowel obstruction is thought possible.

Technique

The aim is to deliver a single continuous column of barium into the small bowel. This is achieved by the patient lying on their right side after the barium has been drunk. Metoclopramide enhances the rate of gastric emptying. If the transit time through the small bowel is found to be slow, the addition of Gastrografin may help to speed it up. If a follow-through examination is combined with a barium meal, glucagon can be used for the duodenal cap views rather than Buscopan because it has a short length of action and does not interfere with the small-bowel transit time.

Images

1. Prone PA images of the abdomen are taken every 15–20 min during the first hour, and subsequently every 20–30 min until the colon is reached. The prone position is used because the pressure on the abdomen helps to separate the loops of small bowel.
2. Each image should be reviewed and spot supine fluoroscopic views, using a compression device or pad if appropriate, may be considered.
3. Dedicated spot views of the terminal ileum are routinely acquired.

Additional images

1. To separate loops of small bowel:
   (a) compression with fluoroscopy
   (b) with X-ray tube angled into the pelvis
   (c) obliques – in particular with the right side raised for terminal ileum views, or
   (d) occasionally with the patient tilted head down.
   (e) pneumocolon.[2] Gaseous insufflation of the colon via a rectal tube after barium arrives in the caecum often results in good-quality double-contrast views of the terminal ileum.
2. Erect image – occasionally used to reveal any fluid levels caused by contrast medium retained within diverticula.

Aftercare

As for barium meal.

Complications

As for barium meal.

References
1. Catena F, Di Saverio S, Kelly MD, et al. Bologna Guidelines for Diagnosis and Management of Adhesive Small Bowel Obstruction (ASBO): 2010

Evidence-Based Guidelines of the World Society of Emergency Surgery. World J Emerg Surg 2011;6:5.

2. Pickhardt PJ. The peroral pneumocolon revisited: a valuable fluoroscopic and CT technique for ileocecal evaluation. Abdom Imaging 2012;37(3):313–25.

SMALL-BOWEL ENEMA

Advantage

This procedure gives better distension and visualization of the proximal small bowel than that achieved by a barium follow-through because rapid infusion of a large continuous column of contrast medium directly into the jejunum. However the degree of distal small bowel distension by small bowel enema and small bowel follow-through methods is usually fairly similar.

Disadvantages

1. Per-nasal/oral intubation may be unpleasant for the patient, and may prove difficult. Some centres routinely use sedation.
2. It is more time-consuming for the radiologist.
3. Potentially higher radiation dose to the patient (screening the tube into position).

Indications and contraindications

These are the same as for a barium follow-through. In some departments it is only performed in the case of an equivocal follow-through.

Contrast medium

1. Single contrast: e.g. E-Z Paque 70% w/v diluted; or Baritop 100% w/v (one 300 ml can made up to 1500 ml with water).
2. 600 ml of 0.5% methylcellulose after 500 ml of 70% w/v barium.[1]

It may be difficult to obtain good distension and double-contrast effect of the distal small bowel and terminal ileum.

Equipment

A choice of tubes is available:

1. Bilbao-Dotter tube (Cook Ltd) with a guidewire (the tube is blind ending). Comes in various sizes and modifications including one variant with an inflatable balloon at the end to prevent reflux into the stomach.
2. Silk tube (E. Merck Ltd). This is a 10-F, 140-cm-long tube. It is made of polyurethane and the stylet and the internal lumen of the tube are coated with a water-activated lubricant to facilitate the smooth removal of the stylet after insertion.

Patient preparation

1. NBM after midnight.
2. Stop antispasmodic drugs 1 day prior to the examination.
3. Consider tetracaine lozenge 30 mg, 30 min before the examination.

Preliminary image

Plain abdominal film is used if a small bowel obstruction is suspected. CT should be considered as it is often a better examination in this scenario.

3

Technique

1. The patient sits on the edge of the X-ray table. If a per-nasal approach is planned, the patency of the nasal passages is checked by asking the patient to sniff with one nostril occluded. The pharynx is anaesthetized with lidocaine spray or Xylocaine gel instilled into a nostril. The Silk tube should be passed with the guidewire pre-lubricated and fully within the tube, whereas for the Bilbao-Dotter tube the guidewire is introduced after the tube tip is in the stomach.
2. The tube is then passed through the nose or the mouth, and brief lateral screening of the neck may be helpful in negotiating the epiglottic region. The patient is asked to swallow with the neck flexed, as the tube is passed through the pharynx. The tube is then advanced into the gastric antrum.
3. The patient then lies down and the tube is passed into the duodenum. Various manoeuvres may be used alone, or in combination, to help this part of the procedure, which may be difficult:
   (a) Lay the patient on his left side so that the gastric air bubble rises to the antrum, thus straightening out the stomach.
   (b) Advance the tube whilst applying clockwise rotational motion (as viewed from the head of the patient looking towards the feet).
   (c) Get the patient to sit up, to try to overcome the tendency of the tube to coil in the fundus of the stomach.
   (d) Metoclopramide (20 mg i.v.) may help.
4. When the tip of the tube has been passed through the pylorus, the guidewire tip is maintained at the pylorus as the tube is passed over it along the duodenum to the level of the ligament of Treitz. The tube is ideally passed beyond the duodenojejunal flexure to diminish the risk of aspiration due to reflux of barium into the stomach.
5. Barium is then run in, ideally with a controllable mechanical pump, or by gravity. Initially start at 50 ml min^{-1} and, with regular initial screening, aim to 'chase' the leading edge of the barium distally to maintain an unbroken column of contrast within the small bowel.

The infusion can usually be increased rapidly to 100 ml min^{-1} depending on the progress of the barium through the bowel. If methylcellulose is used, it is infused continuously, after an initial bolus of 500 ml of barium, until the barium has reached the colon.

6. The tube is then withdrawn, aspirating any residual fluid in the stomach. This is to decrease the risk of aspiration.
7. If the terminal ileum is obscured at the end of the examination it can be helpful to further re-screen the patient after an interval when barium has emptied into the colon as better views may be then obtained. A pneumocolon, as per small bowel follow-through, may also help.

Images

Magnified views of each quadrant recommended with at least one good view of the terminal ileum and an overall view of the abdomen. Fluoroscopic 'grab' images of the examination during the filling phase are also useful as they help record and assess motility.

Modification of technique

In patients with malabsorption, especially if an excess of fluid has been shown on the preliminary image, the volume of barium should be increased (240–260 ml). Compression views of bowel loops should be obtained before obtaining double contrast. Flocculation is likely to occur early. If it is important to obtain images of the duodenum, the catheter tip should be sited proximal to the ligament of Trietz.

Aftercare

The patient should be warned that diarrhoea may occur as a result of the large volume of fluid given.

Complications

1. Aspiration
2. Perforation of the bowel owing to manipulation of the guidewire (very rare).

Reference
1. Ha HK, Park KB, Kim PN, et al. Use of methylcellulose in small bowel follow through examination: comparison with conventional series in normal subjects. Abdom Imaging 1998;23(3):281–5.

Further Reading
Minordi LM, Vecchioli A, Guidi L, et al. Multidetector CT enteroclysis versus barium enteroclysis with methylcellulose in patients with suspected small bowel disease. Eur Radiol 2006;16(7):1527–36.

Nolan DJ. The true yield of the small intestinal barium study. Endoscopy 1997;29(6):447–53.

BARIUM ENEMA

Methods

1. *Double contrast* – the method of choice to demonstrate mucosal pattern.
2. *Single contrast* – uses:
   (a) localization of an obstructing colonic lesion (use water-soluble contrast as surgery or stenting may be required shortly after the procedure)
   (b) children – since it is usually not necessary to demonstrate mucosal pattern
   (c) reduction of an intussusception (see p. 69).

Indication

Suspected large bowel pathology.

N.B. If a tight stricture is demonstrated, only run a small volume of barium proximally to define the upper margin, as otherwise the barium may impact. CTC avoids the risks of barium impaction.

Contraindications

Absolute

1. Toxic megacolon (CT is radiological investigation of choice)
2. Pseudomembranous colitis
3. Recent biopsy[1] via:
   (a) rigid endoscope within previous 5 days (the biopsy forceps used tend to be larger)
   (b) flexible endoscope within previous 24 h (the smaller biopsy forceps only allows superficial mucosal biopsies).

Relative

1. Incomplete bowel preparation – consider if the patient can have extra preparation to return later that day or the next day
2. Recent barium meal – it is advised to wait for 7–10 days
3. Patient frailty.

Contrast medium

1. Polibar 115% w/v 500 ml (or more, as required)
2 Air.

Equipment

Disposable enema tube and pump.

Patient preparation

Many regimens for bowel preparation exist. A suggested regimen is as follows:

For 3 days prior to examination
Low-residue diet.

On the day prior to examination
1. Fluids only
2. Picolax – at 08:00 h and 18:00 h.

Consider admitting the elderly and those with social problems.

On the day of the examination
It is advisable to place diabetics first on the list.

Technique

The double-contrast method:

1. The patient lies on their left side, and the catheter is inserted gently into the rectum. It is taped firmly in position. Connections are made to the barium reservoir and the hand pump for injecting air.
2. An i.v. injection of Buscopan (20 mg) or glucagon (1 mg) is given. Some radiologists choose to give the muscle relaxant half way through the procedure at the end of step (3).
3. The infusion of barium is commenced. Intermittent screening is required to check the progress of the barium. The barium is run to splenic flexure in the left lateral position and then the patient is turned prone. Contrast is then run to the hepatic flexure and is stopped when it tips into the right colon. Gentle puffs of air may be needed to encourage the barium to flow. The patient rolls onto their right and quickly onto their back. An adequate amount of barium in the right colon is confirmed with fluoroscopy. The column of barium within the distal colon is run back out by either lowering the infusion bag to the floor or tilting the table to the erect position.
4. The catheter tube is occluded and air is gently pumped into the bowel to produce the double-contrast effect. CO_2 gas has been shown to reduce the incidence of severe, post enema pain.

Exposures

There is a great variation in views recommended. Fewer films may be taken to reduce the radiation dose. The sequence of positioning enables the barium to flow proximally to reach the caecal pole. Air is pumped in as required to distend the colon.

A suggested sequence of positioning and **films** in a standard over couch image intensifier include:

- **Left lateral rectum**; then roll patient half way back
- **RAO sigmoid**; then roll patient prone and insufflate to distend transverse colon. The patient lifts left side up to obtain

- **LPO sigmoid**, then turn supine
- **AP view(s)** of whole colon
- Raise patient to erect position with dedicated views of both **flexures** with some LAO positioning for splenic flexure and RAO positioning for hepatic flexure. Return patient to supine position
- Over couch views:
  Left lateral decubitus
  Right lateral decubitus
  Prone angled view of rectosigmoid
- Dedicated views of **caecum** and right colon, often with some RAO positioning (sometimes prior to the decubitus films)
- Dedicated views of any pathology encountered.

Aftercare

1. The patient must not drive until any blurring of vision produced by Buscopan has resolved; usually within 30 minutes.
2. Patients should be warned that their bowel motions will be white for a few days after the examination. They may eat normally and should drink extra fluids to avoid barium impaction.

Antibiotic prophylaxis in barium enema[2]

This is not routinely required, but barium enema is identified as the only lower GI intervention with a significant risk of endocarditis in those patients with specific risk factors.

Offer antibiotic prophylaxis to those with:

- previous infective endocarditis
- acquired valvular heart disease with stenosis or regurgitation
- valve replacement
- structural congenital heart disease (but excluding isolated atrial septal defect, fully repaired ventricular septal defect or fully repaired patent ductus arteriosus)
- hypertrophic cardiomyopathy.

Complications[3] (all are rare)

1. Cardiac arrhythmias induced by Buscopan or the procedure itself. This is the most frequent cause of death after barium enema.
2. Perforation of the bowel. The second most common cause of death after barium enema. Often associated with the rectal catheter balloon
3. Transient bacteraemia.
4. Side effects of the pharmacological agents used (see p. 51).
5. Intramural barium.
6. Venous intravasation. This may result in a barium pulmonary embolus, which carries an 80% mortality risk.

References
1. Low VH. What is the current recommended waiting time for performance of a gastrointestinal barium study after endoscopic biopsy of the upper or lower gastrointestinal tract. Am J Roentgenol 1998;170(4):1104–5.
2. NICE. NICE guidance. Antimicrobial prophylaxis against infective endocarditis in adults and children undergoing interventional procedures. NICE Clinical Guidelines 2008;(64) (March 2008).
3. Blakeborough A, Sheridan MB, Chapman AH. Complications of barium enema examinations: a survey of UK Consultant Radiologists 1992 to 1994. Clin Radiol 1997;52(2):142–8.

ENEMA VARIANTS

These variants are less used with the wider availability of CT but may provide extra information in selected cases.

THE 'INSTANT' ENEMA

Indications
1. To identify/confirm the level of suspected large bowel obstruction and to assess the degree of narrowing (e.g. sometimes helpful in stent planning).
2. Rarely, to show the extent and severity of mucosal lesions in active ulcerative colitis.

Contraindications
1. Toxic megacolon
2. Rectal biopsy (as for barium enema)
3. Chronic ulcerative colitis – optical colonoscopy to detect dysplasia and neoplasia in this high-risk group is preferred
4. Crohn's colitis – assessment in this situation is unreliable.

Contrast medium
Water-soluble contrast (e.g. Urografin 150).

Preliminary image
Plain abdominal film – to exclude:

1. Toxic megacolon
2. Perforation.

Technique
1. The contrast medium is run until it flows into an obstructing lesion or dilated bowel loops.
2. Air insufflation is not required – i.e. single contrast technique.

Images

Images are obtained as required; generally to include views of pathology encountered but may include prone, left lateral decubitus and erect films as necessary.

AIR ENEMA

3

Very rarely used.

Indications

Demonstrate extent of ulcerative colitis.

Technique

1. Insert 14–16-F Foley catheter into rectum and inflate balloon (10–20 ml).
2. Take preliminary overcouch anterior posterior (AP) film of abdomen.
3. View film and without the patient moving give relaxant, e.g. Buscopan, and then inflate air (gentle puffs) into catheter lumen.
4. Take AP film of abdomen.

REDUCTION OF AN INTUSSUSCEPTION

This procedure should only be attempted in full consultation with the surgeon in charge of the case and when an anaesthetist with appropriate paediatric training and experience, and with paediatric anaesthetic equipment, is available.[1,2]

Methods

1. Using air and fluoroscopy.[3] Barium is no longer used in the majority of centres as air reduction has the following advantages:
   (a) more rapid reduction, because the low viscosity of air permits rapid filling of the colon
   (b) reduced radiation dose because of the above
   (c) more effective reduction
   (d) in the presence of a perforation, air in the peritoneal cavity is preferable to barium, and gut organisms are not washed into the peritoneal cavity
   (e) there is more accurate control of intraluminal pressure
   (f) less mess, and a dry infant will not lose heat
   (g) less expensive.
2. Using a water-soluble contrast medium and US.

Contraindications

1. Peritonitis, perforation or shock.
2. The pneumatic method should probably not be used in children over 4 years of age as there is a higher incidence of significant lead points which may be missed.[4]
3. Successful reduction is less likely in patients with prolonged symptoms or radiographic signs of obstruction, but this does not preclude an attempt at reduction if the patient is well hydrated and stable.[5]

Patient preparation

1. Sedation is of questionable value, but analgesia is important (e.g. morphine 50 μg kg^{-1} if <1 year or 50–100 μg kg^{-1} if >1 year).
2. Some institutions perform the examination under general anaesthesia. This has the advantage of greater muscle relaxation, which may increase the likelihood of successful reduction, and also enables the child to go to surgery quickly in the event of a failed radiological reduction.
3. Correction of fluid and electrolyte imbalance. The child requires an i.v. line in situ.
4. Antibiotic cover is not routine.

Preliminary investigations

1. Plain abdominal film – to assess bowel distension and to exclude perforation. A right-side-up decubitus film is often helpful in confirming the diagnosis by showing a failure of caecal filling with bowel gas because of the presence of the soft-tissue mass of the intussusception. Normal plain films do not exclude the diagnosis, and the clinical findings and/or history should be sufficient indications.
2. US – should confirm or exclude the diagnosis. Absence of blood flow within the intussusceptum on colour-flow Doppler should lead to cautious reduction.[6] US may identify a lead point; if so, even attempted reduction (to facilitate surgery) should be followed by surgery. If US identifies fluid trapped between the intussusceptum and intussuscipiens, the success rate is significantly reduced.[7]

Contrast medium

1. Air
2. Barium sulphate 100% w/v (now rarely used)
3. Water-soluble contrast, e.g. LOCM 150 or dilute Gastrografin (1 part Gastrografin to 4 or 5 parts water).

Technique

A 16–22-F balloon catheter is inserted into the rectum and the buttocks taped tightly together to provide a seal. It may be necessary to inflate the balloon but if this is done it should be performed under fluoroscopic control so that the rectum is not over distended.

Pneumatic reduction

1. The child is placed in the prone position so that it is easier to maintain the catheter in the rectum and the child is disturbed as little as possible during the procedure.
2. Air is instilled by a hand or mechanical pump and the intussusception is pushed back by a sustained pressure of up to 80 mmHg. Pressure should be monitored at all times and there should be a fail-safe pressure-release valve in the system to ensure that excessive pressures are not delivered.
3. Reduction is successful when there is free flow of air into the distal ileum.
4. If the intussusception does not move after 3 min of sustained pressure, the pressure is reduced and the child rested for 3 minutes. Two further attempts are made increasing the pressure to 120 mmHg for 3 minutes with a 3-minute rest. If the intussusception is still immovable it is considered irreducible and arrangements are made for surgery.
5. The intussusception is only considered completely reduced when the terminal ileum is filled with air. However, it is not uncommon for there to be a persisting filling defect in the caecum at the end of the procedure, with or without reflux of air into the terminal ileum. This is often due to an oedematous ileocaecal valve. In the presence of a soft-tissue caecal mass, a clinically well and stable child should be returned to the ward to await a further attempt at reduction after a period of 2–8 h rather than proceed to surgery. A second enema is often successful at complete reduction or showing resolution of the oedematous ileocaecal valve.[8]
6. When air (or barium) dissects between the two layers of the intussusception – the dissection sign – reduction is less likely.[9]

Ultrasound reduction[10]

1. To facilitate scanning the child must be supine.
2. The intussusception can be identified with US. Rectal saline or Hartmann's solution is run as far as the obstruction and its passage around the colon and the reducing head of the intussusception is monitored by US. The intussusception is reduced when reflux into the terminal ileum is seen.
3. The points regarding failed or incomplete reduction discussed above also apply to this technique.

Barium reduction (now rarely used)

1. Patient positioning is as for the pneumatic method.
2. The bag containing barium is raised 100 cm above the table top and barium run in under hydrostatic pressure. Progress of the column of barium is monitored by intermittent fluoroscopy.

3. If the intussusception does not move after 3 min of sustained pressure, the bag of barium is lowered to table-top height and the child rested for 3 min. If, after three similar attempts, the intussusception is still immovable it is considered irreducible and arrangements are made for surgery.
4. The points regarding failed or incomplete reduction discussed above also apply to hydrostatic reduction.

Images

1. Spot films as required
2. Post-reduction film.

Aftercare

Observation in hospital for 24 h.

Complications

Perforation – for the pneumatic method, if a pump is used without a pressure-monitoring valve, perforation may result in a tension pneumoperitoneum, resulting in respiratory embarrassment. Puncture of the peritoneal cavity with a 'green' 23-G needle may be life-saving.

References

1. The Royal College of Anaesthetists. Guidelines for the Provision of Anaesthetic Services. Guidance on the Provision of Paediatric Anaesthesia. London: Royal College of Anaesthetists; 1999. p. 24–6.
2. The British Association of Paediatric Surgeons. A Guide for Purchasers and Providers of Paediatric Surgeons. London: British Association of Paediatric Surgeons; 1994, revised 1995.
3. Kirks DR. Air intussusception reduction: 'The winds of change'. Pediatric Radiology 1995;25:89–91.
4. Stringer DA, Ein SH. Pneumatic reduction: advantages, risks and indications. Pediatr Radiol 1990;20:475–7.
5. Daneman A, Navarro O. Intussusception Part 2: An update on the evolution of management. Paediatr Radiol 2004;34:97–108.
6. Lim HK, Bae SH, Lee KH, et al. Assessment of reducibility of ileocolic intussusception in children: usefulness of color Doppler sonography. Radiology 1994;191:781–5.
7. Britton I, Wilkinson AG. Ultrasound features of intussusception predicting outcome of air enema. Pediatr Radiol 1999;29:705–10.
8. Gorenstein A, Raucher A, Serour F, et al. Intussusception in children: reduction with repeated, delayed air enema. Radiology 1998;206:721–4.
9. Barr LL, Stansberry SD, Swischuk LE. Significance of age, duration, obstruction and the dissection sign in intussusception. Pediatr Radiol 1990;20:454–6.
10. Khong PL, Peh WC, Lam CH, et al. Ultrasound-guided hydrostatic reduction of childhood intussusception: technique and demonstration. RadioGraphics 2000;20:E1.

CONTRAST ENEMA IN NEONATAL LOW INTESTINAL OBSTRUCTION

The differential diagnosis of low intestinal obstruction in the newborn consists of five conditions which comprise nearly all possible causes. Three involve the colon: Hirschsprung's disease, functional immaturity of the colon (small left colon syndrome, meconium plug syndrome) and colonic atresia. Two involve the distal ileum: meconium ileus and ileal atresia. All infants with low intestinal obstruction require a contrast enema.

Contraindications

Perforation.

Patient preparation

The baby should already have i.v. access and be well hydrated prior to the procedure.

Contrast medium

Dilute ionic contrast medium as is used for cystography, e.g. Urografin 150. This has the advantage of not provoking large fluid shifts and being dense enough to provide satisfactory images. Non-ionic contrast media and barium offer no advantages (and the latter is contraindicated with perforation as a possibility). Infants with meconium ileus or functional immaturity will benefit from a water-soluble contrast enema and so their therapeutic enema commences with the diagnostic study. The non-operative treatment of meconium ileus was first described using the hypertonic agent Gastrografin, which dislodged the sticky meconium by drawing water into the bowel lumen. However, most paediatric radiologists now believe that a hypertonic agent is not necessary for successful treatment.[1]

Technique

If the enema demonstrates that the entire colon is small (a microcolon; <1 cm in diameter) then the diagnosis is likely to be meconium ileus or ileal atresia. (The microcolon of prematurity and total colonic Hirschsprung's disease are alternative rare diagnoses.) For the treatment of meconium ileus, the aim is to run the water-soluble contrast medium into the small bowel to surround the meconium. An attempt should be made to get the contrast medium back into dilated small bowel. If successful, meconium should be passed in the next hour. If no result is seen and the infant's condition deteriorates then surgical intervention will be necessary. If the passage of meconium is incomplete and the clinical condition remains stable, multiple enemas over the succeeding few days will be necessary to ensure complete resolution of the obstruction.

Overall success rate is approximately 50–60%, with a perforation rate of 2%.[1]

Reference

1. Kao SC, Franken Jr EA. Nonoperative treatment of simple meconium ileus: a survey of the Society for Pediatric Radiology. Pediatric Radiol 1995;25(2):97–100.

SINOGRAM

1. A water-soluble contrast medium should be used (e.g. Urografin 150).
2. A preliminary film is taken to exclude the presence of a radio-opaque foreign body.
3. An appropriate-size Foley catheter is then inserted into the orifice of the sinus. The balloon may be inflated inside the sinus to prevent retrograde flow. Alternatively the balloon may be inflated outside the sinus and pushed to the skin using a Spencer-Wells forceps or similar to secure a seal.
4. The contrast medium is injected carefully under fluoroscopic control.
5. Fluoroscopic 'grab' images supplemented by proper exposures are taken as required, including tangential views.

RETROGRADE ILEOGRAM

Indications

To demonstrate anatomy of small bowel in patients with an ileostomy.

Technique

1. Cannulate the ileostomy with an appropriate (16–22-F) Foley catheter. Carefully inflate the balloon at or just inside the stoma.
2. Inject contrast. Dilute barium (Baritop) or water-soluble contrast can be used as a single contrast or as double contrast with either air or water/methyl cellulose (see small bowel enema).
3. Tangential views of the spout of the stoma may be obtained at the end of the examination upon deflation of the balloon.

COLOSTOMY ENEMA

Indications

To demonstrate proximal colon following resection of the rectum.

Technique

1. Cannulate colostomy with a 22–26-F Foley catheter and gently inflate balloon.
2. Infuse barium or water-soluble contrast as for a barium enema.

LOOPOGRAM

Indications

Appropriate in patients following bladder resection to demonstrate anatomy of ileal conduit, ureters and renal pelvicalyceal systems.

Contrast

Low-concentration water-soluble contrast agent (150 mg I ml^{-1}).

Technique

Cannulate ileal conduit with 14–18-F Foley catheter and gently inflate balloon. Inject contrast into ileal conduit. Observe retrograde filling of the renal collecting systems. Stop injecting when adequately distended.

Images

- Plain AP of collecting systems.
- Post filling: AP of collecting systems, two obliques of the kidneys with an additional, often oblique, view of the ureteric – loop anastomosis.

HERNIOGRAM

Indications

1. History suggestive of a hernia with a normal/inconclusive physical examination. Where expertise is available ultrasound, MRI or CT are alternatives.
2. Undiagnosed groin pain.

Contraindications

1. Infancy
2. Pregnancy
3. Intestinal obstruction
4. Allergy to contrast medium.

Patient preparation

The patient is asked to empty their bladder just prior to the examination.

Contrast medium

50–100 ml water-soluble medium (e.g. Omnipaque 300).

Technique

1. The patient lies supine on the X-ray table.
2. An aseptic technique is employed.

3. 5–10 ml of 1% lidocaine is injected into the skin, subcutaneous tissues and peritoneum. The injection site varies between operators; the midline just below the umbilicus is most common, the midpoint of the left lateral rectus muscle is one variation.
4. An 18–22 G spinal needle is introduced into the peritoneal cavity until a 'popping' sensation is felt (as the needle tip passes into peritoneal cavity. Contrast is injected. If the needle is in the correct position a 'spider web' of intraperitoneal contrast outlining the outside of bowel loops is seen. If needle tip is in abdominal wall a bleb is seen and the needle requires repositioning.

Images

1. Prone view
2. Erect films: frontal, obliques, lateral views.

The patient is asked to cough and perform the Valsalva manoeuvre while these are taken. The tube may be angled 25° caudally.

Complications

These are uncommon, and patient admission for observation is all that is usually required:

1. Pain
2. Visceral puncture
3. Vascular puncture
4. Injection into the abdominal wall
5. Haematoma at the injection site
6. Allergy to contrast medium.

Further Reading

Ekberg O. Inguinal herniography in adults: technique, normal anatomy, and diagnostic criteria for hernias. Radiology 1981;138(1):31–6.
Hureibi KA, McLatchie GR, Kidambi AV. Is herniography useful and safe? Eur J Radiol 2011;80(2):e86–90.

EVACUATING PROCTOGRAM

Indications

1. Constipation
2. Suspected pelvic floor weakness – posterior (rectocele/enterocele/ rectal intussuception)
3. Anorectal incontinence – anal manometry and anal US preferred.

Contraindications

Pregnancy.

Contrast medium

Thick barium paste (although commercial pastes are available, this may be satisfactorily prepared with barium powder and proprietary breakfast cereal, e.g. Ready Brek®).

Technique

1. One can of Baritop or equivalent given orally 1 hour prior to examination to opacify small bowel.
2. For female patients, approximately 20–30 ml of water-soluble contrast mixed with US gel are introduced into the vagina through a Foley catheter (not always required).
3. Approximately 120 ml of barium paste (or enough to fill the rectum) are instilled via a bladder syringe.

Films

1. These are taken in a lateral projection with the patient sitting on a commode.
2. Video-recording at rest and during the Valsalva manoeuvre and during pelvic floor contractions.
3. Video-recording during defecation using a maximum of 1-min screening time to minimize patient dose.

Further Reading

Ganeshan A, Anderson EM, Upponi S, et al. Imaging of obstructed defecation. Clin Radiol 2008;63(1):18–26.

COELIAC AXIS, SUPERIOR MESENTERIC AND INFERIOR MESENTERIC ARTERIOGRAPHY

Indications

1. Gastrointestinal haemorrhage
2. Gastrointestinal ischaemia
3. Portal venography. (This is rarely needed except prior to intervention as CT/MR shows PV system well.)
4. Staging tumours prior to (surgical or radiological) intervention. (Again very rarely used since the avent of multislice CT and MRI.)

Contrast medium

LOCM 280 to 370 mg I ml^{-1}.

Equipment

1. Digital fluoroscopy with angiography facility
2. Pump injector
3. Catheter – selective femorovisceral, sidewinder or cobra catheter.

Technique

1. Femoral artery puncture – Seldinger technique
2. Bowel movement causing subtraction artefact can be reduced by using a smooth-muscle relaxant (e.g. Buscopan 10–20 mg) and abdominal compression
3. When performed for gastrointestinal bleeding, provided that the patient is actively bleeding at the time, a blood loss of 0.5–0.6 ml min^{-1} can be demonstrated. The site of active bleeding is revealed by extravasated contrast medium remaining in the bowel on the late films, when intravascular contrast has cleared. Vascular malformations, tumours and varices may be demonstrated.

Coeliac axis

Patient supine; 25–36 ml contrast medium at 5–6 ml s^{-1}.
(Angiography of the pancreas is best achieved by selective injection into the splenic, dorsal pancreatic and gastroduodenal arteries.)

Superior mesenteric artery

Patient supine; 25–42 ml contrast medium at 5–7 ml s^{-1}.

Late-phase visceral arteriography

Patient slightly RPO.

When selective catheterization of the coeliac or SMA has been achieved, delayed venous-phase films will show the portal vein.

N.B. If splenic vein opacification is required, then a late-phase splenic arteriogram is necessary.

Inferior mesenteric artery

If the inferior mesenteric artery is to be examined as part of a procedure which will examine the superior mesenteric artery or coeliac axis as well, e.g. to find the source of gastrointestinal bleeding, then the inferior mesenteric artery should be examined first so that contrast medium in the bladder will not obscure its terminal branches.

Patient 30° LPO (to open the sigmoid loop); 10–20 ml at 4 ml s^{-1}.

ULTRASOUND OF THE GASTROINTESTINAL TRACT

ENDOLUMINAL EXAMINATION OF THE OESOPHAGUS AND STOMACH

Indications

1. Staging of primary malignant disease of the upper gastrointestinal tract or mediastinal pathology, such as suspected lymphadenopathy or mass
2. US-guided biopsy of primary tumours (particularly submucosal tumours), or suspected nodal disease.

Equipment

'Radial' echoendoscope with 5.0–10-MHz 360° transducer for diagnosis.

'Linear' echoendoscope with 5.0–10-MHz transducer for diagnosis and to allow biopsies.

Patient preparation

Conscious sedation is usually required (e.g. with midazolam and/ or fentanyl) and/or the throat anaesthetized with Xylocaine spray.

Technique

Monitoring with a pulse oximeter is required. Patient is placed in left lateral position. The echo-endoscope is passed during endoscopy, either combined with direct vision or blind by an experienced endoscopist. A 360° rotary transducer will provide transverse scans with respect to the long axis of the tube.

Aftercare

The patient should be observed by experienced nursing staff until the effects of any sedation have worn off, in the same manner as for other endoscopic procedures.

TRANSABDOMINAL EXAMINATION OF THE LOWER OESOPHAGUS AND STOMACH

Indications

Not routinely indicated in adults.

HYPERTROPHIC PYLORIC STENOSIS

The typical patient is a 6-week-old male infant presenting with non-bilious projectile vomiting.

Equipment

5–7.5-MHz linear or sector transducer.

Technique

1. The right upper quadrant is scanned with the patient supine. If the stomach is very distended, the pylorus will be displaced posteriorly and the stomach should be decompressed with a nasogastric tube. If the stomach is collapsed, the introduction of some dextrose, by mouth or via a nasogastric tube, will distend the antrum and differentiate it from the pylorus.
2. The pylorus is scanned in its longitudinal and transverse planes and images will resemble an olive and a doughnut, respectively. The

poorly echogenic muscle is easily differentiated from the bright mucosa. Antral peristalsis can be seen and the volume of fluid passing through the pylorus with each antral wave can be assessed.

3. A number of measurements can be made. These include muscle thickness, canal length, pyloric volume and muscle thickness/wall diameter ratio, but there is no universal agreement as to which is the most discriminating parameter.

SMALL BOWEL

Indications

1. In expert hands ultrasound has a useful role in the evaluation of small bowel Crohn's disease, including whether it is present and assessing disease activity. Contrast-enhanced ultrasound and Doppler flow ultrasound may help to evaluate disease activity.
2. In children ultrasound is useful to assess for intussusception.
3. Malrotation of the small bowel may be suspected by alteration of the normal relationship between the superior mesenteric artery and vein. The vein should normally lie anterior and to the right of the artery.

Technique

1. Patient in supine position, fasting for >6 hours helps but is not mandatory.
2. Oral fluids may usefully reduce the air content in the intestine. Graded compression in which the examiner uses the US transducer to squeeze the air away from the area of interest helps.
3. Initially with a 3.5–5-MHz transducer to get an overview, then switch to a curved or linear transducer with frequencies in the range 7.5–14-MHz to focus on pathology.

APPENDIX

Indications

Diagnosis of appendicitis and its complications.

Equipment

5–7.5-MHz linear array transducer.

Patient preparation

None.

Technique

The US transducer is used to apply graded compression to the right lower quadrant of the abdomen. This displaces bowel loops and compresses the caecum. The normal appendix should be compressible and have a maximum diameter of 6 mm. It should also exhibit peristalsis.

LARGE BOWEL

Indications

At present, colonoscopy, CT or barium examinations are first-line imaging investigations, but large-bowel masses can be visualized by US during a routine abdominal scan.

ENDOLUMINAL EXAMINATION OF THE RECTUM AND ANUS

Indications

1. Incontinence and suspected anal sphincter defects
2. Intersphincteric fistula.

Patient preparation

Simple bowel preparation using a small self-administered disposable enema.

Equipment

5–7-MHz radially scanning transducer. A linear transducer can be used but is less satisfactory.

Technique

1. The patient is placed in the left lateral position.
2. A careful digital rectal examination is carried out.
3. The probe is covered with a latex sheath containing contact jelly, and all air bubbles are expelled.
4. More jelly is placed over the latex sheath and the probe is introduced into the rectum.

Aftercare

None.

Further Reading

Endoscopic ultrasound
American Society for Gastrointestinal Endoscopy. Role of endoscopic ultrasonography. Gastrointest Endosc 2000;52(6):852–9.
Weber WA, Ott K. Imaging of esophageal and gastric cancer. Seminars in Oncology 2004;31(4):530–41.

Paediatric GI ultrasound

King SJ. Ultrasound of the hollow gastrointestinal tract in children. Eur Radiol 1997;7(4):559–65.

Misra D, Akhter A, Potts SR, et al. Pyloric stenosis. Is over reliance on ultrasound scans leading to negative explorations. Eur J Ped Surg 1997;7(6):328–30.

Munden MM, Hill JG. Ultrasound of the acute abdomen in children. Ultrasound Clin 2010;5(1):113–35.

Small bowel ultrasound

Fraquelli M, Colli A, Casazza G, et al. Role of US in detection of Crohn disease: meta-analysis. Radiology 2005;236(1):95–101.

Nylund K, Ødegaard S, Hausken T, et al. Sonography of the small intestine. World J Gastroenterol 2009;15(11):1319–30.

Endorectal ultrasound

Beynon J, Feifel GA, Hildebrandt U, et al. An Atlas of Rectal Endosonography. Berlin: Springer-Verlag; 1991.

CT OF THE GASTROINTESTINAL TRACT

Indications

1. Abdominal mass
2. Tumour staging
3. Appendicitis – focused appendiceal CT (FACT)
4. Large and small bowel obstruction
5. Altered bowel habit in the elderly and infirm
6. Location of bleeding
7. Trauma.

Intraluminal contrast agents

Luminal contrast agents may be positive (oral contrast density) or negative (water density). Positive oral contrast (e.g. 25 ml Omnipaque 300 made up to 1 l with water, low in density to avoid artefacts) is universally used in abdominal and pelvic CT to delineate the bowel from pathology which is especially useful in the pelvis. Oral contrast administration is recommended to help assess tumour response using the internationally recognized RECIST criteria. Multislice CT scanners have enabled the acquisition of thin slices (<3 mm) allowing multiplanar reformats and some have suggested that the routine use of intraluminal contrast for all abdominal scanning (especially trauma and follow-up cancer imaging) may not be always feasible or necessary. Nevertheless the detection and characterization of GI pathology is greatly helped by luminal distension produced by luminal contrast agents.

Colonic pathology is best demonstrated on CT by a combination of catharsis, distension with gas and intraluminal contrast (see CT colonography). For those unable to tolerate full catharsis oral contrast given at least 24 h before the examination (e.g. 30 ml Omnipaque 300 given the evening before), 'tags' the faeces and enables obvious colonic pathology to be more easily identified. Divided doses given over 3 days achieve more uniform colon tagging.

'Negative' oral contrast is recommended for the evaluation of oesophageal and stomach pathology. The simplest negative contrast is water and this is adequate for assessing upper GI pathology (i.e. staging oesophageal and gastric tumours with up to 1 l of water as tolerated starting 5–10 minutes before the scan).

Positive oral contrast is contraindicated if the question is whether GI bleeding is present, as it will obscure any bleeding points.

In the small bowel, positive oral contrast generally enables extraluminal pathology (e.g. abscess) and fistulae to be more easily visualized and in general is useful in the post-surgical abdomen. However, negative oral contrast allows mucosal enhancement (important in Crohn's disease) to be more easily seen and not obscured by adjacent positive contrast. As water gets rapidly resorbed, it is not as good for distending the distal small bowel which limits its usefulness. Agents with increased osmolality to avoid resorption are therefore advised. Water–methylcellulose mixtures, polyethylene glycol (the osmotic laxative Klean-Prep®), mannitol (e.g 250 ml mannitol 10% and 750 ml water), locust bean gum (a food additive), Volumen® (a low-density barium-based agent not available in the UK at present) and even milk have been used. In general, better small bowel distension is obtained with a higher volume of fluid and approximately 1½ l drunk gradually over 30 minutes to fill small bowel is usually required, with a larger volume required in some and less in others. Patient encouragement and supervision are important to achieve this. 'Enterography' is the term used to describe this protocol but the same contrast may also be administered via an NJ tube when it is termed 'enteroclysis'. In high-grade intestinal obstruction oral contrast is not necessary as fluid within dilated bowel will act as a negative contrast agent and allow definition of the transition point.

Intravenous contrast

Scans of the colon are generally obtained in portal venous phase (70 s) following i.v. contrast. Modifications depend on the clinical question. In the case of suspected active GI bleeding precontrast, arterial (20–25 s), portal (70 s) and perhaps delayed (150 s) phase contrast should be considered. In the specific case of small bowel evaluation, peak mucosal enhancement is seen at 50 s and this 'enteric' phase is recommended.

COMPUTED TOMOGRAPHIC COLONOGRAPHY

CTC, also known as 'virtual colonoscopy', is the radiological test of choice for the detection of colonic neoplasia of the large bowel due to superior sensitivity and better patient experience compared to barium enema.

Indications

1. Incomplete colonoscopy – can be performed the same day if no biopsies taken. If the patient has had a colonic biopsy then CT colonography should be deferred – a minimum of 1 week though some suggest up to 4 weeks. Tagging the residual colon fluid with, e.g. 30 ml gastrografin 2+ hours before the CTC, helps with interpretation.
2. Patients in high-risk group or who have aversion to colonoscopy.
3. Patients on warfarin when the clinician preference is not to discontinue anticoagulants for colonoscopy.
4. Patients with an obstructing lesion preventing full colonoscopy who require evaluation of the entire colon.
5. It has an evolving role in colorectal cancer screening and in some centres has replaced optical colonoscopy.

Bowel preparation

Full bowel preparation with standard laxatives is used in many centres but the benefits of faecal tagging are increasingly accepted. Three types of preparation may be considered:

1. 'Standard' purgative large-bowel preparation as for barium enema (see above). Diabetic patients may need to be admitted onto the ward for the duration of the bowel preparation.
2. 'Faecal tagging' using water-soluble contrast material in addition to the standard preparation (e.g. an additional 50 ml Gastrografin on the evening before the scan).
3. Faecal tagging alone with no formal bowel prep:
   (a) Low-residue diet for 2 days before test
   (b) Light breakfast and light lunch on the day before the examination, then fast until after the examination
   (c) 100 ml Gastrografin or 150 ml of Omnipaque split in three divided doses on the day before the examination.

Technique

1. Patient to go to toilet immediately before procedure.
2. 20 mg i.v. Buscopan is given (glucagon is not recommended).
3. Patient positioned on their left side and a thin (e.g. Foley) catheter is placed in rectum and gas insufflated. The gas may be air but CO_2 is better tolerated by patients. Gas is best administered by a

dedicated pump. If a pump is available then 1.5–2 l of CO_2 is initially administered, the patient is turned supine and further gas (typically up to 4–6 l) administered. Pumps limit the administered pressure to 25 psi and deliver further gas to maintain this pressure. Manual inflation with a bulb-sized hand pump or alternatively an empty enema bag filled with air/CO_2 and gentle pressure on the enema bag are other options.

4. CT scout performed to check satisfactory gaseous distension of large bowel.
5. CT parameters will depend upon the type of CT scanner available but collimation thickness should be between 1–3 mm. Symptomatic patients typically receive i.v. contrast but asymptomatic patients from cancer screening programmes should not receive i.v. contrast. CT scans may be performed using a low-dose technique (e.g. 80 mA) without i.v. contrast, or using usual diagnostic CT parameters with i.v. iodinated contrast performed in portal phase (70 s delay).
6. Patient is turned prone; further insufflation is usually needed (e.g. 2 l CO_2) and a further low-dose scan performed. If the patient is unable to turn prone they can be scanned in the left lateral position. The supine and prone scans should be reviewed to ensure all areas of the colon are distended on at least one of the acquisitions and if not then consideration of a further low-dose scan after repositioning in a lateral position and extra gas should be made.

Complications

1. Perforations are rare (approximately 1 in 3000 diagnostic CTC examinations in the UK). The operator needs to be trained to identify this at the time of scanning.
2. Discomfort.
3. Adverse reaction to hyoscine or contrast.

Further Reading

Contrast agents

Domjan J, Blaquiere R, Odurny A. Is minimal preparation CT comparable with barium enema in elderly patients with colonic symptom. Clin Radiol 1998;53(12):894–8.

Geffroy Y, Rodallec MH, Boulay-Coletta I, et al. Multidetector CT angiography in acute gastrointestinal bleeding: why, when, and how. RadioGraphics 2011;31(3):E35–46.

Graça BM, Freire PA, Brito JB, et al. Gastroenterologic and radiologic approach to obscure gastrointestinal bleeding: how, why, and when? RadioGraphics 2010;30(1):235–52.

Ilangovan R, Burling D, George A, et al. CT enterography: review of technique and practical tips. Br J Radiol 2012;85(1015):876–86.

Silva AC, Pimenta M, Guimarães LS. Small bowel obstruction: what to look for. RadioGraphics 2009;29(2):423–39.

Slater A, Planner A, Bungay HK, et al. Three-day regimen improves faecal tagging for minimal preparation CT examination of the colon. Br J Radiol 2009;82(979):545–8.

Wittenberg J, Harisinghani MG, Jhaveri K, et al. Algorithmic approach to CT diagnosis of the abnormal bowel wall. RadioGraphics 2002;22(5): 1093–107.

Complications

Burling D, International Collaboration for CT Colonography Standards. CT colonography standards. Clin Radiol 2010;65(6):474–80.

Pickhardt PJ. Missed lesions at CT colonography: lessons learned. Abdom Imaging 2013;38(1):82–97.

Tolan DJ, Armstrong EM, Chapman AH. Replacing barium enema with CT colonography in patients older than 70 years: the importance of detecting extracolonic abnormalities. Am J Roentgenol 2007;189(5): 1104–11.

MAGNETIC RESONANCE IMAGING OF THE GASTROINTESTINAL TRACT

Indications

1. Suspected perianal fistula
2. Local staging of rectal cancer
3. Evaluation of inflammatory bowel disease.

Contraindications

1. Standard MRI contraindications – see Chapter 1
2. Some gadolinium-based contrast agents are contraindicated in patients with known or suspected renal dysfunction – see Chapter 2.

Contrast agents

Contrast agents that can be used to alter the signal intensity within the bowel can be classified as positive contrast agents (high signal on T1 and T2 weighting) or negative agents (low signal on T1 and T2 weighting) but are usually biphasic (high signal on one sequence, low signal on the other). Water is a biphasic agent but is typically resorbed quickly, so a variety of formulations to increase osmolality are employed as discussed earlier on page 83. They include Klean-Prep® or 250 ml of mannitol 10% solution made up to 1 l with water. Air within bowel is a natural contrast agent and is usually sufficient for rectal and anal MRI.

Motion artefacts

The time taken to obtain a scan can be in the order of several minutes if spin echo sequences are used. Consequently, it is important to minimize peristalsis and respiration artefacts. Buscopan or glucagon may be used to try to minimize peristalsis. A prone position or a compression band can be used to help reduce respiratory motion of the anterior abdominal wall. The artefact, which is propagated from the anterior abdominal wall during respiration, is also due to the high signal from fat. Consequently, fat suppression sequences can help to minimize this.

Pulse sequences

The sequences used for imaging the abdomen and gastrointestinal tract will depend on the nature of the clinical problem. Very fast sequences such as breath-hold gradient echo (GE) and single-shot fast-spin echo (SE) sequences may be used to minimize any movement artefact. However, they do suffer from relatively poor contrast resolution. Standard fast-spin echo T1-weighted and T2-weighted sequences (with gadolinium and fat suppression added as necessary) are often used as baseline sequences, but on occasion suffer from movement artefact. The optimal plane of the sequences will be determined by the clinical problem but axial scans are frequently used in the first instance with orthogonal planes (coronal or sagittal) as required.

Techniques

Suspected peri-anal fistula

1. No special patient preparation required, patient scanned supine in MRI scanner.
2. Buscopan not routinely used.
3. The anal canal is angulated forward from the vertical by about 45°. Initial midline sagittal T2 scan to identify the orientation of the canal. Oblique axial and coronal high-resolution scans at right angles, and parallel, to the anal canal complex are obtained to facilitate interpretation. T2W SE (with fat saturation) or short tau inversion recovery (STIR) are particularly useful sequences but T1W SE and occasionally scans following intravenous gadolinium using T1W with fat saturation may also assist.

Local staging of anorectal cancer

1. Patient scanned supine; Buscopan not routinely used.
2. Sagittal T2-weighted SE sequence of central pelvic structures. Large field of view axial T2 scan of the whole pelvis. Use these scans to plan high-resolution 3-mm axial T2W images perpendicular to and also parallel to the long axis of the tumour. Coronal high-resolution scans are useful for low rectal tumours. Diffusion weighted scans may also be useful.
3. Anal cancer staging needs to include the groins.

Small-bowel magnetic resonance enteroclysis

1. Pass Bilbao Dotter tube to DJ flexure using fluoroscopy.
2. Transfer patient to MR scanner and obtain venous access.
3. Scan prone (though some centres scan supine) and obtain 'scout' localizer.
4. Connect Bilbao Dotter tube to enteroclysis pump (situated in control room if not MR compatible). Infuse (80–100 ml min^{-1}) oral contrast under MR fluoroscopy (coronal thick-slab single-shot sequence, e.g. half Fourier acquisition single-shot turbo spin echo (HASTE)) to monitor filling of small bowel to ileocaecal valve. Check for reflux to stomach and slow/stop if significant. Stop infusion when contrast reaches colon.
5. Give Buscopan 20 mg intravenously.
6. Obtain sequences in coronal and transverse axial planes using HASTE, FISP sequences to include one fat-saturated sequence.
7. 3D T1W fat suppressed, e.g. volumetric interpolated breath-hold examination (VIBE) sequences pre-and post-intravenous gadolinium.

Small-bowel magnetic resonance enterography

1. Steadily drink oral contrast (ideally 1.5 l) over 30–45 min and scan immediately.
2. Obtain venous access and give Buscopan 20 mg i.v.
3. Obtain sequences in coronal and axial planes using HASTE, FISP sequences (or manufacturer's equivalent) to include one fat-saturated sequence. Coronal pre-contrast 3D T1W fat suppressed (e.g. VIBE).
4. Give gadolinium-based contrast agent i.v.
5. Obtain fast 3D T1W fat-suppressed (e.g. VIBE) sequences in coronal and axial planes.

Further Reading

Halligan S, Stoker J. Imaging of fistula in ano. Radiology 2006;239(1):18–33.
Shihab OC, Moran BJ, Heald RJ, et al. MRI staging of low rectal cancer. Eur Radiol 2009;19(3):643–50.
Tolan DJ, Greenhalgh R, Zealley IA, et al. MR enterographic manifestations of small bowel Crohn disease. RadioGraphics 2010;30(2):367–84.

RADIONUCLIDE GASTRO-OESOPHAGEAL REFLUX STUDY

Indications

Diagnosis and quantification of suspected gastro-oesophageal reflux.

Contraindications

None.

Radiopharmaceuticals

^{99m}Tc-colloid or ^{99m}Tc-DTPA mixed with:

1. *Adults and older children*: 150–300 ml orange juice acidified with an equal volume of 0.1 M hydrochloric acid.
2. *Infants and young children*: normal milk feed.

Typical adult dose is 10–20 MBq, max. 40 MBq (0.9 mSv ED).

Equipment

1. Gamma-camera
2. Low-energy general purpose collimator
3. Abdominal binder for compression test.

Patient preparation

Nil by mouth for 4–6 h. Infants may be studied at normal feed times.

Technique

Physiological test[1] – adults and older children

1. The liquid containing the tracer is given and washed down with unlabelled liquid to clear residual activity from the oesophagus.
2. The patient lies semi-recumbent with the camera centred over the stomach and lower oesophagus.
3. Dynamic imaging is commenced with 5-s 64 × 64 frames for 30–60 min.

Milk scan[1] – infants and younger children

1. The milk feed is divided into two parts and one mixed with the tracer.
2. The radiolabelled milk is given and washed down with the remaining unlabelled milk.
3. After eructation, the child is placed either supine or prone, according to natural behaviour (although reflux appears to occur more readily in the supine position), with the camera anterior over stomach and oesophagus.
4. Dynamic imaging is commenced with 5-s 64 × 64 frames for 30–60 min.
5. If pulmonary aspiration of feed is suspected, later imaging at 4 h may be performed. The test is specific but not very sensitive for this purpose.

Provocation with abdominal compression[2] – adults and older children

1. The abdominal binder is placed around the upper abdomen.
2. The radiolabelled liquid is given as above.
3. The patient lies supine with the camera centred over the stomach and lower oesophagus.
4. A 30-s image is taken.
5. The pressure in the binder is increased in steps of 20 mmHg up to 100 mmHg, being maintained at each step for 30 s while an image is taken.
6. The test is terminated as soon as significant reflux is seen.

Analysis

1. For dynamic studies, regions are drawn round the stomach and lower, middle and upper oesophagus.
2. Time–activity curves of these regions are produced, from which may be calculated the size, extent, frequency and duration of any reflux episodes.

Additional technique: Oesophageal transit

The reflux study may be combined with a bolus transport investigation by fast-frame (0.2–0.5 s) dynamic imaging during swallowing and the generation of a functional compressed image incorporating information from each frame.

Aftercare

None.

Complications

None.

References

1. Guillet J, Basse-Cathalinat B, Christophe E, et al. Routine studies of swallowed radionuclide transit in paediatrics: experience with 400 patients. Eur J Nucl Med 1984;9:86–90.
2. Martins JC, Isaacs PE, Sladen GE, et al. Gastro-oesophageal reflux scintigraphy compared with pH probe monitoring. Nucl Med Commun 1984;5:201–4.

Further Reading

Heyman S. Paediatric gastrointestinal motility studies. Semin Nucl Med 1995;25:339–47.
Kjellén G, Brudin L, Håkansson HO. Is scintigraphy of value in the diagnosis of gastro-oesophageal reflux disease? Scand J Gastroenterol 1991;26:425–30.

RADIONUCLIDE GASTRIC-EMPTYING STUDY

Indications

1. Investigation of symptoms suggestive of gastroparesis
2. Before or after gastric surgery
3. Investigation of the effects of gastric motility-altering drugs.

Contraindication

High probability of vomiting.

Radiopharmaceuticals

Many radiolabelled meals have been designed for gastric-emptying studies, but as yet no standard has emerged. Emptying rate measured by radiolabelling is influenced by many factors, for example meal bulk, fat content, calorie content, patient position during imaging and labelling stability in vivo. For this reason, so-called 'normal' emptying times need to be taken in the context of the particular meal and protocol used to generate them. It is important that the meal used is physiological and reproducible. For centres new to the technique it is better to use a meal for which published data exist, rather than create yet another formulation with inherently different behaviour.

Both liquid and solid studies may be performed, separately or simultaneously, as a dual isotope study. Liquids have generally shorter emptying times than solids, and tend to follow an exponential emptying pattern. Solids tend to empty linearly after a lag phase. Prolonged solid emptying is highly correlated with prolonged liquid emptying, and there is debate, therefore, as to whether both studies are routinely necessary.[1] Examples of meals used are:

1. *Liquid meal*: Max. 12 MBq ^{99m}Tc-tin colloid (0.3 mSv ED) mixed with 200 ml orange juice, or with milk or formula feed for infants.
2. *Solid meal*: Scrambled egg prepared with max. 12 MBq ^{99m}Tc-colloid (0.3 mSv ED) or ^{99m}Tc-DTPA. Bulk is made up with other non-labelled foods such as bread and milk.
3. *Dual isotope combined liquid and solid meal*:
   (a) *Liquid*: 12 MBq ^{99m}Tc-colloid (0.3 mSv ED) mixed with 200 ml orange juice
   (b) *Solid*: 2 MBq ^{111}In-labelled resin beads (0.7 mSv ED) incorporated into a pancake containing 27 g fat, 18 g protein, 625 calories. Bulk is made up with other non-labelled foods. Only 2 MBq of ^{111}In is suggested (ARSAC max. is 12 MBq, 4 mSv ED) in order to minimize the downscatter into the ^{99m}Tc energy window.

Equipment

1. Gamma-camera, preferably dual-headed
2. Low-energy general purpose collimator for ^{99m}Tc, medium energy for ^{111}In/^{99m}Tc.

Patient preparation

1. Nil by mouth for 8 h
2. No smoking or alcohol from midnight before test
3. Where practical, stop medications affecting gastric motility such as dopaminergic agonists (e.g. metoclopramide, domperidone), cholinergic agonists (e.g. bethanechol), tricyclic antidepressants and anticholinergics for 24 h or more prior to the study, depending upon their biological half-life.

Technique

Imaging from a single projection can cause significant errors due to movement of the meal anteriorly as it transfers to the antrum, thereby altering the amount of tissue attenuation of gamma-photons. The problem is likely to be exacerbated in obese patients. This can largely be overcome by taking pairs of opposing views and calculating the geometric, mean stomach activity in each pair:

1. The patient ingests the meal as quickly as they comfortably can. (If dumping syndrome is suspected, the meal should be eaten in front of the camera with a fast-frame dynamic acquisition running, or the dumping episode may be missed.)
2. The patient is positioned standing.
3. Every 5 min a pair of 1-min anterior and posterior 128 × 128 images is obtained.
4. The patient sits and relaxes between images.
5. A liquid study should be continued for up to 60 min and a solid study for up to 90 min. If it can be seen that the majority of the meal has emptied inside this time, the study may be terminated.
6. If emptying is very slow, later pairs of images may be acquired at intervals of 30–60 min.

Analysis

1. Stomach region of interest is drawn.
2. Stomach time–activity curve is produced, using geometric mean if anterior and posterior imaging performed.
3. Half-emptying time is calculated.
4. Other parameters may be calculated, e.g. lag-phase duration for solid studies, or percentage left in the stomach at various time points.

Additional techniques

1. The small-bowel transit time (SBTT) can be ascertained by continuing imaging at intervals until the caecum is seen. Since the position of the caecum is often not obvious and may be overlain by small bowel, a 12–24-h image can be useful to determine the position of the large bowel.
2. Frequency analysis of fast dynamic scans (1-s frame time) can be used to characterize antral contraction patterns.[2]

Aftercare

None.

Complications

None.

References

1. Siegel JA, Krevsky B, Maurer AH, et al. Scintigraphic evaluation of gastric emptying: are radiolabelled solids necessary. Clin Nucl Med 1989;14:40–6.
2. Urbain J-L, Charkes ND. Recent advances in gastric emptying scintigraphy. Semin Nucl Med 1995;25:318–25.

Further Reading

Maughan RJ, Leiper JB. Methods for the assessment of gastric emptying in humans: an overview. Diabet Med 1996;13(suppl 5):S6–10.

RADIONUCLIDE MECKEL'S DIVERTICULUM SCAN

Indications

Detection of a Meckel's diverticulum as a cause for gastrointestinal bleeding, obstruction or abdominal pain.

Contraindications

1. Barium study in previous 2–3 days (barium causes significant attenuation of gamma photons and may mask a diverticulum).
2. In vivo, labelled red blood cell study in previous few days (due to likelihood of pertechnetate adhering to red cells).
3. Precautions and contraindications to any pre-administered drugs should be observed.

Radiopharmaceuticals

^{99m}Tc-pertechnetate, 200 MBq typical (2.5 mSv ED), 400 MBq max (5 mSv ED). Injected ^{99m}Tc-pertechnetate localizes in ectopic gastric mucosa within a diverticulum.

Equipment

1. Gamma-camera
2. Low-energy general purpose collimator.

Patient preparation

1. Nil by mouth for 6 h, unless emergency
2. It may be possible to enhance detection by prior administration of drugs, e.g. pentagastrin, cimetidine or ranitidine aimed at increasing the uptake of ^{99m}Tc-pertechnetate into gastric mucosa and inhibiting its release into the lumen of the stomach and progression into the bowel.

Technique

1. The bladder is emptied – a full bladder may obscure the diverticulum.
2. The patient lies supine with the camera over the abdomen and pelvis. The stomach must be included in the field of view because diagnosis is dependent on demonstrating uptake of radionuclide in the diverticulum concurrent with uptake by gastric mucosa.
3. Pertechnetate is administered i.v.
4. Dynamic imaging.
5. Posterior and lateral images as required.

Aftercare

None.

Complications

Pre-administered drug sensitivity and side effects.

Further Reading

Elsayes KM, Menias CO, Harvin HJ, et al. Imaging manifestations of Meckel's diverticulum. Am J Roentgenol 2007;189:81–8.
Ford PV, Bartold SP, Fink-Bennett DM, et al. Procedure guidelines for gastrointestinal bleeding and Meckel's diverticulum scintigraphy. J Nucl Med 1999;40:1226–32.

RADIONUCLIDE IMAGING OF GASTROINTESTINAL BLEEDING

Indications

Gastrointestinal bleeding of unknown origin.

Contraindications

1. No active bleeding at time scheduled for study
2. Slow bleeding of less than approximately 0.5 ml min^{-1}
3. Barium study in previous 2–3 days (barium causes significant attenuation of gamma photons and may mask a bleeding site).

Radiopharmaceuticals

1. ^{99m}Tc-labelled red blood cells, 400 MBq max (4 mSv ED). Red cells are pre-treated with a stannous agent. ^{99m}Tc-pertechnetate is added and is reduced by the stannous ions, causing it to be retained intracellularly. Labelling efficiency is important, as false-positive scans can result from accumulations of free pertechnetate. In vitro preparation gives the best labelling efficiency, but is complex and time-consuming. However, commercial kits are available which can reduce the preparation time to around 30 min. In vivo labelling is least efficient, and there is also a compromise in vivo/vitro method where the labelling occurs in the syringe as blood is withdrawn from the patient.[1]
2. ^{99m}Tc-colloid, 400 MBq max (4 mSv ED). This used to be a commonly used alternative to labelled red cells, but studies showed it to be a less sensitive tracer for detecting bleeding sites,[2] hence it is not recommended. Colloids are rapidly extracted from the circulation, so bleeding occurring only within 10 min or so of injection can be detected. It also localizes intensely in liver and spleen, masking upper gastrointestinal bleeding sites.

Equipment

1. Gamma-camera
2. Low-energy general purpose collimator.

Patient preparation

1. In vivo or in vivo/vitro methods: 'Cold' stannous agent (15 g kg^{-1} tin) is administered directly into a vein 20–30 min before the ^{99m}Tc-pertechnetate injection. (Injection via a plastic cannula will result in a poor label.)
2. The patient is asked to empty their bladder before each image is taken. Catheterization is ideal if appropriate.

Technique

1. The patient lies supine.
2. The camera is positioned over the anterior abdomen with the symphysis pubis at the bottom of the field of view.
3. ^{99m}Tc-pertechnetate (in vivo method) or ^{99m}Tc-labelled red cells (in vitro or in vivo/vitro methods) are injected i.v.
4. A 128 × 128 dynamic acquisition is begun immediately with 2-s images for 1 min to help to demonstrate vascular blood pool anatomy, followed by 1-min images up to 45 min. Dynamic imaging permits cinematic viewing of images to detect bleed sites and movement through the bowel.[3]

5. Further 15 × 1-min dynamic image sets are acquired at 1, 2, 4, 6, 8 and 24 h or until bleeding site is detected (imaging much beyond 24 h is limited by radioactive decay).

6. Oblique and lateral views may help to localize any abnormal collections of activity.

Aftercare

None.

Complications

None.

Alternative investigative imaging modalities

1. Catheter angiography

2. Multidetector CT [4]

References

1. Chaudhuri TK. Radionuclide methods of detecting acute gastrointestinal bleeding. Int J Rad Appl Instrum 1991;18(Part B):655–61.
2. Bunker SR, Lull RJ, Tanasescu DE, et al. Scintigraphy of gastrointestinal hemorrhage: superiority of ^{99m}Tc red blood cells over ^{99m}Tc sulfur colloid. Am J Roentgenol 1984;143:543–8.
3. Maurer AH. Gastrointestinal bleeding and cine-scintigraphy. Semin Nucl Med 1996;26:43–50.
4. Laing CJ, Tobias T, Rosenblum DI, et al. Acute gastrointestinal bleeding: emerging role of multidetector CT angiography and review of current imaging techniques. RadioGraphics 2007;27:1055–70.

LABELLED WHITE CELL SCANNING IN INFLAMMATORY BOWEL DISEASE

Described in Chapter 11.

Liver, biliary tract and pancreas

Methods of imaging the hepatobiliary system

1. Plain film
2. Ultrasound (US):
   (a) Transabdominal
   (b) Endoscopic
   (c) Intraoperative
3. CT including:
   (a) Routine 'staging' (portal venous phase) CT
   (b) Triple phase 'characterization' CT
   (c) CT cholangiography
4. MRI
5. Endoscopic retrograde cholangiopancreatography (ERCP)
6. Percutaneous transhepatic cholangiography (PTC)
7. Operative cholangiography
8. Postoperative (T-tube) cholangiography
9. Angiography – diagnostic and interventional
10. Radionuclide imaging:
    (a) Static, with colloid
    (b) Dynamic, with iminodiacetic acid derivatives.

Methods of imaging the pancreas

1. Plain abdominal films
2. US:
   (a) Transabdominal
   (b) Intraoperative
   (c) Endoscopic.
3. CT
4. MRI
5. ERCP
6. Arteriography:
   (a) Coeliac axis
   (b) Superior mesenteric artery.

PLAIN FILMS

May be useful to demonstrate air within the biliary tree or portal venous system, opaque calculi or pancreatic calcification.

ULTRASOUND OF THE LIVER

Indications

1. Suspected focal or diffuse liver lesion
2. Jaundice
3. Abnormal liver function tests
4. Right upper-quadrant pain or mass
5. Hepatomegaly
6. Suspected portal hypertension
7. Staging known extrahepatic malignancy
8. Pyrexia of unknown origin
9. To facilitate the placement of needles for biopsy, etc.
10. Assessment of portal vein, hepatic artery or hepatic veins
11. Assessment of patients with surgical shunts or transjugular intrahepatic portosystemic shunt (TIPS) procedures
12. Follow-up after surgical resection or liver transplant.

Contraindications

None.

Patient preparation

Not imperative, but fasting or restriction to clear fluids only required if the gallbladder is also to be studied.

Equipment

3–5-MHz transducer and contact gel. Selection of the appropriate pre-set protocol and positioning of focal zone will depend upon the type of machine, manufacturer and patient habitus.

Technique

1. Patient supine
2. Time-gain compensation set to give uniform reflectivity throughout the right lobe of the liver
3. Suspended inspiration
4. Longitudinal scans from epigastrium or left subcostal region across to right subcostal region. The transducer should be angled up to include the whole of the left and right lobes
5. Transverse scans, subcostally, to visualize the whole liver
6. If visualization is incomplete, due to a small or high liver, then right intercostal, longitudinal, transverse and oblique scans may

be useful. Suspended respiration without deep inspiration may allow useful intercostal scanning. In patients who are unable to hold their breath, real-time scanning during quiet respiration is often adequate. Upright or left lateral decubitus positions are alternatives if visualization is still incomplete

7. Contrast-enhanced ultrasound of the liver uses microbubble agents to enable the contrast enhancement pattern of focal liver lesions, analogous to contrast-enhanced CT or MRI, to be assessed and thus to characterize them. It requires specific software on the ultrasound machine. The lesion to be interrogated is identified on conventional B mode scanning and then the scanner is switched to low mechanical index (to avoid bursting the bubbles too quickly) contrast-specific scanning mode with a split screen to allow the contrast-enhanced image to be simultaneously viewed with the B mode image. The images are recorded after bolus injection of the contrast agent flushed with saline.

Additional views

Hepatic veins
These are best seen using a transverse intercostal or epigastric approach. During inspiration, in real time, these can be seen traversing the liver to enter the inferior vena cava (IVC). Hepatic vein walls do not have increased reflectivity in comparison to normal liver parenchyma. The normal hepatic vein waveform on Doppler is tri-phasic reflecting right atrial pressures. Power Doppler may be useful to examine flow within the hepatic segment of the IVC since it is angle-independent.

Portal vein
The longitudinal view of the portal vein is shown by an oblique subcostal or intercostal approach. Portal vein walls are of increased reflectivity in comparison to parenchyma. The normal portal vein blood flow is towards the liver. There is usually continuous flow but the velocity may vary with respiration.

Hepatic artery
This may be traced from the coeliac axis, which is recognized by the 'seagull' appearance of the origins of the common hepatic artery and splenic artery. There is normally forward flow throughout systole and diastole with a sharp systolic peak.

Common bile duct
See below in 'Ultrasound of the gallbladder and biliary system'.

Spleen
The spleen size should be measured in all cases of suspected liver disease or portal hypertension. Ninety-five percent of normal adult spleens measure 12 cm or less in length, and less than 7 × 5 cm in thickness. The spleen size is commonly assessed by

'eyeballing' and measurement of the longest diameter.[1] In children, splenomegaly should be suspected if the spleen is more than 1.25 times the length of the adjacent kidney, normal ranges have also been tabulated according to age and sex.[1,2]

References

1. Loftus WK, Metreweli C. Ultrasound assessment of mild splenomegaly: spleen/kidney ratio. Pediatr Radiol 1998;28(2):98–100.
2. Megremis SD, Vlachonikolis IG, Tsilimigaki AM. Spleen length in childhood with US: normal values based on age, sex, and somatometric parameters. Radiology 2004;231(1):129–34.

Further Reading

Claudon M, Dietrich CF, Choi BI, et al. Guidelines and Good Clinical Practice Recommendations for Contrast Enhanced Ultrasound (CEUS) in the Liver-Update 2012: A WFUMB-EFSUMB Initiative in Cooperation With Representatives of AFSUMB, AIUM, ASUM, FLAUS and ICUS. Ultrasound Med Biol 2013;39(2):187–210.

Kono Y, Mattrey RF. Ultrasound of the liver. Radiol Clin North Am 2005;43(5):815–26.

Shapiro RS, Wagreich J, Parsons RB, et al. Tissue harmonic imaging sonography: evaluation of image quality compared with conventional sonography. Am J Roentgenol 1998;171(5):1203–6.

ULTRASOUND OF THE GALLBLADDER AND BILIARY SYSTEM

Indications

1. Suspected gallstones
2. Right upper quadrant pain
3. Jaundice
4. Fever of unknown origin
5. Acute pancreatitis
6. To assess gallbladder function
7. Guided percutaneous procedures.

Contraindications

None.

Patient preparation

Fasting for at least 6 h, preferably overnight. Water may be permitted.

Equipment

3–5-MHz transducer and contact gel. Selection of the appropriate pre-set protocol and positioning of focal zone will depend upon the type of machine, manufacturer and patient habitus. A stand-off may be used for a very anterior gallbladder.

Technique

1. The patient is supine.
2. The gallbladder can be located by following the reflective main lobar fissure from the right portal vein to the gallbladder fossa
3. Developmental anomalies are rare but the gallbladder may be intrahepatic or on a long mesentery. In the absence of a previous cholecystectomy the commonest cause for a non-visualized gallbladder is when a gallbladder packed with stones is mistaken for a gas-filled bowel (usually duodenal) loop.
4. The gallbladder is scanned slowly along its long axis and transversely from the fundus to the neck leading to the cystic duct.
5. The gallbladder should then be re-scanned in the left lateral decubitus or erect positions because stones may be missed if only supine scanning is performed.
6. Visualization of the neck and cystic ducts may be improved by head-down tilt.

The normal gallbladder wall is never more than 3-mm thick.

Additional views

Assessment of gallbladder function
1. Fasting gallbladder volume may be assessed by measuring longitudinal, transverse and antero-posterior (AP) diameters.
2. Normal gallbladder contraction reduces the volume by more than 25%, 30 min after a standard fatty meal. Somatostatin, calcitonin, indometacin and nifedipine antagonize this contraction.

Intrahepatic bile ducts
1. Left lobe: transverse epigastric scan
2. Right lobe: subcostal or intercostal longitudinal oblique.

Normal intrahepatic ducts are visualized with modern scanners. Intrahepatic ducts are dilated if their diameter is more than 40% of the accompanying portal vein branch. There is normally acoustic enhancement posterior to dilated ducts but not portal veins. Dilated ducts have a beaded branching appearance.

Extrahepatic bile ducts
1. The patient is supine or in a lateral position.
2. The upper common duct is demonstrated on a longitudinal oblique, subcostal or intercostal scan running anterior to the portal vein. The right hepatic artery is often seen crossing transversely between the two.
3. The common duct may be followed downwards along its length through the head of the pancreas to the ampulla and, when visualized, transverse scans should also be performed to improve detection of intraduct stones. However, gas in the duodenum often impedes the view of the lower duct.

The segment of bile duct proximal to the junction with the cystic duct (the common hepatic duct) is 4 mm or less in a normal adult; 5 mm is borderline and 6 mm is considered dilated. The lower bile duct (common bile duct) is normally 6 mm or less. Distinction of the common hepatic duct from the common bile duct depends on identification of the junction with the cystic duct. This is usually not possible with US. Colour-flow Doppler enables quick distinction of bile duct from ectatic hepatic artery. In less than one-fifth of patients the artery lies anterior to the bile duct.

Post-cholecystectomy

There is disagreement as to whether the normal common duct dilates after cholecystectomy. Symptomatic patients and those with abnormal liver function tests should have further investigations if the common duct measures more than 6 mm.

Further Reading

Foley WD, Quiroz FA. The role of sonography in imaging of the biliary tract. Ultrasound Q 2007;23(2):123–35.

ULTRASOUND OF THE PANCREAS

Indications

1. Suspected pancreatic tumour
2. Pancreatitis or its complications
3. Epigastric mass
4. Epigastric pain
5. Jaundice
6. To facilitate guided biopsy and/or drainage.

Contraindications

None.

Patient preparation

Nil by mouth, preferably overnight.

Equipment

3–5-MHz transducer and contact gel. Selection of the appropriate pre-set protocol and positioning of focal zone will depend upon the type of machine, manufacturer and patient habitus. A stand-off may be required in thin patients.

Technique

1. The patient is supine.
2. The body of the pancreas is located anterior to the splenic vein in a transverse epigastric scan.

3. The transducer is angled transversely and obliquely to visualize the head and tail.
4. The tail may be demonstrated from a left intercostal view using the spleen as an acoustic window.
5. Longitudinal epigastric scans may be useful.
6. The pancreatic parenchyma increases in reflectivity with age, being equal to liver reflectivity in young adults.
7. Gastric or colonic gas may prevent complete visualization. This may be overcome by left and right oblique decubitus scans or by scanning with the patient erect. Water may be drunk to improve the window through the stomach and the scans repeated in all positions. One cup is usually sufficient. Degassed water is preferable.

4

The pancreatic duct should not measure more than 3 mm in the head or 2 mm in the body.

Endoscopic US (see p. 78) and intraoperative US are useful adjuncts to transabdominal US. EUS may be used to further characterize and biopsy pancreatic solid and cystic lesions. Intraoperative US is used to localize small lesions (e.g. islet cell tumours prior to resection).

Further Reading

Dumonceau JM, Polkowski M, Larghi A, et al. Indications, results, and clinical impact of endoscopic ultrasound (EUS)-guided sampling in gastroenterology: European Society of Gastrointestinal Endoscopy (ESGE) Clinical Guideline. Endoscopy 2011;43(10):897–912.

COMPUTED TOMOGRAPHY OF THE LIVER AND BILIARY TREE

Indications

1. Suspected focal or diffuse liver lesion
2. Staging known primary or secondary malignancy
3. Abnormal liver-function tests
4. Right upper-quadrant pain or mass
5. Hepatomegaly
6. Suspected portal hypertension
7. Characterization of liver lesion
8. Pyrexia of unknown origin
9. To facilitate the placement of needles for biopsy, etc.
10. Assessment of portal vein, hepatic artery or hepatic veins
11. Assessment of patients with surgical shunts or transjugular intrahepatic portosystemic shunt (TIPS) procedures
12. Follow-up after surgical resection or liver transplant.

Contraindications

1. Pregnancy
2. Contraindication to iodinated intravenous (i.v.) contrast medium (contrast-enhanced computed tomography (CECT)) – see Chapter 2.

Technique

Single-phase (portal phase) contrast-enhanced CT

This is the technique for the majority of routine liver CT imaging. The liver is imaged during the peak of parenchymal enhancement, i.e. when contrast-medium-laden portal venous blood is perfusing the liver. This begins about 60–70 s after the start of a bolus injection. Oral contrast may be given but is not necessary if only the liver is being investigated. Slice thickness will depend upon the CT scanner specification but should be 5 mm or less.

Multiphasic contrast-enhanced CT

The fast imaging times of helical/multislice CT enable the liver to be scanned multiple times after a single bolus injection of contrast medium. Most primary liver tumours receive their blood supply from the hepatic artery, unlike normal hepatic parenchyma, which receives 80% of its blood supply from the portal vein. Liver tumours (particularly hypervascular tumours) will therefore enhance strongly during the arterial phase (beginning 20–25 s after the start of a bolus injection) but are of similar or lower density to enhanced normal parenchyma during the portal venous phase (washout). Some tumours are most conspicuous during early-phase arterial scanning (25 s after the start of a bolus injection), others later, during the late arterial phase 35 s after the start of a bolus injection. Thus a patient who is likely to have hypervascular primary or secondary liver tumours should have an arterial phase scan as well as a portal venous phase CT scan (see above). Early and late arterial phase with portal venous phase is appropriate for patients with suspected hepatocellular cancer (triple phase). In general, late arterial and portal venous scans are appropriate to investigate suspected hypervascular metastases. Some centres, however, also use a 'delayed' or 'equilibrium' phase scan at 180 seconds to help identify and characterize primary liver tumours (quadruple phase). Terminology may be potentially confusing as some centres may consider a triple phase scan to include arterial, portal and delayed scans. Non-contrast examinations have limited usefulness.

Haemangiomas often show a characteristic peripheral nodular enhancement and progressive centripetal 'fill-in'. After the initial dual- or triple-phase protocol, delayed images at 5 and 10 min are obtained through the lesion.

COMPUTED TOMOGRAPHIC CHOLANGIOGRAPHY

Magnetic resonance (MR) cholangiography is non-invasive but sometimes fails to display the normal intrahepatic ducts. Multidetector CT cholangiography can be useful in this instance. With this technique the biliary tree is opacified using an i.v. cholangiographic agent. Isotropic data from 0.625 mm section thickness slices can be reconstructed to provide high-resolution three-dimensional images. Insufficient opacification may be seen with excessively dilated ducts.

Contraindications

Allergy to iodinated contrast agents.

Indications

1. Screening for cholelithiasis
2. Pre-operative screening of anatomy
3. Suspected traumatic bile-duct injury
4. Other biliary abnormalities, e.g. cholesterol polyps, adenomyomatosis and congenital abnormalities.

Technique

1. Patient fasted for at least 6 h.
2. 100 ml i.v. cholangiographic agent, e.g. meglumine iotroxate (biliscopin R) infused for 50 min as a biliary contrast[1] or iodipamide meglumine 52% – 20 ml diluted with 80 ml of normal saline infused over 30 min.[2]
3. CT scan should be obtained at least 35 min after infusion of contrast agent.

References
1. Hyodo T, Kumano S, Kushihata F, et al. CT and MR cholangiography: advantages and pitfalls in perioperative evaluation of biliary tree. Br J Radiol 2012;85(1015):887–96.
2. Schindera ST, Nelson RC, Paulson EK, et al. Assessment of the optimal temporal window for intravenous CT cholangiography. Eur Radiol 2007;17(10):2531–7.

Further Reading
Francis IR, Cohan RH, McNulty NJ, et al. Multidetector CT of the liver and hepatic neoplasms: effect of multiphasic imaging on tumor conspicuity and vascular enhancement. Am J Roentgenol 2003;180(5):1217–24 [Erratum in Am J Roentgenol 2003;181(1):283].
Oto A, Tamm EP, Szklaruk J. Multidetector row CT of the liver. Radiol Clin North Am 2005;43(5):827–48.

COMPUTED TOMOGRAPHY OF THE PANCREAS

Indications

1. Epigastric pain
2. Obstructive jaundice
3. Suspected pancreatic malignancy
4. Acute pancreatitis and its complications
5. Chronic pancreatitis and its complications.

Contraindications

1. Pregnancy
2. Contraindication to iodinated intravenous contrast medium – see Chapter 2.

Technique

1. Negative (e.g. water) oral contrast is generally preferred but positive (e.g. iodinated) may be given if necessary to opacify distal bowel loops. Positive oral contrast agent is contraindicated if CT angiography is to be performed. Volume and timing of oral contrast agent will depend upon whether opacification of distal bowel loops is required.
2. Venous access is obtained.
3. The patient is scanned supine and a scout view is obtained.
4. A non-contrast-enhanced examination can be performed initially if detection of subtle calcification is required.
5. The volume of i.v. contrast used will depend upon the type of scanner. Faster acquisition will allow a smaller volume of contrast, generally 100 ml or less. The timing of the scan in relation to i.v. contrast will depend upon the clinical question. Pancreatic phase enhancement (40 s after commencement of bolus injection) is necessary for optimum contrast differences between pancreatic adenocarcinoma and normal pancreatic tissue, with portal venous phase scans included in the protocol to investigate hepatic metastatic disease. Islet cell tumours and their metastases may show avid enhancement on arterial phase scans and become isodense with normal pancreatic tissue on portal phase scans. A portal phase scan is generally necessary to investigate flow and the relationship of the tumour to the portal vein.
6. The volume and strength of the i.v. contrast will depend upon the speed of the scanner.
7. Slice thickness should be 3 mm or less.

Further Reading

Fletcher JG, Wiersema MJ, Farrell MA, et al. Pancreatic malignancy: value of arterial, pancreatic, and hepatic phase imaging with multi-detector row CT. Radiology 2003;229(1):81–90.

Goshima S, Kanematsu M, Kondo H, et al. Pancreas: optimal scan delay for contrast-enhanced multi-detector row CT. Radiology 2006;241(1):167–74.

MAGNETIC RESONANCE IMAGING OF THE LIVER

Indications

1. Lesion characterization following detection by CT or US
2. Lesion detection, particularly prior to hepatic resection for hepatic metastatic disease.

Magnetic resonance imaging (MRI) is rapidly emerging as the imaging modality of choice for detection and characterization of liver lesions. There is high specificity with optimal lesion-to-liver contrast and characteristic appearances on differing sequences and after contrast agents. Focal lesions may be identified on most pulse sequences. Most metastases are hypo- to isointense on T1 and iso- to hyperintense on T2-weighted images. However, multiple sequences are usually necessary for confident tissue characterization. The timing, degree and nature of tumour vascularity form the basis for liver lesion characterization based on enhancement properties. Liver metastases may be hypo- or hyper-vascular.

Magnetic resonance imaging pulse sequences

Common pulse sequences are:

1. T1-weighted spoiled gradient echo (GRE). This has replaced the conventional spin-echo sequence. In and out of phase scans are used to investigate patients with suspected fatty liver.
2. Magnetization-prepared T1-weighted GRE. A further breath-hold technique with very short sequential image acquisition.
3. T1-W GRE fat-suppressed volume acquisition. This sequence can be obtained rapidly following i.v. gadolinium.
4. T2-weighted spin echo (SE). T2-weighted fast spin-echo (FSE; General Electric) or turbo spin-echo (TSE; Siemens).

Compared with conventional T2-weighted SE images, FSE/TSE images show:

1. Fat with higher signal intensity
2. Reduced magnetic susceptibility effects which are of advantage in patients with embolization coils, IVC filters, etc., but disadvantageous after injection of superparamagnetic oxide contrast agent
3. Increased magnetization transfer which may lower signal intensity for solid liver tumours. These sequences may be obtained with fat suppression.

Fat suppression:

1. Decreases the motion artifact from subcutaneous and intra-abdominal fat

2. Increases the dynamic range of the image
3. Improves signal-to-noise and contrast-to-noise ratios of focal liver lesions.

Very heavily T2-weighted sequences can be used to show water content in bile ducts, cysts and some focal lesions. These may be obtained as:

1. Gradient echo breath-hold sequences (e.g. fast imaging with steady state precession (FISP), fast imaging employing steady state acquisition (FIESTA)) or
2. breath-hold very fast spin echo, e.g. half Fourier acquisition single-shot turbo spin echo (HASTE) or
3. non-breath-hold respiratory gated sequences used for magnetic resonance cholangiopancreatography (MRCP).

Fat suppression is also used to allow better delineation of fluid-containing structures.

Short tau inversion recovery (STIR) also suppresses fat, which has a short T1 relaxation time. Other tissues with short T1 relaxation (haemorrhage, metastases and melanoma) are also suppressed.

Diffusion weighted imaging

This very rapidly acquired sequence forms an image based on the microscopic motion of water molecules and may potentially help to detect extra liver lesions and help better characterize them in conjunction with other sequences.

Contrast-enhanced magnetic resonance liver imaging

Gadolinium-enhanced T1-weighted MRI

These probably do not increase sensitivity for focal abnormalities but may help in tissue characterization. When used in conjunction with spoiled GRE sequences it is possible to obtain images during the arterial phase (ideal for metastatic disease and hepatocellular carcinoma), portal phase (hypovascular malignancies) and equilibrium phase (cholangiocarcinoma, slow-flow haemangiomas and fibrosis). Hepatic arterial phase and fast spin-echo T2-weighted sequences are the most sensitive sequences for the detection of hepatic metastases of neuroendocrine tumours.

Liver-specific contrast agents

Standard gadolinium extracellular agents are commonly used for liver MRI as described above, but other contrast agents have been developed to enhance the distinction between normal liver and lesions, especially malignant lesions. These are mostly used in patients who are potentially suitable for major liver surgery, e.g. resection or transplantation:

1. Hepato-biliary agents (e.g. Gadoxetic acid (Primovist®); gadobenate dimeglumine (Multihance®)) are taken up by normal hepatocytes and excreted by normal liver into the bile. The normal liver shows increased signal on T1-weighted sequences for a prolonged period which varies according to the particular agent. Metastases, and other lesions not containing normal-functioning hepatocytes, show as a lower signal than the background liver. Lesions containing hepatocytes will enhance to varying extents. High signal contrast can be seen in the bile ducts which has clinical usefulness. These agents are also excreted by the kidneys. Further details cany be found in Chapter 2.

2. Reticuloendothelial (RE) cell agents (also called super paramagnetic iron oxides, SPIO) are not currently available as they have been withdrawn from the market for commercial reasons. They are taken up by the RE or Kuppfer cells in normal liver giving a decrease in signal on T2- and especially T2*-weighted sequences. They can also be used with T1-weighted sequences for characterization. On T2*-weighted images, malignant lesions without RE cells show as higher signal than the background normal liver. Examination with a SPIO agent may be combined with dynamic gadolinium enhancement in order to maximize the detection and characterization of metastases (and benign lesions) in a patient being considered for surgical resection of metastases. The same combination can be used in a patient with cirrhosis to maximize diagnosis and characterization of HCC vs dysplastic or regenerative nodules.

Magnetic resonance angiography

Contrast-enhanced spoiled GRE images may be obtained to give information with respect to the hepatic artery, portal vein and hepatic venous system.

MAGNETIC RESONANCE CHOLANGIOPANCREATOGRAPHY (MRCP)

Indications

1. Investigation of obstructive jaundice
2. Suspected biliary colic/bile duct stones
3. Suspected chronic pancreatitis
4. Suspected sclerosing cholangitis
5. Investigation of jaundice or cholangitis in patients who have undergone biliary enteric anastomosis
6. Prior to ERCP/PTC.

Contraindications

Those that apply to MRI – see Chapter 1.

Technique

MRCP is a non-invasive technique which uses heavily T2-weighted images to demonstrate the intra- and extrahepatic biliary tree and pancreatic duct. Most commonly used to demonstrate the presence of stones and the level and cause of obstruction, especially combined with cross-sectional MRI, in cases of tumour or suspected tumour.

MAGNETIC RESONANCE IMAGING OF THE PANCREAS

Indications

1. Staging of pancreatic tumours
2. Suspected islet cell tumour
3. Other indications are similar to CT, although CT is generally preferred because of availability, cost and time implications.

Technique

Typical sequences in the axial plane include:

1. T1-weighted fat-suppressed gradient-echo. Normal pancreas hyperintense to normal liver.
2. T1-weighted spoiled gradient-echo (SPGR, GE Medical Systems; fast low-angle shot (FLASH), Siemens). Normal pancreas isointense to normal liver.
3. T2 weighted turbo-spin echo.
4. Gadolinium-enhanced T1-weighted fat-suppressed spoiled gradient echo (GRE). Images are obtained immediately after the injection of contrast medium, after 45 s, after 90 s and after 10 min. Normal pancreas hyperintense to normal liver and adjacent fat on early images, fading on later images.
5. The polypeptide hormone secretin may be given slowly i.v. over one minute to temporarily distend the pancreatic ducts. This can help better assess pancreatic ductal anomalies and also provide information about the exocrine function of the gland.

Further Reading

Bartolozzi C, Battaglia V, Bargellini I, et al. Contrast-enhanced magnetic resonance imaging of 102 nodules in cirrhosis: correlation with histological findings on explanted livers. Abdom Imaging 2013;38(2):290–6.

Catalano OA, Sahani DV, Kalva SP, et al. MR imaging of the gallbladder: a pictorial essay. Radiographics 2008;28(1):135–55.

Kele PG, van der Jagt EJ. Diffusion weighted imaging in the liver. World J Gastroenterol 2010;16(13):1567–76.

Lee NK, Kim S, Lee JW, et al. Biliary MR imaging with Gd-EOB-DTPA and its clinical applications. Radiographics 2009;29(6):1707–24.

Sandrasegaran K, Lin C, Akisik FM, et al. State-of-the-art pancreatic MRI. Am J Roentgenol 2010;195(1):42–53.

Ward J, Robinson PJ, Guthrie JA, et al. Liver metastases in candidates for hepatic resection: comparison of helical CT and gadolinium – and SPIO-enhanced MR imaging. Radiology 2005;237(1):170–80.

ENDOSCOPIC RETROGRADE CHOLANGIOPANCREATOGRAPHY

Diagnostic endoscopic retrograde cholangiopancreatography (ERCP) has been largely replaced by non-invasive investigations, e.g. CT, MRI supplemented by endoscopic ultrasound. With the advances in non-invasive imaging of the biliary tree and pancreas, over 90% of ERCP procedures are performed with therapeutic (interventional) intent. ERCP is performed by physicians most commonly, but surgeons and radiologists do perform this procedure.

Indications

1. Management of bile duct stones
2. Management of benign and malignant biliary strictures
3. Evaluation of ampullary lesions
4. Diagnostic cholangiography in patients unsuitable/intolerant of MRCP and in whom endoscopic ultrasound is inconclusive or unavailable
5. Treatment and evaluation of chronic pancreatitis
6. Investigation of diffuse biliary disease, e.g. sclerosing cholangitis
7. Post-cholecystectomy syndrome.

Contraindications

1. Oesophageal obstruction; pyloric stenosis/gastric or duodenal obstruction
2. Previous gastric surgery that prevents access to the duodenum
3. Severe cardiac/respiratory disease.

Contrast medium

Pancreas
LOCM 240/300 mg I ml^{-1}.

Bile ducts
LOCM 150 mg I ml^{-1}; dilute contrast medium ensures that calculi will not be obscured.

Equipment

1. Side-viewing endoscope
2. Polythene catheters
3. Fluoroscopic unit with spot film facilities.

Patient preparation

1. Nil orally for 4–6 h prior to procedure
2. Premedication (see Chapter 18)
3. Antibiotic cover for patients with biliary obstruction, pseudocyst or high risk of endocarditis.

Preliminary image

Prone AP and left anterior oblique (LAO) of the upper abdomen, to check for opaque gallstones and pancreatic calcification/calculi.

Technique

The patient is sedated until conscious sedation is achieved. The pharynx may also be anaesthetized with 50–100 mg Xylocaine spray. The patient then lies in the left/prone position and the endoscope is introduced. The ampulla of Vater is located and a polythene catheter prefilled with contrast medium is inserted into the ampulla, having ensured that all air bubbles are excluded. A small test injection of contrast under fluoroscopic control is made to determine the position of the cannula. It is important to avoid over-filling of the pancreatic duct. If it is desirable both to opacify the biliary tree and the pancreatic duct, the latter should be cannulated first. If there is evidence of biliary obstruction, a sample of bile should be sent for culture and sensitivity.

Images

Pancreas (using fine focal spot)
Prone, both posterior obliques.

Bile ducts
1. Early filling images to show calculi:
    (a) Prone – straight and posterior obliques
    (b) Supine – straight, both obliques; Trendelenburg to fill intrahepatic ducts; semi-erect to fill lower end of common bile duct and gallbladder
2. Images following removal of the endoscope, which may obscure the duct
3. Delayed images to assess the gallbladder and emptying of the common bile duct.

Aftercare

1. Nil orally until conscious and sensation has returned to the pharynx (usually <1 hour)
2. Pulse, temperature and blood pressure half-hourly for 6 h
3. Maintain antibiotics if there is biliary or pancreatic obstruction
4. Serum/urinary amylase if pancreatitis is suspected.

Complications

Due to the contrast medium

1. Acute pancreatitis – more likely with large volumes, high-pressure injections
2. Allergic reactions – rare.

Due to the technique

Local

Damage by the endoscope, e.g. rupture of the oesophagus, damage to the ampulla, proximal pancreatic duct and distal common duct.

Distant

Bacteraemia, septicaemia, aspiration pneumonitis, hyperamylasaemia (approximately 70%). Acute pancreatitis (0.7–7.4%).

INTRA-OPERATIVE CHOLANGIOGRAPHY

Indications

During cholecystectomy or bile duct surgery, to avoid surgical exploration of the common bile duct. This technique has been replaced in some centres by pre-operative MRCP and/or EUS.

Contraindications

None.

Contrast medium

High osmolar contrast material (HOCM) or low osmolar contrast material (LOCM) 150, i.e. low iodine content so as not to obscure any calculi; 20 ml.

Equipment

1. Operating table with CR/DR available or a film cassette tunnel
2. Mobile X-ray machine.

Patient preparation

As for surgery.

Technique

The surgeon cannulates the cystic duct with a fine catheter. This is prefilled with contrast medium to exclude air bubbles which might simulate calculi.

Images

1. After 5 ml have been injected
2. After 20 ml have been injected. Contrast medium should flow freely into the duodenum. Spasm of the sphincter of Oddi is a

fairly frequent occurrence and may be due to anaesthetic agents or surgical manipulation. It can be relieved by glucagon, propantheline or amyl nitrite.

The criteria for a normal operative choledochogram were given by Le Quesne[1] as:

1. Common bile duct width not greater than 12 mm
2. Free flow of contrast medium into the duodenum
3. The terminal narrow segment of the duct is clearly seen
4. There are no filling defects
5. There is no excess retrograde filling of the hepatic ducts.

POSTOPERATIVE (T-TUBE) CHOLANGIOGRAPHY

Indications

1. To exclude biliary tract calculi where (a) operative cholangiography was not performed, or (b) the results of operative cholangiography are not satisfactory or are suspect
2. Assessment of biliary leaks following biliary surgery.

Contraindications

None.

Contrast medium

HOCM or LOCM 150 mg I ml^{-1}; 20–30 ml.

Equipment

Fluoroscopy unit with spot film device.

Patient preparation

Antibiotics may be considered if previous cholangitis or if immunosuppressed (e.g. liver transplant).

Preliminary image

Coned supine PA of the right side of the abdomen.

Technique

1. The examination is performed on or about the 10th postoperative day, prior to removing the T-tube.
2. The patient lies supine on the X-ray table. The drainage tube is clamped off near to the patient and cleaned thoroughly with antiseptic.
3. A 23G needle, extension tubing and 20 ml syringe are assembled and filled with contrast medium (e.g. a butterfly needle). After all air bubbles have been expelled the needle is inserted into the

tubing between the patient and the clamp. The injection is made under fluoroscopic control, the total volume depending on duct filling. In the case of recent biliary anastomosis (i.e. liver transplant) only a small volume of contrast (approximately 10 ml), gently injected, is required.

Images

Fluoroscopic 'grab' images during filling are frequently useful. PA and oblique exposures when satisfactory opacification of biliary system.

Aftercare

None.

Complications

Due to the contrast medium

The biliary ducts do absorb contrast medium and cholangiovenous reflux can occur with high injection pressures. Adverse reactions are, therefore, possible, but the incidence is small.

Due to the technique

Injection of contrast medium under high pressure into an obstructed biliary tract can produce septicaemia.

PERCUTANEOUS TRANSHEPATIC CHOLANGIOGRAPHY

Indications

1. Prior to therapeutic intervention, e.g. biliary drainage procedure to relieve obstructive jaundice, or to drain infected bile
2. Place a percutaneous biliary stent
3. Dilate a postoperative stricture
4. Stone removal (see below)
5. To facilitate ERCP by rendezvous technique
6. Rarely for diagnostic purposes only.

Contraindications

1. Bleeding tendency:
   (a) Platelets less than $100 \times 10^9 \; l^{-1}$
   (b) Prothrombin time >2 s more than control.
      If patient requires urgent procedure then platelet transfusion and FFP can be used to correct. Vitamin K will correct abnormal prothrombin time due to biliary obstruction.
2. Biliary tract sepsis except to control the infection by drainage.

Contrast medium

LOCM 150 mg I ml^{-1}; 20–60 ml.

Equipment

1. Fluoroscopy unit with digital spot film device (tilting table optional)
2. Chiba needle (a fine, flexible 22G needle, 15–20-cm long)
3. Appropriate catheters and wire for drainage or interventional procedure planned.

Patient preparation

1. Haemoglobin, prothrombin time and platelets are checked, and corrected if necessary
2. Prophylactic antibiotics, e.g. ciprofloxacin 500–750 mg oral before and after procedure
3. Nil by mouth or clear fluids only for 4 h prior to the procedure
4. Ensure patient well hydrated, by i.v. fluids if necessary
5. Sedation (i.v.) and analgesia with oxygen and monitoring.

Preliminary imaging

US to confirm position of liver and dilated ducts.

Technique

1. The patient lies supine. Using US a spot is marked over the right or left lobe of the liver as appropriate. On the right side this is usually intercostal between mid and anterior axillary lines. For the left lobe this is usually subcostal to the left side of the xiphisternum in the epigastrium.
2. Using aseptic technique the skin, deeper tissues and liver capsule are anaesthetized at the site of the mark.
3. During suspended respiration the Chiba needle is inserted into the liver, but once it is within the liver parenchyma the patient is allowed shallow respirations. It is advanced into the liver with real-time US or fluoroscopy control.
4. The stilette is withdrawn and the needle connected to a syringe and extension tubing prefilled with contrast medium. Contrast medium is injected under fluoroscopic control while the needle is slowly withdrawn. If a duct is not entered at the first attempt, the needle tip is withdrawn to approximately 2–3 cm from the liver capsule and further passes are made, directing the needle tip more cranially, caudally, anteriorly or posteriorly until a duct is entered. The incidence of complications is not related to the number of passes within the liver itself and the likelihood of success is directly related to the degree of duct dilatation and the number of passes made.
5. Excessive parenchymal injection should be avoided and when it does occur it results in opacification of intrahepatic lymphatics.

Injection of contrast medium into a vein or artery is followed by rapid dispersion.

6. If the intrahepatic ducts are seen to be dilated, bile should be aspirated and sent for microbiological examination. (The incidence of infected bile is high in such cases.)
7. Contrast medium is injected to outline the duct system and allow access for a guidewire or selection of an appropriate duct for drainage.
8. Care should be taken not to overfill an obstructed duct system because septic shock may be precipitated.
9. For diagnostic PTC only the needle is removed after suitable images have been recorded.

Images

Contrast medium is denser than bile and the sequence of duct opacification is, therefore, gravity-dependent and determined by the site of injection and the position of the patient.

Using the undercouch tube with the patient *horizontal*:

1. PA
2. LAO
3. RAO
4. If on a non-tilting table, rolling the patient onto the left side will fill the left ducts and common duct above an obstruction.

When the above images have shown an obstruction at the level of the porta hepatis, a further image after the patient has been tilted towards the erect position for 30 min may show the level of obstruction to be lower than originally thought.

Delayed images

Images taken after several hours, or the next day, may show contrast medium in the gallbladder if this was not achieved during the initial part of the investigation.

Aftercare

Bed rest, pulse and blood pressure measurement half-hourly for 6 h.

Complications

Morbidity approximately 3%; mortality less than 0.1%.

Due to the contrast medium
Allergic/idiosyncratic reactions – very uncommon.

Due to the technique
Local
1. Puncture of extrahepatic structures – usually no serious sequelae
2. Intrathoracic injection

3. Cholangitis

4. Bile leakage – may lead to biliary peritonitis (incidence 0.5%). More likely if the ducts are under pressure and if there are multiple puncture attempts. Less likely if a drainage catheter is left in situ. (See 'Biliary drainage' below)

5. Subphrenic abscess

6. Haemorrhage

7. Shock – owing to injection into the region of the coeliac plexus.

Generalized

Bacteraemia, septicaemia and endotoxic shock. The likelihood of sepsis is greatest in the presence of choledocholithiasis because of the higher incidence of pre-existing infected bile.

Reference

1. Patey DH, Le Quesne LP, Whiteside CG, et al. Discussion on cholangiography. Proc R Soc Med 1960;53:851–60.

Further Reading

Canlas KR, Branch MS. Role of endoscopic retrograde cholangiopancreatography in acute pancreatitis. World J Gastroenterol 2007;13(47):6314–20.

EXTERNAL BILIARY DRAINAGE

This is achieved following transhepatic cannulation of the biliary tree as described above. The procedure may be performed to improve jaundice or sepsis prior to surgery or as a further percutaneous intervention.

INTERNAL BILIARY DRAINAGE

This can be achieved following transhepatic (as above) or endoscopic cannulation of the biliary tree. A percutaneous drainage catheter may allow internal or external drainage with sideholes above and below the point of obstruction. At ERCP an endoprosthesis or stent is placed to drain bile from above a stricture or to prevent obstruction by a stone in the duct.

Indications

1. Malignant biliary stricture

2. Benign stricture following balloon dilatation.

Contraindications

As for percutaneous transhepatic cholangiography (PTC).

Contrast media

LOCM 200 mg I ml^{-1}; 20–60 ml.

Equipment

1. Wide-channelled endoscope for introduction of endoprosthesis by ERCP
2. A biplane fluoroscope facility is useful but not essential for transhepatic puncture
3. Set including guidewires, dilators and endoprosthesis.

Patient preparation

See percutaneous transhepatic cholangiography above.

Technique

Transhepatic

1. A percutaneous transhepatic cholangiogram is performed.
2. A duct in the right lobe of the liver that has a horizontal or caudal course to the porta hepatis is usually chosen. This duct is studied on US to judge its depth and then a 22G Chiba needle is inserted into the duct under US or fluoroscopic guidance. A coaxial introducer system is used over a 0.018 guidewire to allow 0.035 wire and catheter access into the bile ducts. If the duct is not successfully punctured, the Chiba needle is withdrawn but remains within the liver capsule allowing a further puncture attempt. Once a 0.035 wire is established in the bile duct a sheath can be inserted, e.g. 7-F. Bile can be drained through the side arm of the sheath while a catheter is manipulated over the wire. For internal drainage or stent insertion the wire and catheter must be passed through the stricture into the duodenum or postoperative jejunal loop. For external drainage, a suitable catheter can be inserted over the wire after the sheath is withdrawn. A variety of wires and catheters may be needed to cross difficult strictures. Failing this, external drainage is instituted and a further attempt is made to pass the stricture a few days later.
3. An internal/external catheter may be placed across the stricture and secured to the skin with sutures.
4. A metal biliary stent may be positioned and deployed across a malignant stricture to facilitate internal drainage of bile. Balloon dilatation may be required before or after stent deployment in some cases. A temporary external drainage tube may be left in place for 24–48 h.

Endoscopic

1. Cholangiography following cannulation of the biliary tree
2. Endoscopic sphincterotomy
3. A guidewire is placed via the channel of the endoscope through the sphincter and pushed past the stricture using fluoroscopy to monitor progress
4. Following dilatation of the stricture the endoprosthesis (plastic stent) is pushed over the guidewire and sited with its side-holes above and below the stricture. Metal biliary stents can also be placed at ERCP when appropriate.

Aftercare

1. As for percutaneous transhepatic cholangiography
2. Antibiotics for at least 3 days
3. An externally draining catheter should be regularly flushed through with normal saline and exchanged at 3-monthly intervals. (It is rare to leave a drain in situ for such a long period.)

Complications

1. As for PTC, ERCP and sphincterotomy
2. Sepsis – particularly common with long-term, externally draining catheters
3. Dislodgement of catheters, endoprostheses
4. Blockage of catheters/endoprostheses
5. Perforation of bile duct above the stricture on passage of guidewires.

PERCUTANEOUS EXTRACTION OF RETAINED BILIARY CALCULI (BURHENNE TECHNIQUE)

Indications

Retained biliary calculi seen on the T-tube cholangiogram (incidence 3%).

Contraindications

1. Small T-tube (<12-F)
2. Tortuous T-tube course in soft tissues
3. Acute pancreatitis
4. Drain in situ (cross connections exist between the drain tract and the T-tube tract).

Contrast medium

HOCM or LOCM 150 mg I ml^{-1} (low-density contrast medium is used to avoid obscuring the calculus).

Equipment

1. Fluoroscopy unit with spot film device
2. Steerable catheter system with wire baskets.

Patient preparation

1. Admission to hospital on the day prior to the procedure
2. Prophylactic antibiotics and pre-medication 1 h prior to the procedure
3. Analgesia during the procedure.

Technique

1. The patient lies supine on the X-ray table. A PTC is performed if a biliary drainage catheter is not already in situ.
2. The drainage catheter is removed over a guidewire and a sheath inserted in to the ducts (7 or 8-F).
3. Contrast is injected to identify stones and strictures.
4. If there is a stricture, advance a biliary manipulation catheter and guidewire (0.035) across it. Commence balloon dilatation over the guidewire (e.g. 8, 10 and possibly 12 mm).
5. Attempt to dislodge stones with balloons into the Roux loop.
6. If this is unsuccessful pass Dormier basket through sheath and attempt to catch the stone in the basket.
7. Advance the basket into the Roux loop and release the stone into the loop.
8. Remove the basket.
9. Pass the guidewire, remove the sheath and place the biliary drainage catheter.
10. Intermittently inject the contrast media to clarify the position of the stones.

Aftercare

1. Pulse and blood pressure half-hourly for 6 h
2. Bed rest for 4–6 h.

Complications

Due to the contrast medium

1. Allergic reactions – rare
2. Pancreatitis.

Due to the technique

1. Fever
2. Perforation of the T-tube tract.

Further Reading

Complications

Burke DR, Lewis CA, Cardella JF, et al. Society of Interventional Radiology Standards of Practice Committee: Quality improvement guidelines for percutaneous transhepatic cholangiography and biliary drainage. J Vasc Interv Radiol 2003;14(9 Pt 2):S243–6 [Republished from J Vasc Interv Radiol 1997;8(4):677–81].

Uberoi R, Das N, Moss J, et al. British Society of Interventional Radiology: Biliary Drainage and Stenting Registry (BDSR). Cardiovasc Intervent Radiol 2012;35(1):127–38.

ANGIOGRAPHY

COELIAC AXIS AND SUPERIOR MESENTERIC

Indications

1. Suspected haemorrhage/haemobilia prior to intervention (embolization of bleeding point or aneurysm)
2. Prior to embolization and intervention, e.g. embolization, chemo-embolization, radio-embolization of tumours
3. Suspected polyarteritis nodosa
4. Demonstration of portal venous system (when cross-sectional imaging is insufficient). This indication is rare with modern imaging.

Technique

See Chapter 3, page 77.

RADIONUCLIDE IMAGING OF LIVER AND SPLEEN

Indications

1. To assess liver for space-occupying lesions – essentially no longer performed because of greater utility of CT, MR and US
2. To characterize a focal liver lesion as possible focal nodular hyperplasia (these lesions contain Kupffer cells and hence take up colloid; other liver masses will be manifest as photopenic lesions)
3. To detect splenunculi (ectopic splenic tissue)
4. Assessment of liver function (displacement of activity of spleen and bone marrow).

Contraindications

None.

Radiopharmaceuticals

^{99m}Tc tin or sulphur colloid 80 MBq (ED 1 mSv), for SPECT 200 MBq (ED 2 mSv). Cleared by phagocytosis into the reticuloendothelial cells, where it is retained. Spleen is demonstrated as well as liver.

Equipment

1. Gamma-camera
2. Low-energy general purpose collimator.

Patient preparation

None.

Technique

1. Patient lies supine
2. Image at 20 min post injection
3. Images anterior with costal margin markers, posterior, left and right laterals.

500 kilocounts are used for each view. SPECT can be used when necessary.

An additional technique is first-pass dynamic flow study, which may occasionally be performed to improve differential diagnosis of liver masses.

Aftercare

None.

Complications

None.

Alternative investigative imaging modalities

1. Multidetector CT
2. MRI with reticuloendothelial contrast agent
3. [18]FDG-PET for investigation of primary or secondary malignancy (see Chapter 11)
4. Platelet or denatured red-cell scan for splenunculi.

Further Reading

Harding LK, Notghi A. Gastrointestinal tract and liver. In: Sharp PF, Gemmell HG, Murray AD, editors. Practical Nuclear Medicine, 3rd ed. London: Springer-Verlag; 2005. p. 273–304.

RADIONUCLIDE HEPATOBILIARY AND GALLBLADDER RADIONUCLIDE IMAGING

Indications

1. Suspected acute cholecystitis
2. Assessment of gallbladder, common bile duct and sphincter of Oddi function[1,2]
3. Assessment of neonatal jaundice where biliary atresia is considered

4. Suspected bile leaks after trauma or surgery[3]
5. Investigation of biliary drainage.

Contraindications

None.

Radiopharmaceuticals

[99m]Tc-trimethylbromo-iminodiacetic acid (TBIDA) or other iminodiacetic acid (IDA) derivative; 80 MBq typical (1 mSv ED), 150 MBq max (2 mSv ED). ^{99m}Tc-pertechnetate 10 MBq (0.13 mSv ED) to demonstrate stomach outline.

These ^{99m}Tc-labelled IDA derivatives are rapidly cleared from the circulation by hepatocytes and secreted into bile in a similar way to bilirubin;[4] this allows the assessment of biliary drainage and gallbladder function. A number have been developed with similar kinetics, but the later ones, such as TBIDA, have high hepatic uptake and low urinary excretion, giving better visualization of the biliary tract at high bilirubin levels than the early agents.

Equipment

1. Gamma-camera
2. Low-energy general purpose collimator.

Patient preparation

1. Nil by mouth for 4–6 h
2. For the investigation of biliary atresia, infants are given phenobarbital orally 5 mg kg^{-1} day^{-1} in two divided doses for 3–5 days prior to the study to enhance hepatic excretion of radiopharmaceutical.

Technique

The imaging protocol depends upon the clinical question being asked. A dynamic study should be performed where it is important to visualize the progress of the bile in detail, e.g. post-surgery:

1. The patient lies supine with the camera anterior and liver at the top of the field of view.
2. The radiopharmaceutical is injected i.v.

Images

1. 1-min 128×128 dynamic images are acquired for 45 min after injection.
2. 30–45 min post-injection when the gallbladder is well visualized, a liquid fatty meal (e.g. 300 ml full cream milk) is given through a straw to stimulate gallbladder contraction and imaging continued

for a further 45 min. A gallbladder ejection fraction can be calculated.
3. If the gallbladder and duodenum are not seen, static images are obtained at intervals of up to 4–6 h.
4. If images are suggestive of reflux, 100–200 ml of water is given through a straw to diffuse any activity in the stomach and thereby differentiate it from nearby bowel activity. Four min before the end of imaging, 100 ml of water containing 10 MBq ^{99m}Tc-pertechnetate may be given to delineate the stomach.
5. If no bowel activity is seen by 4–6 h and it is important to detect any flow of bile at all, e.g. in suspected biliary atresia, a 24-h image should be taken.

Additional techniques

Cholecystokinin (CCK) and morphine provocation[1]

Pharmacological intervention can be used in combination with TBIDA scanning to improve diagnosis of diseases affecting the gallbladder, common bile duct or sphincter of Oddi. CCK causes gallbladder contraction and sphincter of Oddi relaxation. An i.v. infusion of CCK is given over 2–3 min when the gallbladder is visualized 30–45 min after TBIDA administration. Dynamic imaging is continued for a further 30–40 min.

Quantitative measures of gallbladder ejection fraction and emptying rate can be calculated. It has been suggested that a slow CCK infusion over 30–60 min may improve specificity.[5]

Morphine causes sphincter of Oddi contraction. In a clinical setting of suspected acute cholecystitis, if the gallbladder is not observed by 60 min, an infusion of 0.04 mg kg^{-1} over 1 min can be given and imaging continued for a further 30 min. Continued non-visualization of the gallbladder up to 90 min is considered to confirm the diagnosis. Morphine provocation has also found success in diagnosis of elevated sphincter of Oddi basal pressure.[2]

Quantitative analysis

Some investigators have calculated liver function parameters from dynamic studies, e.g. in order to attempt to differentiate between transplant rejection and hepatocyte dysfunction.

Aftercare

None.

Complications

Monitor for adverse reactions to CCK and morphine.

References

1. Krishnamurthy S, Krishnamurthy GT. Cholecystokinin and morphine pharmacological intervention during ^{99m}Tc-HIDA cholescintigraphy: a rational approach. Semin Nucl Med 1996;26(1):16–24.

2. Thomas PD, Turner JG, Dobbs BR, et al. Use of ^{99m}Tc-DISIDA biliary scanning with morphine provocation for the detection of elevated sphincter of Oddi basal pressure. Gut 2000;46(6):838–41.
3. Rayter Z, Tonge C, Bennett C, et al. Ultrasound and HIDA: scanning in evaluating bile leaks after cholecystectomy. Nucl Med Commun 1991;12(3):197–202.
4. Krishnamurthy GT, Turner FE. Pharmacokinetics and clinical application of technetium 99m-labeled hepatobiliary agents. Semin Nucl Med 1990;20(2):130–49.
5. Ziessman HA. Cholecystokinin cholescintigraphy: victim of its own success? Q J Nucl Med 1999;40(12):2038–42.

Further Reading

Harding LK, Notghi A. Gastrointestinal tract and liver. In: Sharp PF, Gemmell HG, Murray AD, editors. Practical Nuclear Medicine, 3rd ed. London: Springer-Verlag; 2005. p. 273–304.

INVESTIGATION OF SPECIFIC CLINICAL PROBLEMS

THE INVESTIGATION OF LIVER TUMOURS

Investigation

This falls into three stages:

1. Detection
2. Characterization of the tumour
3. Assessment for surgical resection or staging for chemotherapy.

The clinical context and proposed management course usually determine the extent of investigation. Liver metastases are much commoner than primary liver cancers. Benign haemangiomas are also common, being present in 5–10% of the population. Other benign liver lesions, except cysts, are less common.

The clinical data correlated with the radiological investigations usually enable the character of a liver tumour to be determined with a high degree of probability. This can be confirmed with image-guided or surgical biopsy when appropriate. Many surgeons are averse to pre-operative biopsy in a patient with a potentially resectable/curable lesion because of the small risk of disseminating malignant cells and the possibility of misleading sampling error. If biopsy is performed, it is sometimes important to sample the 'normal' liver as well as the lesion. The presence of cirrhosis may have a major impact on management. Hepatic resection is an established procedure for the management of selected hepatic metastases and primary liver tumours. Imaging is used to assess the number and location of tumours.

Ultrasound

Often the first modality to detect an unsuspected focal liver lesion or lesions, but no longer appropriate for screening all patients for liver metastases.

Computed tomography

Widely used for general screening and staging. The remainder of the abdomen and chest may also be imaged for full staging.

Magnetic resonance imaging

Very useful for determining the nature of an unknown liver lesion and for characterizing and staging patients who are considered to be suitable for surgical resection based on CT findings.

4

THE INVESTIGATION OF JAUNDICE

The aim is to separate haemolytic causes of jaundice from obstructive jaundice or hepatocellular jaundice. Clinical history and examination are followed by biochemical tests of blood and urine, and haematological tests.

Investigations

Obstructive jaundice

US is the primary imaging investigation. The presence of dilated ducts suggests obstructive jaundice. The bile ducts, gallbladder and pancreas should be examined to determine the level and cause of obstruction. MRCP or CT is often required to confirm the cause of the obstruction. If the suspected cause is tumour, a CT or MRI scan is performed to stage the tumour. MRCP is a non-invasive method of imaging the ducts to demonstrate the presence of stones and the level and cause of obstruction, especially combined with cross-sectional MRI in cases of tumour or suspected tumour. Endoscopic ultrasound also can be very helpful in cases where the diagnosis is in doubt after cross-sectional imaging and to confirm or exclude small tumours or very small stones.

ERCP and/or PTC for higher level obstruction should be reserved for those cases where a non-operative management strategy has been determined or in cases with severe jaundice requiring drainage before definitive treatment.

Non-obstructive jaundice

When US shows no dilated ducts and hepatocellular jaundice is suspected, liver biopsy is considered. There may be other US evidence of parenchymal liver disease or signs of portal hypertension.

If obstructive jaundice is still suspected despite the US result, then MRCP is required. Extrahepatic obstruction may be present in the absence of duct dilatation, and patients with primary sclerosing cholangitis or widespread intrahepatic metastases may have obstruction without duct dilatation.

THE INVESTIGATION OF PANCREATITIS

US can be the first investigation, but in acute pancreatitis the presence of a sentinel loop of bowel will often obscure the pancreas and prevent good visualization. Even if the pancreas is seen, it can appear normal in acute pancreatitis. It is important to check for gallstones and biliary dilatation.

CT is the next investigation. If not known to have chronic pancreatitis or gallstones, a plain scan to look for these may be considered. Scans of the pancreas should then be obtained during both pancreatic and portal venous phase enhancement to enable identification of non-perfused areas of pancreas and characterize peripancreatic collections.

PANCREATIC PSEUDOCYSTS

Initial investigation can be with US. Pseudocysts can occur anywhere in the abdomen or pelvis or even the thorax. The spleen and left kidney provide acoustic windows to visualize the region of the tail of the pancreas.

CT scanning may also be performed if bowel loops prevent adequate visualization and should always be performed prior to radiologically guided intervention to prevent drainage of a pseudoaneurysm. (During ultrasonography supposed fluid collections can be interrogated with colour or duplex Doppler.). Pseudocysts can also be drained by endoscopic ultrasound.

Further Reading

Burns PN, Wilson SR. Focal liver masses: enhancement patterns on contrast-enhanced images – concordance of US scans with CT scans and MR images. Radiology 2007;242(1):162–74.

Hussain SM, Semelka RC. Hepatic imaging: comparison of modalities. Radiol Clin North Am 2005;43(5):929–47.

Rubens DJ. Hepatobiliary imaging and its pitfalls. Radiol Clin North Am 2004;42(2):257–78.

Siddiqi AJ, Miller F. Chronic pancreatitis: ultrasound, computed tomography, and magnetic resonance imaging features. Semin Ultrasound CT MR 2007;28(5):384–94.

Wilson SR, Kim TK, Jang HJ, et al. Enhancement patterns of focal liver masses: discordance between contrast-enhanced sonography and contrast-enhanced CT and MRI. Am J Roentgenol 2007;189(1):W7–12.

Urinary tract

Methods of imaging the urinary tract

1. Plain film radiography
2. Excretion urography (IVU)
3. Ultrasound (US)
4. Computed tomography (CT):
   (a) CT for urological diagnosis and urological cancer staging
   (b) CT for characterization of renal lesion
   (c) CT adrenals
   (d) CT KUB (kidneys, ureters, bladder)
   (e) CT urography (CTU)
   (f) CT angiography.
5. Magnetic resonance imaging (MRI):
   (a) MR for characterization of renal lesion
   (b) MR prostate
   (c) MR bladder
   (d) MR urography
   (e) MR adrenals
   (f) MR angiography.
6. Micturating cystography and cystourethrography
7. Ascending urethrography
8. Retrograde pyeloureterography
9. Percutaneous renal procedures:
   (a) Biopsy
   (b) Cyst puncture
   (c) Antegrade pyelography
   (d) Nephrostomy
   (e) Percutaneous nephrolithotomy.
10. Arteriography
11. Venography
12. Conduitogram
13. Radionuclide imaging:
    (a) Static renography
    (b) Dynamic renography
    (c) Radionuclide cystography – direct and indirect.

PLAIN FILM RADIOGRAPHY

Indications

Predominantly to evaluate renal tract calcifications – recognizing that CT is significantly more sensitive (>98% compared to 60% for plain films).

Technique

As for preliminary films for excretion urography (below).

INTRAVENOUS EXCRETION UROGRAPHY (IVU)

The technique is less frequently used than in the past and is now largely replaced by CT, MRI or US.

Indications

1. Haematuria
2. Renal colic (see variation)
3. Recurrent urinary tract infection
4. Loin pain
5. Suspected urinary tract pathology.

Contraindications

See Chapter 2 – general contraindications to intravenous (i.v.) water-soluble contrast media and ionizing radiation. In patients with contrast medium allergies alternative modalities such as ultrasound or MR can be considered. Patients with impaired renal function, particularly those with diabetes should be prepared with oral or intravenous hydration, or an alternative imaging modality considered. See Chapter 2.

Contrast medium

Low osmolar contrast material (LOCM) 300–370 mg I ml^{-1}.

Adult dose
50–100 ml.

Paediatric dose
1 ml kg^{-1}.

Patient preparation

1. No food for 5 h prior to the examination. Dehydration is not necessary and does not improve image quality.
2. The routine administration of bowel preparation has been shown not to improve the diagnostic quality of the examination.

Preliminary images

Supine, full-length anterior posterior (AP) of the abdomen, in inspiration. The lower border of the cassette is at the level of the symphysis pubis and the X-ray beam is centred in the mid-line at the level of the iliac crests.

If necessary, the location of overlying opacities may be further determined by:

- supine AP film of the renal areas, in expiration. The X-ray beam is centred in the mid-line at the level of the lower costal margin or
- 35° posterior oblique views (side of interest towards the film) or
- tomography of the kidneys.

The examination should not proceed further until these images have been reviewed by the radiologist or radiographer and deemed satisfactory.

5

Technique

Venous access is established. The gauge of the cannula/needle should allow the injection to be given rapidly as a bolus to maximize the density of the nephrogram.

Images

1. *Immediate film*. AP of the renal areas. This film is exposed 10–14 s after the injection (approximate 'arm-to-kidney' time). It aims to show the nephrogram at its most dense, i.e. the renal parenchyma opacified by contrast medium in the renal tubules. Tomography may assist in evaluation of the renal outline or possible masses (or ultrasound if subsequently available).
2. *5-min film*. AP of the renal areas. This film gives an initial assessment of pathology – specifically the presence or absence of obstruction before administering compression.

   A compression band is then applied positioned midway between the anterior superior iliac spines, i.e. precisely over the ureters as they cross the pelvic brim. The aim is to produce pelvicalyceal distension. Compression is contraindicated:
   (a) after recent abdominal surgery
   (b) after renal trauma
   (c) if there is a large abdominal mass or aortic aneurysm
   (d) when the 5-min film shows already distended calyces indicative of obstruction.
3. *10-min film*. AP of the renal areas. There is usually adequate distension of the pelvicalyceal systems with opaque urine by this time. Compression is released when satisfactory demonstration of the pelvicalyceal system has been achieved. If the compression film is inadequate the compression should be checked and repositioned

if necessary and a further 50 ml of contrast medium administered and the film after 5 minutes.

4. *Release film.* Supine AP abdomen taken immediately after release of compression. This film is taken to show the ureters. If this film is satisfactory, the patient is asked to empty their bladder.

5. *After micturition film.* Full-length supine AP abdomen. The aims of this film are to assess bladder emptying, to demonstrate drainage of the upper tracts, to aid the diagnosis of bladder tumours, to confirm ureterovesical junction calculi and, uncommonly, to demonstrate a urethral diverticulum in females.

Additional images

1. 35° posterior obliques of the kidneys, ureters or bladder – for equivocal collecting system lesions or localization of calculi.
2. Tomography – if renal outlines are not well seen.
3. Prone abdomen following the release film – may improve visualization of distal ureters by making them more dependent.
4. Delayed films at increasing (doubling of time intervals) up to 24 h after injection in renal obstruction.

Variation

Renal colic – a limited study may be performed: preliminary films; 20-min full length (no compression); post-micturition full length; delayed films up to 24 hours as required to show level and cause of obstruction.

Further Reading

Amis ES. Epitaph for the urogram. Radiology 1999;213:639–40.
Becker JA, Pollack HM, McClennan BL. Urography survives. Radiology 2001;218:299–300.
Webb JAW. Imaging in haematuria. Clin Radiol 1997;52:167–71.

ULTRASOUND OF THE URINARY TRACT

Indications

1. Renal mass lesion
2. Renal parenchymal disease
3. Renal obstruction/loin pain
4. Haematuria
5. Hypertension
6. Renal cystic disease
7. Renal size measurement
8. Bladder outflow obstruction
9. Urinary tract infection

10. Bladder tumour
11. Following renal transplant:
    (a) Obstruction
    (b) Patency of vessels
    (c) Perirenal collections.
12. To guide needle placement in interventional procedures
13. Renal vascular studies.

Contraindications

None.

Patient preparation

Kidneys only – none.

Kidneys and bladder – prehydrate with oral fluids, e.g. 500–1000 ml 1 h before scan, patient attends with a full bladder. This may have the disadvantage of making the collecting systems appear mildly hydronephrotic pre-micturition.

Equipment

3.5–5-MHz transducer.

Technique

1. Patient supine, right (RAO) and left anterior oblique (LAO) positions or lateral for kidneys. The kidneys are scanned longitudinally in an oblique coronal plane supplemented by transverse sections perpendicular to the axis. The right kidney may be scanned through the liver and posteriorly in the right loin. The left kidney is harder to visualize anteriorly, but can be visualized from a lateral approach. In difficult cases the patient should lie on their side with a pillow under the left loin to widen the space between the rib cage and pelvis.
2. The length of the kidney measured by US is 1–2 cm smaller than that measured at excretion urography because there is no geometric magnification. With US measurement, care must be taken to ensure that the true longitudinal lengthwise measurement is obtained. The range of lengths of the normal kidneys is 9–12 cm, and the difference between each kidney should be less than 1–2 cm.
3. The bladder is scanned suprapubically in transverse and longitudinal planes. Measurements taken of the three orthogonal diameters before and after micturition enable an approximate volume to be calculated by multiplying the three diameters and applying a conversion factor. (A conversion factor is usually pre-programmed into modern ultrasound machines.)

4. Renal transplants are usually located in the right or left iliac fossa. These usually lie fairly superficially and are easy to evaluate using oblique planes and gentle pressure to displace overlying bowel loops.

5. The native or transplant kidneys can be evaluated for vascular pathology using Doppler techniques.
   - Renal artery stenosis is diagnosed by direct Doppler interrogation of the main renal arteries from a transabdominal approach. Elevated peak systolic velocities greater than 200 cm s^{-1} are suggestive of a >50% stenosis. Alternatively, as the main renal arteries in the native kidneys are often hard to visualize, the intrarenal arteries can be evaluated from a flank approach for downstream changes in waveform – the *tardusparvus* pattern;[1] a slow rise (*tardus*) to a reduced peak (*parvus*) producing a prolonged acceleration time (a value >70 ms is indicative of a severe stenosis).
   - Renal vein thrombosis is diagnosed by absent colour Doppler venous flow, direct visualization of thrombus within the distended vein, and a raised resistive index with reversal of arterial diastolic flow within the intrarenal arteries.

Reference
1. Kotval PS. Doppler waveform parvus and tardus: a sign of proximal flow obstruction. J Ultrasound Med 1989;8:435–40.

Further Reading
Bih L-I, Ho C-C, Tsai S-J, et al. Bladder shape impact on the accuracy of ultrasonic estimation of bladder volume. Arch Phys Med Rehabil 1998;79:1553–6.

Sidhu R, Lockhart ME. Imaging of renovascular disease. Semin Ultrasound, CT and MRI 2009;30(4):271–88.

COMPUTED TOMOGRAPHY OF THE URINARY TRACT

Indications
1. Renal colic/renal stone disease
2. Renal tumour
3. Renal/perirenal collection
4. Loin mass
5. Staging and follow-up of renal, collecting system or prostatic cancer (local staging of prostatic cancer is performed using thin-section MRI)
6. Investigation of renal tract obstruction
7. CT angiography may be used to assess renal vessels for suspected renal artery stenosis or arterio-venous fistula or malformation.

Techniques

Standard diagnostic CT

This technique is used to stage and follow-up known renal-tract malignancy or to investigate non-specific signs attributed to the renal tract. Examination of the thorax in addition to the abdomen and pelvis is usually performed where pulmonary metastatic disease or mediastinal nodal spread is a possibility:

1. Venous access is obtained
2. Patient lies supine
3. Scanogram of chest, abdomen and pelvis as appropriate
4. 100 ml i.v. LOCM given
5. Scans obtained approximately 70 s (portal venous phase) after i.v. contrast (arterial phase scans of the liver (20–25 s after i.v. contrast) may be appropriate in those patients with suspected metastatic renal cancer who may have hypervascular liver metastases.)

Renal lesion characterization CT

This is used to assess renal cysts or masses identified on another imaging modality such as ultrasound.

Pre- and post-i.v. contrast scans are obtained through the kidneys in order to assess precontrast attenuation and subsequent enhancement patterns. Many practitioners advise the post-contrast scan be performed at 100 seconds (nephrographic phase) to prevent small intraparenchymal lesions being obscured by corticomedullary differentiation.

Adrenal lesion characterization CT

Indication: adrenal mass is suspected or needs characterization.

Technique: Unenhanced CT of the abdomen to enable measurement of attenuation of any adrenal mass.

A value <10 HU is highly specific for a benign (lipid-rich) adenoma, and is often the only test required. This may, however, be supplemented when necessary by washout CT; re-measurement of the adrenal density in Hounsfield units at 15 min following i.v. contrast. Benign adenomas (whether or not lipid-rich) typically show rapid washout of contrast; an *absolute percentage washout* (APW) >60% or *relative percentage washout* (RPW) >40%, on delayed images, is highly specific for a benign lesion.

$$APW = \frac{(\text{density at 70 s} - \text{density at 15 min})}{(\text{density at 70 s} - \text{precontrast density})} \times 100$$

$$RPW = \frac{(\text{density at 70 s} - \text{density at 15 min})}{(\text{density at 70 s})} \times 100$$

Densities of lesion (in HU) measured pre and post i.v. contrast administration

(Alternatively chemical shift MRI may be used for characterization.)

CT KUB

Plain CT (commonly referred to as CT KUB – kidneys, ureters, bladder) is useful to assess possible stone disease. It is used in many centres as the primary investigation of renal colic (replacing plain KUB radiograph):

1. No intravenous or oral contrast is given.
2. Patient supine. (Some authorities advise prone scanning to differentiate if stones are impacted at the vesicoureteric junction or have passed into the bladder.)
3. A low-radiation-dose technique is used to scan from the top of the kidneys to include the bladder base with a slice thickness of 5 mm or less, as determined by CT scanner. (Due to the low-dose nature of the scan and the absence of i.v. and oral contrast, the scan has a very limited role in identifying pathology other than renal tract calculus disease and should not be used indiscriminately for investigation of non-specific abdominal pain.)

CT urogram (CTU)

This technique uses a combination of unenhanced, nephrographic and delayed scans following i.v. contrast to sequentially allow examination of renal parenchyma and collecting systems.

Suggested protocol:

1. An oral water load of 500–1000 ml 30–60 minutes before injection is recommended to ensure a diuresis and collecting system dilatation. No positive oral contrast
2. Patient supine
3. Initial low-dose unenhanced scans of urinary tract (CT KUB) to determine if renal tract calculus disease is present
4. Low osmolar contrast material (LOCM) 300 mg I ml^{-1} 100 ml is given as bolus intravenously
5. Thin-section (usually 1 mm) scans are obtained from diaphragm to lower poles of kidneys during nephrographic/parenchymal enhancement phase (100 s following start of bolus injection). Alternatively, scan may instead be acquired during the portal venous phase (70 s) but normal corticomedullary differentiation may make small tumours difficult to appreciate
6. Delayed thin-section (1 mm) scans are acquired from upper pole of kidneys to bladder base 20 min after contrast injection, to examine collecting systems and ureters
7. Source images are reviewed along with multiplanar reconstructions. Post-processing with maximum-intensity projections and surface-shaded displays may be helpful, especially for demonstration.

Variations

The nephrographic phase may be omitted if the scan is specifically for urothelial tumour or collecting system assessment.

Some protocols use diuretics or use abdominal compression bands to achieve collecting system distension.

Radiation dose is a significant consideration for a triple-phase CTU (compared to an IVU) but newer iterative reconstruction techniques increasingly available are reducing the differential. Some authorities advocate the use of a split bolus technique, i.e. 50 ml of i.v. contrast 10–15 min before scanning, with a further 50 ml at the time of the scan, to achieve demonstration of the nephrographic and pyelographic phases with the same acquisition with consequent radiation dose saving.

CT angiography

Indications

1. Renal artery stenosis
2. Renal artery aneurysm, arteriovenous malformation, dissection or thrombosis
3. Delineation of vascular anatomy prior to laparoscopic surgery, e.g. nephrectomy, pyeloplasty.

Technique

1. No oral iodinated contrast used
2. Scan from the upper pole of the kidneys to the aortic bifurcation. Modern scanners are fast enough to produce high-quality studies of the whole abdomen
3. Narrow collimation (1 mm)
4. 100–150 ml i.v. contrast medium (LOCM 300) injected at 3–4 ml s^{-1}
5. Use of bolus tracking/triggering devices or timing test injections is recommended to ensure appropriate timing. Otherwise scans are initiated after a preset empiric delay of 20–25 s from start of contrast material injection
6. Source axial scans are supplemented by multiplanar reconstructions and maximum intensity projection and volume-rendered surface-shaded display postprocessing.

Further Reading

Adrenal Lesion Characterization CT

Johnson PT, Horton KM, Fishman EK. Adrenal imaging with multidetector CT: evidence-based protocol optimization and interpretive practice. RadioGraphics 2009;29:1319–31.

Technique

Low G, Dhliwayo H, Lomas DJ. Adrenal neoplasms. Clin Radiol 2012;67(10):988–1000.

O'Regan KN, O'Connor OJ, McLoughlin P, et al. The role of imaging in the investigation of painless hematuria in adults. Semin Ultrasound, CT and MRI 2009;30(4):258–70.

Van Der Molen AJ, Cowan NC, Mueller-Lisse UG, et al. CT urography working group of the European Society of Urogenital Radiology (ESUR). CT urography: definition, indications and techniques. A guideline for clinical practice. Eur Radiol 2008;18(1):4–17.

MAGNETIC RESONANCE IMAGING OF THE URINARY TRACT

Indications

1. Local staging of prostatic cancer
2. Local staging of bladder cancer
3. Staging of pelvic lymph nodes
4. Renal mass
5. Screening of patients with von Hippel–Lindau disease or their relatives, or other genetic conditions
6. MR urography where intravenous or CT urography contraindicated
7. MR angiography: potential living related donors, suspected renal artery stenosis.

Technique

Technique will be tailored to the clinical indication. MR of the kidneys and upper abdomen will generally include T1 and T2 weighted sequences in axial and coronal planes with or without fat saturation; with pre and post contrast T1 weighted imaging at 30 and 70 seconds. MRI of the abdomen and pelvis can be obtained to assess retroperitoneal lymphadenopathy as part of the staging investigations for patients with bladder and prostate cancer but CT is often used for this purpose with MRI reserved for local staging.

MAGNETIC RESONANCE IMAGING OF THE PROSTATE

Technique/example protocol

1. Patient supine. Phased array body coil. The best images will be obtained with an endorectal coil, but many authorities do not use these. 1.5T or 3T scanners are both used. 3T scanners afford better signal-to-noise ratio but may be subject to more artefacts, notably susceptibility
2. Antiperistaltic drugs (hyoscine butyl-bromide or glucagon are recommended)
3. T1W and T2W axial scans whole pelvis
4. Thin-section (3–4 mm) small field of view T1-weighted spin echo (SE) scans in axial plane orthogonal to the axis of the prostate to evaluate for post-biopsy haemorrhage

5. Thin-section (3–4 mm) small field of view T2-weighted spin echo (SE) scans in transverse, sagittal and coronal planes orthogonal to the axis of the prostate
6. Multiparametric MRI – there is increasing use of the following functional studies:
   (a) Diffusion weighted imaging values 0, 100 and 800–1400 s/mm^2 with apparent diffusion coefficient (ADC) map
   (b) Dynamic contrast-enhanced (DCE) T1W imaging
   (c) MR spectroscopy – citrate, creatine, choline.

Further Reading

Barentsz JO, Richenberg J, Clements R, et al. ESUR prostate MR guidelines. Eur Radiol 2012;22(4):746–57.

MAGNETIC RESONANCE UROGRAPHY

Indications

1. To demonstrate the collecting system/determine level of obstruction in a poorly functioning/obstructed kidney
2. Urinary tract obstruction unrelated to urolithiasis. Suspected renal colic from underlying calculus is better imaged with CT KUB
3. Congenital anomalies
4. Renal transplant donor assessment (combined with MR angiography).

Technique

The two most common MR urographic techniques are:

- static fluid-sensitive urography using heavily T2-weighted MRI techniques to visualize fluid-filled structures (equivalent to magnetic resonance cholangio-pancreatography (MRCP))
- excretory MR urography using T1-weighted sequences post gadolinium enhancement.

1. Patient supine with an empty bladder for comfort. If the bladder is of interest, a moderately full bladder may be preferred.
2. Scout views are obtained.
3. Static MR urography may be performed prior to excretory urography. Thick-slab, single-shot, fast-spin echo or a similar thin-section technique, e.g. half-Fourier rapid acquisition with relaxation enhancement; single-shot, fast-spin echo; single-shot, turbo-spin echo. 3D respiratory triggered sequences may be used to obtain thin-section data sets that may be further post-processed.
4. Oral or intravenous hydration, compression or diuretics may be used to enhance collecting system distension.
5. Excretory MR urography: a gadolinium-based contrast agent is administered i.v. using a dose of 0.1 mmol gadolinium kg^{-1} body

weight. The collecting systems are imaged during the excretory phase (10–20 min) using a breath-hold, three-dimensional gradient echo, T1-weighted sequence. Fat suppression will improve the conspicuity of the ureters. T2* effects from a high concentration of contrast agent may reduce the signal intensity of urine and potentially obscure small masses within the collecting system. This can be overcome by using a lower volume of i.v. contrast but may compromise soft-tissue imaging.

Further Reading

Leyendecker JR, Barnes CE, Zagoria RJ. MR urography: techniques and clinical applications. RadioGraphics 2008;28(1):23–46.

Nikken JJ, Krestin GP. MRI of the kidney – state of the art. Eur Radiol 2007;17(11):2780–93.

MAGNETIC RESONANCE IMAGING OF THE ADRENALS

Indications

Characterization of adrenal mass.

Technique

Chemical shift imaging: based on a high proportion of intracellular lipid causing alteration of the local magnetic environment within the voxel and hence resonant frequency of protons. Lipid-rich benign adenomas can be shown to lose signal on opposed phase T1W imaging compared to in-phase studies. This is highly specific.

Alternative: unenhanced CT can be used to characterize an adrenal mass as malignant (see above) or FDG-PET can be used to characterize an adrenal mass as malignant (see Chapter 11).

Further Reading

Low G, Dhliwayo H, Lomas DJ. Adrenal neoplasms. Clin Radiol 2012;67(10):988–1000.

MAGNETIC RESONANCE RENAL ANGIOGRAPHY

Indications

1. Possible renal artery stenosis
2. Number and disposition of renal arteries
   (a) Pre surgery
   (b) Renal transplant donors.

Technique

1. Three-dimensional spoiled gradient echo sequences before and following i.v. injection (2 ml s^{-1}) of 0.1 mmol kg^{-1} gadolinium.
2. A saline flush (20 ml) at the same rate is given.

3. Accurate timing of injection is determined by bolus tracking with ROI (region of interest) positioned over abdominal aorta.
4. The scan is triggered when signal intensity at the ROI reaches a preset value.
5. Source imaging is supplemented by post processing with multiplanar reconstructions and maximum-intensity projections.

Alternative non-contrast MR angiographic techniques

Time-of-flight and phase contrast angiography are of limited application in this context in comparison to contrast-enhanced studies.

Further Reading

Soulez G, Pasowicz M, Benea G, et al. Renal artery stenosis evaluation: diagnostic performance of gadobenate dimeglumine-enhanced MR angiography – comparison with DSA. Radiology 2008;247(1):273–85.

MICTURATING CYSTOURETHROGRAPHY

Indications

1. Vesicoureteric reflux
2. Study of the urethra during micturition
3. Bladder leak post surgery or trauma
4. Urodynamic studies, e.g. for incontinence.

Contraindications

Acute urinary tract infection.

Contrast medium

High osmolar contrast material (HOCM) or LOCM 150 mg I ml^{-1}.

Equipment

1. Fluoroscopy unit with spot film device and tilting table
2. Video recorder (for urodynamics)
3. Bladder catheter.

Patient preparation

The patient empties their bladder prior to the examination.

Preliminary image

Coned view of the bladder.

Technique

To demonstrate vesico-ureteric reflux (this indication is almost exclusively confined to children):

1. Using aseptic technique the bladder is catheterized. Residual urine is drained.
2. Contrast medium (LOCM 150 mg I ml^{-1}) is slowly injected or dripped in with the patient supine and bladder filling is observed by intermittent fluoroscopy. It is important that early filling is monitored by fluoroscopy in case the catheter is malpositioned, e.g. in the distal ureter or vagina.
3. Intermittent monitoring is also necessary to identify transient reflux. Any reflux should be recorded.
4. The catheter should not be removed until the radiologist is confident that the patient will be able to micturate, the patient does not tolerate further infusion or until no more contrast medium will drip into the bladder.
5. Older children and adults are given a urine receiver but smaller children should be allowed to pass urine onto absorbent pads on which they can lie. Children can lie on the table but adults will probably find it easier to micturate while standing erect. In infants and children with a neuropathic bladder, micturition may be accomplished by suprapubic pressure.
6. Spot images are taken during micturition and any reflux recorded. A video recording may be useful. The lower ureter is best seen in the anterior oblique position of that side. Boys should micturate in an oblique or lateral projection, so that spot films can be taken of the entire urethra.
7. Finally, a full-length view of the abdomen is taken to demonstrate any undetected reflux of contrast medium that might have occurred into the kidneys and to record the post-micturition residue.
8. Lateral views are helpful when fistulation into the rectum or vagina are suspected.
9. Oblique views are needed when evaluating for leaks.
10. Stress views are used for urodynamic studies.

Aftercare

1. No special aftercare is necessary, but patients and parents of children should be warned that dysuria, possibly leading to retention of urine, may rarely be experienced. In such cases a simple analgesic is helpful and children may be helped by allowing them to micturate in a warm bath.
2. Most children will already be receiving antibiotics for their recent urinary tract infection – the dose will usually be doubled for 3 days, starting on the day prior to the procedure. Children not already on antibiotics will also usually be prescribed a 3-day course (often trimethoprim).

Complications

1. Urinary tract infection
2. Catheter trauma may lead to dysuria, frequency, haematuria and urinary retention
3. Complications of bladder filling, e.g. perforation from overdistension – prevented by using a non-retaining catheter, e.g. Jacques
4. Catheterization of vagina or an ectopic ureteral orifice
5. Retention of a Foley catheter.

ASCENDING URETHROGRAPHY IN THE MALE

5

Indications

1. Stricture
2. Urethral trauma
3. Fistulae or false passage
4. Congenital abnormalities.

Contraindications

1. Acute urinary tract infection
2. Recent instrumentation.

Contrast medium

LOCM 200–300 mg I ml^{-1} 20 ml. Pre-warming the contrast medium will help reduce the incidence of spasm of the external sphincter.

Equipment

1. Fluoroscopy unit and spot film device
2. Foley catheter 8-F.

Patient preparation

Consent.

Preliminary image

Coned supine postero-anterior (PA) of bladder base and urethra.

Technique

1. Patient supine
2. The catheter is connected to a 50 ml syringe containing contrast medium and flushed to eliminate air bubbles
3. Using aseptic technique the tip of the catheter is inserted so that the balloon lies in the fossa navicularis (i.e. immediately proximal to the meatus within the glans) and its balloon is inflated with 2–3 ml of water to anchor the catheter and occlude the meatus

4. Contrast medium is injected under fluoroscopic control and steep (30–45°) oblique films taken. Gentle traction on the catheter is used to straighten the penis over the ipsilateral leg and prevent urethral overlap or foreshortening from obscuring pathology.

Depending on the clinical indication, ascending urethrography may be followed by descending micturating cystourethrography to demonstrate the proximal urethra and bladder, assuming there is no contraindication to bladder catheterization, e.g. false passage, stricture. It may be possible to fill the bladder retrogradely via the urethral catheter if the patient is able to relax the bladder neck (and thus avoid bladder catheterization).

Aftercare

None.

Complications due to the technique

1. Acute urinary tract infection
2. Urethral trauma
3. Intravasation of contrast medium, especially if excessive pressure is used to overcome a stricture.

Further Reading

Kawashima A, Sandler CM, Wasserman NF, et al. Imaging of urethral disease: a pictorial review. RadioGraphics 2004;24:S195–216.

RETROGRADE PYELOURETEROGRAPHY

Indications

1. Demonstration of the site and nature of an obstructive lesion
2. Demonstration of the pelvicalyceal system and potential urothelial abnormalities after previous indeterminate imaging.

Contraindications

Acute urinary tract infection.

Contrast medium

HOCM or LOCM 150–200 mg I ml^{-1} (i.e. not too dense to obscure small lesions) 10 ml.

Equipment

Fluoroscopy unit.

Patient preparation

As for surgery.

Preliminary image

Full-length supine antero-posterior (AP) abdomen when the examination is performed in the X-ray department.

Technique

In the operating theatre

The surgeon catheterizes the ureter via a cystoscope and advances the ureteric catheter to the desired level. Contrast medium is injected under fluoroscopic control and spot films are exposed. Technique and imaging as below. Some form of hard copy or soft copy recording is recommended – ideally to the hospital PACS system.

In the X-ray department

1. With ureteric catheter(s) in situ, the patient is transferred from the operating theatre to the X-ray department.
2. Urine is aspirated and, under fluoroscopic control, contrast medium is slowly injected. Care should be taken to eliminate air bubbles before injection (as these may mimic pathology such as tumour or calculus. About 3–5 ml is usually enough to fill the pelvis but if the patient complains of pain or fullness in the loin, the injection should be terminated before this.
3. Images are taken as the catheter is withdrawn. These should include frontal and oblique projections.

Aftercare

1. Post-anaesthetic observations
2. Prophylactic antibiotics may be used.

Complications

1. Pyelosinus extravasation and pyelotubular reflux due to over-filling may result in pain, fever and rigors
2. Introduction of infection
3. Damage or perforation of the ureters or renal pelvis.

CONDUITOGRAM

Indications

1. To evaluate for development of upper tract tumour
2. Suspected stricture at anastomosis of ureter and ileal urinary conduit
3. Suspected narrowing of conduit.

Contrast

LOCM or HOCM 150 mg I ml^{-1}.

Technique

1. The patient should be advised to bring a spare stoma bag or one should be available.
2. A urinary catheter is chosen tailored to the size of the stoma. (Although larger catheters may pass more easily, a smaller catheter may be needed.)
3. The catheter is flushed with contrast medium and a syringe or giving set with contrast medium is connected. It is very important to exclude air bubbles which can be confused for upper tract tumours.
4. The conduit is then catheterized using a sterile technique.
5. The catheter balloon is inflated and minimal traction applied to the catheter to occlude the stoma.
6. Contrast is instilled under fluoroscopic control into the lumen of the conduit.
7. AP and oblique views are taken as appropriate, of sufficient number to demonstrate the whole pelvicalyceal systems and ureters.

PERCUTANEOUS RENAL CYST PUNCTURE AND BIOPSY

Indications

1. Diagnostic biopsy: unexplained renal failure, mass, etc.
2. Renal cyst puncture to relieve local symptoms attributable to a cyst.

Contraindications

1. Bleeding diathesis
2. The possibility of renal hydatid disease.

Equipment

Ultrasound or CT guidance.

Patient preparation

Pre-medication or sedation may be needed.

Technique

Insertion of the needle can be controlled by either ultrasonography or CT:

1. The patient is placed in the prone position, or as appropriate depending on patient habitus and position of lesion.
2. The kidney, mass or cyst is located directly with US or CT or indirectly, after opacification of the kidneys with i.v. contrast medium. The optimum site for puncture is marked on the skin.

For renal biopsy in the investigation of parenchyma disease the lower pole of the left kidney is often preferred.

3. The skin and subcutaneous tissues are infiltrated with 1% lidocaine.
4. The needle is passed directly into the lesion during suspended respiration. US or CT are used to monitor the path of the needle. For cyst puncture the stilette is removed and the cyst contents are aspirated and examined.
5. For biopsy, the biopsy needle is deployed following confirmation of needle position with imaging.

Complications

- Bleeding – perinephric or haematuria
- Arteriovenous fistula
- Pseudoaneurysm.

PERCUTANEOUS ANTEGRADE PYELOGRAPHY AND NEPHROSTOMY

This is the introduction of a drainage catheter into the collecting system of the kidney.

Indications

1. Renal tract obstruction
2. Pyonephrosis
3. Prior to percutaneous nephrolithotomy
4. Ureteric or bladder fistulae: external drainage, i.e. urinary diversion may allow closure.

Contraindications

Uncontrolled bleeding diathesis.

Contrast medium

As for percutaneous renal puncture.

Equipment

1. Puncturing needle: coaxial needle/catheter set or sheathed 18G needle
2. Drainage catheter: at least 6-F pigtail with multiple side holes
3. Guidewires: conventional J-wire ± extra stiff wire
4. US and/or fluoroscopy – usually used in combination.

Patient preparation

1. Fasting for 4 h
2. Premedication as required
3. Prophylactic antibiotic.

Technique

Patient position

Patient lies prone oblique with a foam pad or pillow under the abdomen to present the kidney optimally.

Identifying the collecting system prior to the definitive procedure

1. Freehand or with a biopsy needle attachment; US guidance is the most common method for localizing the kidney and guiding the initial needle puncture into the collecting system.
2. Excretion urography, if adequate residual function and a non-dilated system using a parallax technique.
3. Occasionally retrograde injection through an ileal conduit or a ureteric catheter may be used to demonstrate the target collecting system.

Site/plane of puncture

A point on the posterior axillary line is chosen below the twelfth rib. Having identified the mid/lower pole calyces with US or contrast, the plane of puncture is determined. This will be via the soft tissues and renal parenchyma avoiding direct puncture of the renal pelvis, so that vessels around the renal pelvis will be avoided and the drainage catheter will gain some purchase on the renal parenchyma. There is a relatively avascular plane between the ventral and dorsal parts of the kidney which affords the ideal access.

Techniques of puncture, catheterization

The skin and soft tissues are infiltrated with local anaesthetic using a spinal needle.

Puncture may then be made using one of the following systems (depending on preference):

1. *An 18G sheathed needle, or Kellett needle,* using the Seldinger technique for catheterization. Contrast injection is used to confirm successful siting of the needle and for preliminary demonstration of the pelvicalyceal system. On occasion air is used as a negative contrast medium to enable targeting of a posterior non-dependent calyx. Upon successful puncture a J-guidewire is inserted and coiled within the collecting system; the sheath is then pushed over the wire, which may be exchanged for a stiffer wire. Dilatation is then performed to the size of the drainage catheter, which is then inserted. Care must be taken not to kink the guidewire within the soft tissues. Sufficient guidewire should be maintained within the collecting system, ideally with the wire in the upper ureter to maintain position and, if kinking does occur, the kinked portion of the wire can be withdrawn outside the skin.

2. *Coaxial needle puncture systems* using a 22/21G puncturing needle that takes a 0.018 guidewire. This affords a single puncture with a fine needle, with insertion of a three-part coaxial system to allow insertion of 0.035 guidewire and then proceed as in (1) above.

3. *The trocar-cannula system*, in which direct puncture of the collecting system is made with the drainage catheter already assembled over a trocar. On removal of the trocar the drainage catheter is advanced further into the collecting system.

Having successfully introduced the catheter, it is securely fixed to the skin and drainage commenced.

Antegrade pyelography is rarely performed as an isolated procedure; usually it is undertaken following placement of, and via, a nephrostomy catheter as above. Oblique and AP images are taken with gentle introduction of water-soluble contrast medium. Semi-erect films may be necessary to encourage contrast medium down the ureters to show the site and nature of obstruction. Post nephrostomy studies are best performed after a delay of 1–2 days to allow the patient to recover and be able to cooperate, blood clot to resolve, and infected systems to be drained.

Aftercare

1. Bed rest for 4 h
2. Pulse, blood pressure and temperature half-hourly for 6 h
3. Analgesia
4. Urine samples sent for culture and sensitivity.

Complications

1. Septicaemia
2. Haemorrhage
3. Perforation of the collecting system with urine leak
4. Unsuccessful drainage
5. Injury to adjacent organs such as lung, pleura, spleen or colon
6. Later catheter dislodgement.

Further Reading

Dyer RB, Regan JD, Kavanagh PV, et al. Percutaneous nephrostomy with extensions of the technique: step by step. RadioGraphics 2002;22:503–25.

PERCUTANEOUS NEPHROLITHOTOMY

This is the removal of renal calculi through a nephrostomy track. It is often reserved for large complicated calculi which are unsuitable for extracorporeal shock-wave lithotripsy.

Indications

1. Removal of renal calculi
2. Disintegration of large renal calculi.

Contraindications

Uncontrolled bleeding diathesis.

Contrast medium

As for percutaneous renal puncture.

Equipment

1. Puncturing needle (18G): Kellett (15–20 cm length) or equivalent
2. Guidewires, including hydrophilic and superstiff
3. Track dilating equipment; Teflon dilators (from 7-F–30-F), metal coaxial dilators or a special angioplasty-type balloon catheter
4. US machine
5. Fluoroscopy facilities with rotating C arm if possible.

Patient preparation

1. Full discussion between radiologist/urologist concerning indications, etc.
2. Imaging (IVU, CT KUB, CTU) to demonstrate position of calculus and relationship to calyces
3. General anaesthetic
4. Coagulation screen
5. Two units of blood cross matched
6. Antibiotic cover
7. Premedication
8. Bladder catheterization, as large volumes of irrigation fluid will pass down the ureter during a prolonged procedure.

Technique

Pre-procedure planning may include a CT KUB and CTU to localize stones and to choose most appropriate access.

Patient position

As for a percutaneous nephrostomy, usually prone (see p. 147).

Methods of opacification of the collecting system

1. Retrograde ureteric catheterization for demonstration and distension of the collecting system may be achieved. In addition, a retrograde occlusion balloon catheter in the ureter will prevent large fragments of stone passing down the ureter
2. Intravenous excretion urography
3. Antegrade pyelography; this also enables distension of the collecting system.

Puncture of the collecting system

A lower pole posterior calyx is ideally chosen if the calculus is situated in the renal pelvis. Otherwise the calyx in which the calculus is situated is usually punctured. Special care must be taken if puncturing above the twelfth rib because of the risk of perforating the diaphragm and pleura. Puncture is in an oblique plane from the posterior axillary line through the renal parenchyma. Puncture of the selected calyx is made using a combination of US and a rotating C-arm fluoroscopic facility. On successful puncture a guidewire is inserted through the cannula and as much wire as possible is guided into the collecting system. The cannula is then exchanged for an angled catheter and the wire and catheter are manipulated into the distal ureter. At this stage full dilatation may be performed (single-stage) or a nephrostomy tube left in situ with dilatation later (two-stage procedure).

Dilatation

This is carried out under general anaesthesia. It is performed using Teflon dilators from 7-F to 30-F, which are introduced over the guidewire. Alternatively, metal coaxial dilators or a special angioplasty balloon (10 cm long) are used. A sheath is inserted over the largest dilator or balloon through which the nephroscope is passed followed by removal of the calculus or disintegration.

Removal/disintegration

Removal of calculi of less than 1 cm is possible using a nephroscope and forceps. Larger calculi must be disintegrated using an ultrasonic or electrohydraulic disintegrator.

Aftercare

1. A large bore soft non-locking straight nephrostomy tube (sutured) is left in for 24 hours following the procedure.
2. Patient care is usually determined by the anaesthetist/urologist.
3. Plain radiograph of renal area to ensure that all calculi/fragments have been removed.

Complications

Immediate

1. Failure of access, dilatation or removal
2. Perforation of the renal pelvis on dilatation
3. Inadvertent access to renal vein and IVC
4. Haemorrhage. Less than 3% of procedures should require transfusion. Rarely, balloon tamponade of the tract or embolization may be required

5. Damage to surrounding structures, i.e. diaphragm, colon, spleen, liver and lung
6. Problems related to the irrigating fluid.

Delayed
1. Pseudo-aneurysm of an intrarenal artery
2. Arterio-venous fistula.

RENAL ARTERIOGRAPHY

Indications
1. Renal artery stenosis prior to angioplasty or stent placement. Diagnostic arteriography has been replaced generally by MR or CT angiography (MRA or CTA).
2. Assessment of living related renal transplant donors – replaced generally by MRA or CTA.
3. Embolization of vascular renal tumour prior to surgery.
4. Haematuria particularly following trauma, including biopsy. This may precede embolization.
5. Prior to prophylactic embolization of an angiomyolipoma (AML) or therapeutic embolization of a bleeding AML.

Contrast medium

Flush aortic
LOCM 300/320 mg I ml^{-1}, 45 ml at 15 ml s^{-1}.

Selective renal artery injection
LOCM 300 mg I ml^{-1}, 10 ml at 5 ml s^{-1}, or by hand injection.

Equipment
1. Digital fluoroscopy unit
2. Pump injector
3. Catheters:
    (a) Flush aortic injection – pigtail 4-F
    (b) Selective injection – Sidewinder or Cobra catheter.

Technique
1. Femoral artery puncture
2. Flush aortography.

The catheter is placed proximal to the renal vessels (i.e. approximately T12) and AP and oblique runs are performed (the oblique run demonstrating the renal origins). Selective catheterization as required is used for optimal demonstration of intrarenal vessels, and prior to interventional procedures.

STATIC RENAL RADIONUCLIDE SCINTIGRAPHY

Indications

1. Assessment of individual renal function
2. Investigation of urinary tract infections, particularly in children for scarring
3. Assessment of reflux nephropathy for scarring
4. Identification of horseshoe, solitary or ectopic kidney
5. Differentiation of a pseudotumour due to a hypertrophied column of Bertin from a true tumour.

Contraindications

Pregnancy.

Radiopharmaceuticals

^{99m}Tc-dimercaptosuccinic acid (DMSA), 80 MBq max (0.7 mSv ED), which is bound to plasma proteins and cleared by tubular absorption. DMSA is retained in the renal cortex, with an uptake of 40–65% of the injected dose within 2 h, and no significant excretion during the imaging period. DMSA gives the best morphological images of any renal radiopharmaceutical and is used for assessment of scarring. It also gives the most accurate assessment of differential renal function.

Equipment

Gamma-camera with a low-energy high-resolution collimator.

Patient preparation

None.

Technique

1. The radiopharmaceutical is administered i.v.
2. Images are acquired at any time 1–6 h later. Imaging in the first hour is to be avoided because of free ^{99m}Tc in the urine.

Images

1. Posterior, right (RPO) and left posterior oblique (LPO) views. Anterior images in cases of suspected pelvic or horseshoe kidney and severe scoliosis, or if relative function is to be calculated by geometric mean method.
2. Zoomed or pinhole views may be useful in children.

Analysis

Relative function is best calculated from the geometric mean of posterior and anterior computer images. A single posterior view is often used, but this requires assumptions about kidney depth (unless depth information is available to enable attenuation correction).

Additional techniques

1. Single photon emission computed tomography (SPECT) – in the assessment of scarring and renal masses/'pseudotumours'.
2. ^{99m}Tc-mercaptoacetyltriglycine (MAG-3) (max. 100 MBq, 0.7 mSv ED) may be considered as a possible alternative to DMSA; it gives inferior kidney visualization, but has the advantage of additional dynamic assessment of excretion in the same study and a lower radiation dose.
3. Fast dynamic frames with motion correction may be useful to reduce movement artefact, particularly in young children.

Aftercare

None.

Complications

None.

Further Reading

Blaufox MD. Procedures of choice in renal nuclear medicine. J Nucl Med 1991;32:1301–9.

Hilson AJ. Functional renal imaging with nuclear medicine. Abdom Imaging 2003;28:176–9.

DYNAMIC RENAL RADIONUCLIDE SCINTIGRAPHY

Indications

1. Evaluation of obstruction
2. Assessment of renal function following drainage procedures to the urinary tract
3. Assessment of perfusion in acute native or transplant kidney failure
4. Demonstration of vesicoureteric reflux
5. Assessment of renal transplantation
6. Renal trauma
7. Diagnosis of renal artery stenosis.

Contraindications

None.

Radiopharmaceuticals

1. ^{99m}Tc-MAG-3 (mercaptoacetyltriglycine), 100 MBq max (0.7 mSv ED); (200 MBq max (1 mSv ED) for first-pass blood flow imaging). Highly protein-bound, it is mainly cleared by tubular secretion (80%), but with around 20% glomerular filtration. It is now the radiopharmaceutical of choice owing to better image quality, particularly in patients with impaired renal function (compared with ^{99m}Tc-diethylene triaminepentacetic acid (DTPA)).
2. ^{99m}Tc-DTPA, 150 MBq typical (1 mSv ED), 300 MBq max (2 mSv ED); (800 MBq max (5 mSv ED) for first-pass blood flow imaging). This is cleared by glomerular filtration. There is a lower kidney/background ratio than MAG-3 resulting in poorer image quality and noisier clearance curves.
3. ^{123}I-orthoiodohippurate (hippuran). This is almost entirely cleared by tubular secretion. It is not in common clinical use now.

5

Equipment

Gamma-camera with a low-energy general purpose collimator.

Patient preparation

1. The patient should be well hydrated with around 500 ml of fluid immediately before administration of tracer.
2. The bladder should be voided before injection.

Technique

1. The patient lies supine or sits reclining with their back against the camera.
2. The radiopharmaceutical is injected i.v. and image acquisition is started simultaneously.
3. Perform dynamic acquisition with 10–15 s frames for 30–40 min. (For quantitative perfusion studies, e.g. in the transplanted kidney, 1–2 s frames over the first minute are acquired.)
4. If poor drainage is seen from one or both kidneys after 10–20 min, a diuretic (furosemide 40 mg) is administered slowly during imaging. Imaging should be continued for at least a further 15 min. Since maximum diuresis does not occur until 15 min after administration of furosemide, as an alternative it may be given 15 min before the radiopharmaceutical (the so-called 'F – 15' renogram), which can be useful after equivocal standard 'F + 20' studies.
5. If significant retention in the kidneys is apparent at the end of the imaging period, the patient is asked to void and walk around for a minute, then a further short image is taken.

Images

1. All posterior
2. 2–5-min images for duration of study.

Analysis

The following information is produced using standard computer analysis:

1. Kidney time–activity ('renogram') curves (background-subtracted)
2. Relative function figures.

Additional figures are sometimes calculated:

3. Perfusion index, especially in renal transplant assessment
4. Parenchymal and whole kidney transit times.

Additional techniques

1. Pre- and 1 h post-captopril (25–50 mg) study for diagnosis of renal artery stenosis (RAS). Radionuclide techniques have the advantage of showing the functional effect of a stenotic renal artery, as opposed to the anatomical demonstration as provided by angiographic techniques. This, therefore, helps identify patients in whom RAS is the cause of hypertension (renovascular). The patient should, ideally, stop diuretic and ACE inhibitor medication 3–5 days prior to the test. The renogram curves post-captopril are compared with the baseline study to look for a deterioration.
2. In direct micturating cystography following renography to demonstrate vesicoureteric reflux. The bladder must not have been emptied and the kidneys should be reasonably clear of activity. Continuous dynamic 5-s images are acquired for 2 min before and up to 3 min after micturition, with generation of bladder and kidney time–activity curves.
3. Glomerular filtration rate (GFR) measurement and individual kidney GFR can be performed with DTPA studies by taking blood samples for counting. GFR is measured using a non-imaging technique with ^{51}Cr EDTA.

Aftercare

1. The patient should be warned that the effects of diuresis may last a couple of hours. The patient may experience postural hypotension when standing erect at the end of the procedure.
2. If captopril has been administered, blood pressure should be monitored until it has returned to baseline level.
3. Normal radiation safety precautions (see Chapter 1).

Complications

None, except after captopril, when care must be taken in patients with severe vascular disease to avoid hypotension and renal failure.

Further Reading

Blaufox MD. Procedures of choice in renal nuclear medicine. J Nucl Med 1991;32:1301–9.

Hilson AJ. Functional renal imaging with nuclear medicine. Abdominal Imaging 2003;28:176–9.

Taylor A, Nally J, Aurell M, et al. Consensus report on ACE inhibitor renography for detecting renovascular hypertension. J Nucl Med 1996;37:1876–82.

Woolfson RG, Neild GH. The true clinical significance of renography in nephro-urology. Eur J Nucl Med 1997;24(5):557–70.

5

DIRECT RADIONUCLIDE MICTURATING CYSTOGRAPHY

Indications

Vesicoureteric reflux.

Contraindications

Acute urinary tract infection.

Radiopharmaceuticals

^{99m}Tc-*pertechnetate*, 25 MBq max (0.3 mSv ED), administered into the bladder.

Equipment

Gamma-camera with a low-energy general purpose collimator.

Technique

This examination is most frequently performed on children.

The technique requires catheterization and is similar to that for MCU but enables continuous imaging and is a lower dose investigation. It is not commonly used however.

Aftercare

As for conventional cystography.

Complications

As for conventional cystography.

Alternative

Indirect radionuclide cystography may be performed after conventional radionuclide renography (see 'Dynamic renal scintigraphy'), or radiographic cystography (see above).

Further Reading

Johnson PT, Horton KM, Fishman EK. Optimizing detectability of renal pathology with MDCT: Protocols, pearls, and pitfalls. Am J Roentgenol 2010;194(4):1001–12.

Mandell GA, Eggli DF, Gilday DL, et al. Procedure guideline for radionuclide cystography in children. J Nucl Med 1997;38:1650–4.

Reproductive system

Methods of imaging the female reproductive system

1. Plain abdominal film
2. Hysterosalpingography
3. Ultrasound (US) – transabdominal/transvaginal
4. Computerized tomography (CT)
5. Magnetic resonance imaging (MRI)
6. Minimally invasive procedures including biopsies, cyst drainage, angiography, fibroid embolization
7. PET-CT.

Methods of imaging the male reproductive system (scrotum and testes)

1. US
2. MRI
3. Radionuclide imaging
4. Venography (including embolization of varices) and angiography.

Further Reading

Akin O, Mironov S, Pandit-Taskar N, et al. Imaging of uterine cancer. Radiol Clin North Am 2007;45(1):167–82.

Barakat RR, Hricak H. What do we expect from imaging. Radiol Clin North Am 2002;40(3):521–6, vii.

Fütterer JJ, Heijmink SW, Spermon JR. Imaging the male reproductive tract: current trends and future directions. Radiol Clin North Am 2008;46(1):133–47, vii.

Hedgire SS, Pargaonkar VK, Elmi A, et al. Male pelvic imaging. Radiol Clin North Am 2012;50(6):1015–226.

HYSTEROSALPINGOGRAPHY

Indications

1. Infertility
2. Recurrent miscarriages: investigation of suspected incompetent cervix, suspected congenital anomaly

3. Following tubal surgery, post sterilization to confirm obstruction and prior to reversal of sterilization
4. Assessment of the integrity of a caesarean uterine scar (rare).

Contraindications

1. During menstruation
2. Pregnancy or unprotected intercourse during the cycle
3. A purulent discharge on inspection of the vulva or cervix, or diagnosed pelvic inflammatory disease (PID) in the preceding 6 months
4. Contrast sensitivity (relative).

Contrast medium

High osmolar iodinated contrast material (HOCM) or low osmolar iodinated contrast material (LOCM) 270/300 mg I ml^{-1} 10–20 ml.

Equipment

1. Fluoroscopy unit with spot film device
2. Vaginal speculum
3. Vulsellum forceps
4. Hysterosalpingography balloon catheter 5-F to 7-F. In patients with narrow cervix or stenosis of cervical os, Margolin HSG cannula may be used. It has a silicone tip and provides tight occlusion of the cervix for contrast injection.

Patient preparation

1. The patient should abstain from intercourse between booking the appointment and the time of the examination, unless she uses a reliable method of contraception and the appointment is made before day 21, *or* the examination can be booked between the 4th and 10th days in a patient with a regular 28-day cycle.
2. Apprehensive patients may need premedication.
3. Consent should be obtained.[1]

Technique

1. The patient lies supine on the table with knees flexed, legs abducted.
2. The vulva can be cleaned with chlorhexidine or saline. A disposable speculum is then placed using sterile jelly and the cervix is exposed.
3. The cervical os is identified using a bright light and the HSG catheter is inserted into the cervical canal. It is usually not necessary to use a Vulsellum forceps to hold the cervix with a forceps, but occasionally this may be necessary. The catheter should be left within the lower cervical canal if cervical incompetence is suspected.

4. Care must be taken to expel all air bubbles from the syringe and cannula, as these would otherwise cause confusion in interpretation. Contrast medium is injected slowly into the uterine cavity under intermittent fluoroscopic observation.
5. Spasm of the uterine cornu may be relieved by intravenous (i.v.) glucagon if there is no tubal spill bilaterally.

N.B. Opiates increase pain by stimulating smooth muscle contraction.

Images

The radiation dose should be kept as low as possible. Intermittent screening should be performed to the minimal requirement. Images should demonstrate:

1. Endometrial cavity, demonstrating or excluding congenital abnormalities or filling defects
2. Full view of the tubes demonstrating spill. If occluded, show the extent and level of block
3. If there is abnormal loculation of contrast, a delayed view may be useful.

Aftercare

1. It must be ensured that the patient is in no serious discomfort nor has significant bleeding before she leaves.
2. The patient must be advised that she may have spotting or occasionally bleeding per vagina for 1–2 days and pain which may persist for up to 2 weeks.
3. Prophylactic antibiotics are routinely given in several centres and is good practice.

Complications

Due to the contrast medium
Allergic phenomena – especially if contrast medium is forced into the circulation.

Due to the technique
1. Pain may occur at the following times:
    (a) When using the speculum
    (b) During insertion of the cannula or inflation of balloon, some patients may have develop vasovagal syncope – 'cervical shock'
    (c) With tubal distension proximal to a block
    (d) With distension of the uterus if there is tubal spasm
    (e) With peritoneal irritation during the following day, and up to 2 weeks.
2. Bleeding from trauma to the uterus or cervix
3. Transient nausea, vomiting and headache

4. Intravasation of contrast medium into the venous system of the uterus results in a fine lace-like pattern within the uterine wall. When more extensive, intravasation outlines larger veins. It is of little significance when water-soluble contrast medium is used. Intravasation may be precipitated by: direct trauma to the endometrium, timing of the procedure near to menstruation or curettage, tubal occlusion or congenital abnormalities
5. Infection – which may be delayed. Occurs in up to 2% of patients and is more likely when there is a previous history of pelvic infection.

ULTRASOUND OF THE FEMALE REPRODUCTIVE SYSTEM

This can be performed transabdominal (TA) and/or transvaginal (TV).

Indications

1. Pelvic mass
2. Pregnancy – normal and suspected ectopic
3. Precocious puberty or delayed puberty
4. Pelvic pain
5. Assessment of tubal patency
6. In assisted fertilization techniques
7. Postmenopausal bleeding
8. Menstrual problems, location on IUD
9. Ovarian cancer screening.

Contraindications

None.

Patient preparation

1. Transabdominal scan – full bladder
   Transvaginal scan – empty bladder
2. Patient consent.[1]

It is advisable to always have a chaperone.

Equipment

TA – 4–10-MHz curvilinear transducers TV 9–13-MHz endovaginal transducers.

Reporting gynaecological ultrasound

The following format may be useful to assess the female reproductive system:

1. Uterine size in three dimensions, note on any congenital anomalies, presence of fibroids (include size and location) or adenomyosis
2. Three-dimensional ovarian measurements and volume. Presence of features including polycystic ovaries, significant cysts or mass lesions. Colour Doppler is useful in the assessment of complex adnexal mass lesions helping to differentiate retracted clot from solid components with blood supply
3. Comment on adnexae for extra-ovarian lesions
4. Examine the cul-de-sac for presence of endometriotic deposits or mass lesions. Note presence of free fluid or ascites.

Several software enhancements are available to improve resolution. Tissue harmonic imaging is useful for interrogation of difficult patients. 3D and 4D ultrasound are also currently widely available and mainly used in obstetric imaging. In gynaecology, 3D endometrial imaging may be useful, but generally adds little clinical value.

6

Contrast medium

Galactose monosaccharide microparticles (Echovist) were used as a specific contrast agent in the assessment of tubal patency; spillage of the microparticles into the peritoneal cavity infers patency. However, this product has been withdrawn recently. Sonovue (sulphur hexafluoride microbubbles) is not currently licensed for intrafallopian use.[2] Hence fluoroscopic hysterosalpingography remains the most reliable and safe investigation currently.

References
1. General Medical Council. Consent: Patients and Doctors Making Decisions Together. London: General Medical Council; 2008.
2. Killick S, Allison G, Parker P. The use of Sonovue for HyCoSy: UK experience to date. Ultrasound 2011;19:6–10.

Further Reading
Ascher SM, Reinhold C. Imaging of cancer of the endometrium. Radiol Clin North Am 2002;40(3):563–76.
Bates J. Practical Gynaecological Ultrasound. 2nd ed. Cambridge: Cambridge University Press; 2006.
Bhatt S, Ghazale H, Dogra VS. Sonographic evaluation of ectopic pregnancy. Radiol Clin North Am 2007;45(3):549–60.
Funt SA, Hann LE. Detection and characterization of adnexal masses. Radiol Clin North Am 2002;40(3):591–608.

ULTRASOUND OF THE SCROTUM

Indications
1. Suspected testicular tumour
2. Suspected epididymo-orchitis

3. Hydrocele
4. Acute torsion. In boys or young men in whom this clinical diagnosis has been made and emergency surgical exploration is planned, US should not delay the operation. Although colour Doppler may show an absence of vessels in the ischaemic testis, it is possible that partial untwisting resulting in some blood flow could lead to a false-negative examination
5. Suspected varicocele
6. Scrotal trauma.

Contraindications

None.

Patient preparation

Explanation of procedure and verbal consent is usually obtained.

Equipment

7.5–15-MHz transducer. Linear array for optimum imaging.

Technique

1. Secure environment with patient privacy protected.
2. Patient supine with legs together. Some operators support the scrotum on a towel draped beneath it or in a gloved hand.
3. Both sides are examined with longitudinal and transverse scans enabling comparison to be made.
4. Real-time scanning enables the optimal oblique planes to be examined.
5. In comparing the 'normal' with the 'abnormal' side, the machine settings should be optimized for the normal side, especially for colour Doppler. They should not be changed until both sides have been compared using the same image settings.
6. Patient should also be scanned standing upright and a Valsalva manoeuvre can be performed if a varicocele is suspected.
7. Testicular size and volume, echogenicity and presence of focal lesions to be noted. Epididymes are seen posterolaterally. Presence of cysts and inflammatory changes needs to be noted. Also look for hydrocele evident as free fluid outside the testes in the tunica.

Further Reading

Kim W, Rosen MA, Langer JE, et al. US MR imaging correlation in pathologic conditions of the scrotum. RadioGraphics 2007;27(5):1239–53.

Pearl MS, Hill MC. Ultrasound of the scrotum. Semin Ultrasound CT MR 2007;28(4):225–48.

CT OF THE REPRODUCTIVE SYSTEM

Indications

1. Staging ovarian, endometrial and cervical cancers.
2. To evaluate causes of raised CA125 levels.
3. In postoperative settings such as evaluation for intestinal obstruction or collections.

Technique

CT staging is usually performed with oral and i.v. contrast. Local staging in endometrial and cervical cancers is better performed with MRI. CT of thorax, abdomen and pelvis is indicated in endometrial cancers with advanced local disease, aggressive histology and in sarcomas. Local staging in cervical cancer is also performed with MRI, but CT of abdomen may be indicated in assessment of cephalad extent of nodal disease. CT of abdomen and pelvis is generally used for staging of ovarian cancer, but is of limited value in characterization of ovarian lesions, where MRI is more useful.

MAGNETIC RESONANCE IMAGING OF THE REPRODUCTIVE SYSTEM

Indications

1. Staging of cervical and endometrial cancer
2. Characterization of complex ovarian mass
3. Suspected Müllerian tract anomalies
4. Investigation of endometriosis
5. Staging of ovarian cancer (although CT is often necessary)
6. Assessment of pelvic floor
7. Scrotal MR can be used, generally after US, to further characterize a mass as intra- or extra-testicular and to determine the location of intra-abdominal undescended testis
8. Localization and morphology of uterine fibroids prior to consideration for uterine artery embolization.

Artifacts

Artifact from small-bowel peristalsis and, to a lesser extent, colonic peristalsis can occasionally be a problem in the pelvis and i.v. Buscopan 20 mg can be used to minimize this. Respiratory motion artifact is less of a problem in the pelvis than in the upper and mid abdomen. Movement from anterior abdominal wall fat can be suppressed using a saturation band.

Pulse sequences

For midline structures (uterus, cervix and vagina) sagittal T2-weighted spin-echo sequences can be supplemented with further axial sequences angled to regions of interest as required. Inclined axial images perpendicular to the long axis of the uterus or the long axis of the cervix are helpful for uterine and cervical abnormalities respectively. This technique is also mandatory for accurate local staging of uterine and cervical cancers.

The ovaries can be assessed with axial and coronal T1-weighted and T2-weighted spin-echo sequences. T1-weighted fat-saturated sequences are used to identify haemorrhage (e.g. within endometriomas) and to help characterize fat-containing masses.

Perfusion imaging of the uterus can be used to assess the effectiveness of uterine fibroid therapy.

MRI is also used to measure the pelvic outlet in pelvimetry in order to avoid ionizing radiation.

Scrotal MR is generally performed with the scrotum supported as in US, using a surface coil. High-resolution axial, sagittal and coronal T2-weighted spin echo scans are obtained with a T1-weighted scan to identify haemorrhage. Large field-of-view (FOV) scans should be performed to assess the inguinal canal for the presence of a hernia. Gadolinium i.v. can be given if necessary to assess perfusion. Scans should include the pelvis and kidneys if an undescended testis is being investigated.

GYNAECOLOGICAL MALIGNANCY

There are two commonly used staging systems for gynaecological cancers, namely Fédération Internationale de Gynécologie et d'Obstétrique (FIGO) and TNM; the former is recommended for use in current UK practice.[1]

CERVICAL CANCER

Initial diagnosis is made on clinical history, examination and biopsy. Regular cervical smears are recommended in disease prevention.

Staging

MRI is the technique of choice for staging of cervical cancer though it is of limited use in clinical stage less than 1B1. If the tumour is more than 4 cm, then it is staged as 1B2, and not suitable for surgery and would warrant radiotherapy. If there is spread of tumour outside the pelvis, CT scan may be necessary to evaluate distant metastatic disease. PET-CT may be useful if extensive pelvic exenteration surgery is needed. (The FIGO system does not consider lymph node status in staging so the presence of lymph nodes should be indicated in the final report.)

MRI sequences

1. Axial T1W – whole pelvis (slice thickness 5–7 mm)
2. Axial, coronal and sagittal T2W high resolution (3-mm slices).

Use of intravenous Buscopan or the other antiperistaltic agent may be useful to reduce artefacts from bowel movements.

Additional sequences may be necessary and be varied according to local protocol.

The presence of regional nodes – paracervical, parametrial, internal iliac, obturator, common iliac, external iliac, presacral, lateral sacral – should be assessed.

Follow-up

Clinical and imaging follow-up as appropriate and according to local protocol.

If recurrence is suspected, local spread is best assessed by MRI. More extensive and distant spread is assessed by CT. Treatment decisions are usually made in multi-disciplinary meetings.

UTERINE CARCINOMA

Uterine cancer presents usually as postmenopausal bleeding. Initial evaluation is performed with ultrasound to assess endometrial thickness. Endometrial thickness greater than 4 mm in postmenopausal women warrants further investigation with hysteroscopy and biopsy.

MRI staging should be performed in biopsy-positive cases for local staging. However, in more histologically aggressive tumours, a CT scan of the thorax, abdomen and pelvis is necessary to assess for distant metastatic spread.

MRI staging

A surface coil is used for pelvic imaging. Intravenous Buscopan or other antiperistaltic agent may be given if necessary.

Suggested sequences are:

1. Axial and sagittal high-resolution 3-mm slices with small FOV
2. Axial T2 whole pelvis 5 mm thickness
3. Axial T1W whole pelvis 5–7 mm thickness
4. T1W fat-saturated GRE sagittal and axial dynamic at 30, 60 and 180 s post-i.v. gadolinium
5. Diffusion-weighted imaging may improve the overall staging accuracy.

Follow-up

Clinical and imaging follow-up in accordance with local protocol. The optimal imaging strategy should be determined following discussion in multi-disciplinary meetings.

OVARIAN CANCER

Ultrasound is the initial mode of investigation in evaluation of ovarian mass lesion. Most of the simple cysts may be characterized by transvaginal ultrasound.

Indeterminate cysts on ultrasound can be characterized by MR imaging. Additional fat saturated T1-W sequence may be useful in characterizing dermoid cysts, due to their fat content. Haemorrhagic cysts, which have high T1 signal, do not show suppression on fat-saturated sequences. Malignant cysts typically contain solid components that show post-contrast enhancement.

Highly raised CA125 levels suggest the possibility of metastatic disease and would warrant a CT scan.

Typical spread of ovarian cancer is to the omentum, retroperitoneal nodes and surface liver deposits. Diagnosis can be obtained by omental biopsy. It is not recommended to biopsy ovarian masses percutaneously, due to the risk of dissemination of disease into the peritoneum.

Reference

1. McCluggage G, Hirschowitz L, Ganesan R, et al. Which staging system to use for gynaecological cancers: a survey with recommendations for practice in the UK. J Clin Pathol 2010;63(9):768–770.

Further Reading

Lewin SN. Revised FIGO staging system for endometrial cancer. Clin Obstet Gynecol 2011;54(2):215–18.

Pecorelli S. Revised FIGO staging for carcinoma of the vulva, cervix and endometrium. Int J Gynecol Obstet 2009;105(2):103–4.

Pecorelli S, Zigliani L, Odicino F, et al. Revised FIGO staging for carcinoma of the cervix. Int J Gynaecol Obstet 2009;105(2):107–8.

OMENTAL BIOPSY

Percutaneous omental biopsy has significantly reduced the need for diagnostic laparotomy and laparoscopic biopsies. Omental biopsy is usually best performed under ultrasound guidance or CT guidance. This can be performed as a day case or with overnight hospitalization.

Patient preparation

Full blood count and clotting needs should be performed to exclude coagulopathy. If patient has ascites, it should be drained.

This allows better visualization of the omental mass and also makes the biopsy easier.

Written consent should be obtained. Risk of bleeding and injury to bowel should be explained.

Technique

The procedure can be performed under local anaesthesia. The largest and most superficial omental mass is chosen for biopsy. With ultrasound omental mass can be confused with bowel and procedure should be performed by an experienced radiologist. Omental mass is more hypoechoic than bowel, shows colour Doppler flow and on compression would not show peristalsis. (Correlation with recent CT imaging is often very helpful and if unsure, procedure should be performed under CT guidance.)

Procedure performed with an 18G Trucut biopsy needle. Usually 2–3 passes can be made to ensure adequate specimen. Care should be exercised to avoid injury to the small bowel as sometimes the tumour can be fixed to the bowel.

Aftercare

Patient need to be under observation for at least 6 h post procedure.

Further Reading

Brown MA, Martin DR, Semelka R. Future directions in MR imaging of the female pelvis. Magn Reson Imaging Clin N Am 2006;14(4):431–7.

Burn PR, McCall JM, Chinn RJ, et al. Uterine fibroleiomyoma: MR imaging appearances before and after embolization of uterine arteries. Radiology 2000;214(3):729–34.

Coakley FV. Staging ovarian cancer: role of imaging. Radiol Clin North Am 2002;40(3):609–36.

Hamm B, Forstner R, Kim ES, et al. MRI and CT of the female pelvis. J Nucl Med 2008;49(5):862.

Humphries PD, Simpson JC, Creighton SM, et al. MRI in the assessment of congenital vaginal anomalies. Clin Radiol 2008;63(4):442–8.

Martin DR, Salman K, Wilmot CC. MR imaging evaluation of the pelvic floor for the assessment of vaginal prolapse and urinary incontinence. Magn Reson Imaging Clin N Am 2006;14(4):523–35.

Que Y, Wang X, Liu Y, et al. Ultrasound-guided biopsy of greater omentum: an effective method to trace the origin of unclear ascites. Eur J Radiol 2009;70(2):331–5.

Scheidler J, Heuck AF. Imaging of cancer of the cervix. Radiol Clin North Am 2002;40(3):577–90.

Spencer JA, Swift SE, Wilkinson N, et al. Peritoneal carcinomatosis: image-guided peritoneal core biopsy for tumor type and patient care. Radiology 2001;221(1):173–7.

Spencer JA, Weston MJ, Saidi SA, et al. Clinical utility of image-guided peritoneal and omental biopsy. Nat Rev Clin Oncol 2010;7(11):623–31.

6

Respiratory system

Methods of imaging the respiratory system

1. Plain films
2. Computed tomography (CT)
3. Radionuclide imaging (V/Q scans)
4. Ultrasound (US) – for pleural and chest wall disease
5. Magnetic resonance imaging (MRI)
6. Positron emission tomography (PET).

Further Reading
Hansell DM, Lynch DA, Page H, et al. Technical considerations. In: Imaging of Diseases of the Chest. 5th ed. London: Elsevier; 2009. p. 1–37.

COMPUTED TOMOGRAPHY OF THE THORAX

Indications

1. In the assessment of pulmonary masses, chest wall or pleural disease
2. For the staging and follow-up of malignancy in the chest
3. In the assessment (characterisation, quantification and follow-up) of diffuse lung disease
4. Evaluation of known/suspected thoracic vascular assessment (congenital or acquired – pulmonary embolus, aortic dissection, arteriovenous malformation, etc.)
5. In the assessment of airways disease, bronchiectasis and large airway stenosis.
6. Evaluation for thoracic manifestations of known extrathoracic disease
7. Trauma of the chest
8. Performing CT-guided intervention, e.g. lung, pleura or chest wall mass biopsy, bronchial stent insertion, pleural collection drainage, radiofrequency ablation, etc.

Contraindications

Where i.v. contrast medium is to be administered, the presence of impaired renal function, nephrotoxic drugs, and history of previous reaction to i.v. iodinated contrast media must be evaluated.

Technique

1. **Volume scan** – usually performed with intravenous contrast enhancement at a rate of 3–5 ml s^{-1} with a delay of 25–40 s. However, bolus tracking software can be used to trigger the scan more precisely to coincide with optimal contrast enhancement of specific structures, e.g. mediastinum, aorta in suspected aortic dissection or pulmonary artery in suspected pulmonary embolism. (Delayed imaging at 60 s can be useful in cases of large pleural effusion to assess for underlying soft tissue pleural thickening.)
2. **High-resolution scan.** Non-contrast scan obtained on full inspiration either:
   (a) 1 mm slices at 10 to 20 mm intervals or
   (b) Volume acquisition through the lungs with reconstruction of contiguous 1 mm slices:
      • Spatial resolution should be maximized using the smallest field of view possible.
      • Use a high-resolution (high spatial resolution) 'bone' algorithm to reconstruct images.
      • A volume acquisition with reconstruction of contiguous slices has the benefit of post-processing capabilities, e.g. multiplanar reformatting can help to illustrate the cranio-caudal distribution of lung changes.
      • Additional expiratory images can be performed in suspected air-trapping and airways disease.
      • Additional prone images are indicated to differentiate reversible-dependent change from early interstitial fibrosis.

Further Reading

Beigelman-Aubry C, Hill C, Brillet P-Y, Grenier PA. MDCT of the airways: technique and normal results. Radiol Clin North Am 2009;47(2):185–201.

Webb WR, Muller NL, Naidich DP. Technical aspects of high-resolution computed tomography of lung disease. In: High-Resolution CT of the Lung. 4th ed. Lippincott Williams and Wilkins; 2008. p. 1–41.

COMPUTED TOMOGRAPHY-GUIDED LUNG BIOPSY

Indications

1. Investigation of a new or progressing pulmonary opacity when other diagnostic techniques such as bronchoscopy have failed to make a diagnosis.

2. Investigation of a new lung/pleural/chest wall lesion in a patient with known malignancy.
3. To obtain material for culture when other techniques have failed to identify the causative organism in a patient with persistent consolidation.

All biopsies should be planned after case discussion at a multi-disciplinary meeting with a respiratory physician, radiologist, surgeon and oncologist where the balance of benefit versus risk can best be assessed. Central lesions are preferably biopsied transbronchially either by standard bronchoscopy (where there is endobronchial disease) or, if extrabronchial, by transbronchial needle aspiration (TBNA) either 'blind' or with endoscopic ultrasound guidance (EBUS).

Contraindications

Contraindications are not absolute but should be carefully evaluated by the relevant multi-disciplinary team.

1. Vascular: bleeding diatheses (including conditions that affect platelet function such as chronic renal failure), patient on anticoagulants, significant pulmonary arterial or venous hypertension.
2. Respiratory: contralateral pneumonectomy (unless the lesion is pleurally based and lung tissue will not be traversed), presence of significant emphysema (particularly bullous disease) or significantly impaired respiratory function such that pneumothorax would not be tolerated. (An FEV_1 of <1 l or <35% predicted is often used as lower limit cut-off for biopsy.) Air travel should not be undertaken within 6 weeks following the procedure.
3. Suspected hydatid disease.
4. Uncooperative patient (including intractable cough).

Equipment

1. Sampling needle:
   - Fine needle aspiration can be performed if there is an on-site cytopathology service. Usually use 20 or 22G needles. Different needles vary by the profile of the needle tip and include Chiba (with a bevelled tip which allows straightforward cytological sample aspiration) and those with modified tips which allow 'cutting' to obtain small histological fragments as well as aspiration (suitable for more fibrous lesions), e.g. Franseen® (Cook Medical™) and Westcott® (Becton-Dickinson Medical™).
   - Cutting needle biopsy needles are larger gauge (usually 18 or 20G) and obtain a solid core of tissue for histological examination. They usually have adjustable throw of the

7

specimen notch for precise sampling of the lesion. Types include Temno® and Quick-Core® (Cook Medical™). Coaxial needle biopsy systems can be used as these stabilize the cutting needle, allowing resampling without re-puncturing the pleura, aid re-angling of the cutting needle and allow accurate preplanning of depth of passes.

2. Full resuscitation equipment including equipment for pleural aspiration and chest drain insertion.

Staff should be prepared for recognition and treatment of complications of pneumothorax, vasovagal episodes, haemoptysis and (very rarely) air embolus.

Patient preparation

1. Sedative premedication should be avoided if possible as the patient must remain cooperative so that a consistent breathing pattern can be maintained during the procedure.
2. The procedure can routinely be performed on an outpatient basis with observation for 4–6 hours post procedure, but a bed should be available in case of complications. Particularly frail patients, those with frail carers or dependants, or those living alone should be admitted overnight following the procedure.
3. Clotting screen (ideally INR ≤1.4 and platelets $> 100 \times 10^9$ l^{-1}). There is no clear evidence that aspirin should be discontinued pre-biopsy but consensus suggests clopidogrel should be stopped 5 days prior to procedure.[1]
4. Pulmonary function tests (spirometry).

Aftercare

1. Close observation post procedure for at least 1 h in a supervised ward or recovery area, with the patient lying in puncture-site-down position (which should be possible for all but anterior approach interventions). (A limited CT at the end of the procedure will have determined if a pneumothorax or parenchymal bleed is present.)
2. Departmental PA chest X-ray at approximately 1–4 h post procedure. If a pneumothorax has developed (or progressed) then the further management will depend on the size of the pneumothorax and clinical condition of the patient. Small pneumothoraces in asymptomatic patients may be observed; larger pneumothoraces in symptomatic patients will require aspiration or chest drain insertion.
3. High-risk and frail patients, particularly those with pre-existing impairment of respiratory function, are best routinely admitted overnight.

Complications[2-4]

Usually occur early following the procedure:

1. Pneumothorax in 20%. However, chest drain insertion is necessary in only a small minority (about 3%). The incidence of pneumothorax is increased if:
   - the operator is inexperienced
   - a larger gauge needle is used
   - there is an increased number of needle passes made
   - there is a greater pleura to lesion depth
   - smaller lesions are biopsied
   - the needle traverses a fissure
   - the patient is coughing (precipitated by haemorrhage/haemoptysis).
2. Local pulmonary haemorrhage (10%)
3. Haemoptysis (2–5%)
4. Other complications, such as haemothorax, implantation of malignant cells along the needle track, spread of infection and air embolism, are all extremely rare
5. The current documented death rate is 0.15%.

References

1. Malloy PC, Grassi CJ, Kundu A, et al. Consensus guidelines for periprocedural management of coagulation status and hemostasis risk in percutaneous image-guided interventions. J Vasc Interv Radiol 2009;20(7):240–9.
2. Gohari A, Haramati LB. Complications of CT scan-guided lung biopsy: lesion size and depth matter. Chest 2004;126(3):666–8.
3. Yeow K-M, Su I-H I-Hao, Pan K-T, et al. Risk factors of pneumothorax and bleeding: multivariate analysis of 660 CT-guided coaxial cutting needle lung biopsies. Chest 2004;126(3):748–54.
4. Manhire A, Charig M, Clelland C, et al. BTS Guidelines: Guidelines for radiologically guided lung biopsy. Thorax 2003;58(11):920–36.

Further Reading

Anderson JM, Murchison J, Patel D. CT-guided lung biopsy: factors influencing diagnostic yield and complication rate. Clin Radiol 2003;58(10):791–7.

Birchard KR. Transthoracic needle biopsy. Semin Intervent Radiol 2011;28(1):87–97.

Aviram G, Schwartz DS, Meirsdorf S, et al. Transthoracic needle biopsy of lung masses: a survey of techniques. Clin Radiol 2005;60(3):370–4.

Richardson CM, Pointon KS, Manhire AR, et al. Percutaneous lung biopsies: a survey of UK practice based on 5444 biopsies. Br J Radiol 2002;75(897):731–5.

METHODS OF IMAGING PULMONARY EMBOLISM

1. *Plain film chest radiograph.* The initial chest radiograph is often normal. Various signs have been described in association with

pulmonary embolism but, overall, the chest radiograph is neither specific nor sensitive. It may, however, usefully identify other pathology producing the clinical picture including infection, pneumothorax and rib fracture.

2. *Ventilation/perfusion (V/Q) radionuclide scanning.* The technique is described later in this chapter. Interpretation of V/Q images is not straightforward and there are a number of causes for the typical V/Q mismatch. Interpretive criteria divide results into normal, very-low and low-probability, intermediate (or indeterminate) probability and high probability groups. Specificity and sensitivity are such that pulmonary embolism is virtually excluded in the 'normal' group and is very likely (85–90%) in the high probability group. A significant proportion of patients, however, are placed in the indeterminate/intermediate risk group where specificity is poor and further imaging with CTPA is usually required.

3. *Doppler ultrasound* of pelvic and leg veins to detect deep vein thrombosis.

4. *Multidetector CT pulmonary angiography* (CTPA) to diagnose pulmonary emboli down to subsegmental level. Will also assess for presence of secondary right heart strain and for presence of other pathology in the chest. Can be complemented with a CT venography sequence performed at the same examination as CTPA.[1]

5. *Pulmonary arteriography* was traditionally the 'gold standard' and will detect most pulmonary emboli but has been superseded by multidetector CTPA.

6. *MR angiography* has yet to find a role in the routine investigation of suspected PE but clearly may be of great benefit in patients where ionizing radiation exposure or the use of iodinated contrast media is relatively contraindicated.

RADIONUCLIDE LUNG VENTILATION/ PERFUSION (V/Q) IMAGING

Indications

1. Suspected pulmonary embolism
2. Assessment of perfusion and ventilation abnormalities, e.g. in congenital cardiac or pulmonary disease, e.g. cardiac shunts, pulmonary arterial stenosis, arteriovenous malformations, etc.
3. Quantitative assessment of right-to-left shunting (perfusion only)
4. Quantitative assessment of differential perfusion and ventilation before lung cancer, lung transplant or lung volume reduction surgery[1,2]
5. Evaluate causes of pulmonary hypertension (to exclude chronic thromboembolism).

Contraindications (to perfusion imaging)

1. Right-to-left shunt – because of the risk of cerebral emboli
2. Severe pulmonary hypertension.

Neither of these are absolute contraindications (indeed, perfusion imaging can be used for assessment of shunts), and it may be considered acceptable to reduce the number of particles administered in these cases.

Radiopharmaceuticals

Perfusion

^{99m}Tc ($T_{1/2}$ 6 h, photopeak 140 keV) labelled macroaggregated albumin particles (MAA), 100 MBq max (1 mSv ED), 10–40 μm in diameter which occlude small lung vessels (<0.5% of total capillary bed). The biologic half-life of the MAA in the lungs is 1.5–3 h.

Ventilation

1. ^{81m}Kr (krypton) gas, 6000 MBq max (0.2 mSv ED). Ideal generator-produced agent with a short $T_{1/2}$ of 13 s and a γ-energy of 190 keV. Simultaneous dual isotope ventilation and perfusion imaging is possible because of different γ-energy to ^{99m}Tc. Wash-in and wash-out studies are not possible. Expensive and limited availability
2. ^{99m}Tc-Technegas, 40 MBq max (0.6 mSv ED).[3] Ultrafine Tc labelled carbon particles, 5–20 nm in size. No simultaneous ventilation and perfusion imaging. Longer residence time in lungs than aerosols, so SPECT and respiration-gated studies possible. Similar diagnostic efficacy to krypton. Expensive dispensing system
3. ^{99m}Tc-DTPA, aerosol, 80 MBq max (0.4 mSv ED). Simultaneous ventilation and perfusion imaging not possible. Cheap and readily available alternative to krypton, but less suitable in patients with chronic obstructive airways disease or chronic asthma because clumping of aerosol particles is likely
4. ^{133}Xe (xenon) gas, 400 MBq max (0.4 mSv ED) diluted in 10 l and re-breathed for 5 min. Long $T_{1/2}$ of 5.25 days and a γ-energy of 81 keV. Ventilation must precede perfusion study because low γ-energy would be swamped by scatter from ^{99m}Tc. Wash-in and wash-out studies are possible. Poor-quality images and rarely used.

Equipment

1. Gamma-camera, preferably multi-headed for SPECT
2. Low-energy general purpose collimator
3. Gas dispensing system and breathing circuit for ventilation.

Patient preparation

1. For ventilation, familiarization with breathing equipment
2. A current chest X-ray is required to assist with interpretation.

7

Technique

Perfusion

1. The injection may be given in the supine, semirecumbent or sitting position (N.B. MAA particle uptake is affected by gravity)
2. The syringe is shaken to prevent particles settling
3. A slow i.v. injection is given directly into a vein (particles will stick to a plastic cannula) over about 10 s. Avoid drawing blood into the syringe as this can cause clumping
4. The patient must remain in position for 2–3 min while the particles become fixed in the lungs
5. Imaging may begin immediately, preferably in the sitting position.

Ventilation

^{81m}Kr gas

This is performed at the same time as the perfusion study, either by dual isotope acquisition or swapping energy windows at each patient position:

1. The patient is positioned to obtain identical views to the perfusion images and asked to breathe normally through the mouthpiece.
2. The air supply attached to the generator is turned on and imaging commenced.

^{99m}Tc-DTPA aerosol

This scan is performed before the perfusion study, which may follow immediately unless there is clumping of aerosol particles in the lungs, in which case it is delayed for 1–2 h:

1. A DTPA kit is made up with approx. 600 MBq ^{99m}Tc ml^{-1}
2. ^{99m}Tc-DTPA is drawn into a 5 ml syringe with 2 ml air, then injected into the nebulizer and flushed through with air
3. The patient is positioned initially with their back to the camera, sitting if possible
4. The nose-clip is placed on the patient who is asked to breathe normally through the mouthpiece. The air supply is turned on to deliver a rate of 10 l min^{-1}
5. After reaching a sufficient count rate the air supply is turned off. The patient should continue to breathe through the mouthpiece for a further 15 s
6. The nose-clip is removed and the patient is given a mouth wash and then imaging is commenced.

Images

Anterior, posterior, left and right posterior obliques.

Since perfusion and ventilation images are directly compared, it is important to have identical views for each. Foam wedges between the patient's back and the camera assist accurate oblique positioning.

Additional techniques

1. SPECT imaging appears to significantly improve the specificity of the technique by reducing the number of intermediate probability scans.
2. Standardized interpretation of images can improve the clinical effectiveness of V/Q scans, and criteria have been published which are widely used.[4,5]

Aftercare

None.

Complications

Care should be taken when injecting MAA not to induce respiratory failure in patients with severe pulmonary hypertension. In these patients, inject very slowly.

COMPUTED TOMOGRAPHY IN THE DIAGNOSIS OF PULMONARY EMBOLI

7

Technique

The technique will depend on individual CT scanner technology. Individual CT manufacturers will recommend specific scanning protocols including delivery of i.v. contrast medium. CT will not only identify the presence of thrombus but allow assessment of secondary right heart strain.[1]

Computed tomography pulmonary angiography – enhanced scan of pulmonary arterial system[1]

1. Volume of contrast medium – 100–150 ml or when dual phase injector is used, 60–80 ml of contrast medium followed by saline chase of 30–50 ml
2. Delay:
   (a) Preset delay of approximately 15–25 s for depending on scanner type
   OR preferably
   (b) Bolus tracking. A ROI (region of interest) is positioned over the pulmonary artery at the level of the carina. After commencing the injection a 'tracker scan' monitors the contrast density within the pulmonary artery and the scan is then triggered when the density at the ROI reaches a preset value – usually 100–120 HU.
3. Rate of injection – 4 ml s^{-1}:
   • Contrast delivery aiming optimally for main pulmonary artery enhancement of 350 HU

4. Scan from lowest hemidiaphragm to lung apex. Caudocranial scanning may reduce respiratory motion artifact at the lung bases though this is less of an issue with faster multislice scanners

5. Image review and post-processing[2] – images should be reviewed at three settings:

   (a) Mediastinal window (window width/window level e.g. 400/40 HU)
   (b) Pulmonary embolism-specific window (e.g. 700/100 HU – adjusted to remove contrast 'glare')
   (c) Lung window (e.g. 1500/–500 HU).

Multiplanar reformatted images through the longitudinal axis of a vessel can be helpful to overcome difficulties encountered on axial sections of obliquely oriented arteries, aiding confidence in diagnosis or exclusion of thrombus. If there is no evidence of pulmonary embolism, then need to carefully determine presence of other possible causes of patient's clinical picture.

PULMONARY ARTERIOGRAPHY

Indications

1. Demonstration of pulmonary emboli and other peripheral abnormalities, e.g. arteriovenous malformations, when less invasive investigations have been non-diagnostic.
2. Planning and performing therapeutic procedures such as catheter-directed thrombolysis or catheter embolectomy (in patients who cannot receive systemic thrombolysis due to bleeding risk and where surgical embolectomy is contraindicated).

Contraindications[1]

These include the general contraindications to any form of arteriography such as contrast allergy, renal failure and bleeding diatheses. There are more specific relative contraindications to diagnostic pulmonary arteriography:

1. Elevated right ventricular end-diastolic pressure (>20 mmHg) and/ or elevated pulmonary artery pressure (>70 mmHg) – where the mortality rate is increased to 2–3% (compared to a documented mortality rate of 0.2–0.5% where pressures are not elevated). Selective arteriography is advised if the results of arteriography are essential to patient management.
2. Left bundle branch block – right heart catheterization may induce complete heart block. Insertion of temporary pacemaker may be indicated prior to the procedure.

Contrast medium

Low osmolar contrast material (LOCM) 370 mg I ml^{-1}; 0.75 ml kg^{-1} at 20–25 ml s^{-1} (max. 40 ml).

Equipment

1. Fluoroscopy unit on a C- or U-arm, with digital subtraction facilities
2. Pump injector
3. Catheter: pigtail (coiled end, end hole and 12 side holes; see Fig. 8.3).

Technique

The Seldinger technique is used via the right femoral vein. The catheter is introduced via an introducer sheath. The catheter tip is sited, under fluoroscopic control, to lie 1–3 cm above the pulmonary valve. Pulmonary pressures should routinely be measured during the procedure; lower injection rates are advised if the pressures are raised.

Additional techniques

1. If the entire chest cannot be accommodated on one field of view, the examination can be repeated by examining each lung. The catheter is advanced to lie in each main pulmonary artery in turn. For the right lung the patient, or the tube, is turned 10° RAO and for the left lung 10° LAO.
2. 40° caudal-cranial view: this view is optimal for the visualization of the bifurcation of the right and left pulmonary arteries, the pulmonary valve, annulus and trunk. With this manoeuvre the pulmonary trunk is no longer foreshortened and is not superimposed over its bifurcation.

Complications

The rate of minor complications is 1–3%. These include respiratory distress, major dysrhythmias, contrast reactions and renal failure. The current documented mortality rate is 0.2–0.5%.

For further details regarding general complications related to catheter techniques see Chapter 9, page 213.

MAGNETIC RESONANCE OF PULMONARY EMBOLI

A combination of real-time MR (SSFPS – steady-state free precession sequences), MR perfusion imaging (fat 3D gradient-echo sequences) and contrast-enhanced MR angiography (CE-MRA) can be used to detect pulmonary emboli.[1] Single-centre studies have shown CE-MRA detecting PE with sensitivities of 77–100% and specificities of 95–100%; there is, however, significant variation in results with high levels of technically inadequate scans and sensitivities as low as 45% in some institutions. The place of MR imaging in diagnosing PE is still evolving but, with the additional benefit of performing lower-limb MR-venography during the same examination, may produce a highly sensitive combined investigation for thromboembolic disease.[2]

References

Methods of Imaging Pulmonary Embolism
1. Krishan S, Panditaratne N, Verma R, et al. Incremental value of CT venography combined with pulmonary CT angiography for the detection of thromboembolic disease: systematic review and meta-analysis. Am J Roent 2011;196(5):1065–72.

Complications
1. Beckles MA, Spiro S, Colis G, Rudd R. The physiologic evaluation of patients with lung cancer being considered for resectional surgery. Chest 2003;123(suppl):105S–14S.
2. Wang SC, Fischer KC, Slone RM, et al. Perfusion scintigraphy in the evaluation for lung volume reduction surgery: correlation with clinical outcome. Radiology 1997;205(1):243–8.
3. Win T, Tasker AD, Groves AM, et al. Ventilation-perfusion scintigraphy to predict postoperative pulmonary function in lung cancer patients undergoing pneumonectomy. Am J Roent 2006;187(5):1260–5.
4. Howarth DM, Lan L, Thomas PA, et al. ^{99m}Tc Technegas ventilation and perfusion lung scintigraphy for the diagnosis of pulmonary embolus. J Nucl Med 1999;40(4):579–84.
5. Freitas JE, Sarosi MG, Nagle CC, et al. Modified PIOPED criteria used in clinical practice. J Nucl Med 1995;36(9):1573–8.

Computed Tomography Pulmonary Angiography – Enhanced Scan of Pulmonary Arterial System
1. Furlan A, Aghayev A, Chang C-CH, et al. Short-term mortality in acute pulmonary embolism: clot burden and signs of right heart dysfunction at CT pulmonary angiography. Radiology 2012;265(1):283–93.
2. Wittram C. How I do it: CT pulmonary angiography. Am J Roent 2007;188(5):1255–61.

Complications
1. Gotway MB, Reddy GP, Dawn SK. Pulmonary thromboembolic disease. In: Webb WR, Higgins CB, editors. Thoracic Imaging: Pulmonary and Cardiovascular Radiology. Philadelphia: Lippincott Williams & Wilkins; 2005. p. 609–29.

Magnetic Resonance of Pulmonary Emboli
1. Kluge A, Luboldt W, Bachmann G. Acute pulmonary embolism to the subsegmental level: diagnostic accuracy of three MRI techniques compared with 16-MDCT. Am J Roent 2006;187(1):W7–W14.
2. Stein PD, Chenevert TL, Fowler SE. Gadolinium-enhanced magnetic resonance angiography for pulmonary embolism: a multicenter prospective study (PIOPED III). Ann Intern Med 2010;152(7):434–43.

Further Reading

Methods of Imaging Pulmonary Embolism

Roy PM, Colombet I, Durieux P, et al. Systematic review and meta-analysis of strategies for the diagnosis of suspected pulmonary embolism. Br Med J 2005;331(7511):259.

Stein PD, Woodard PK, Weg JG, et al. Diagnostic pathways in acute pulmonary embolism: recommendations of the PIOPED II investigators. Radiology 2007;242(1):15–21.

Complications

Parker JA, Coleman RE, Grady E, et al. SNM Practice Guideline for Lung Scintigraphy 4.0. J Nucl Med Technol 2012;40(1):57–65.

Sostman HD, Stein PD, Gottschalk A, et al. Acute pulmonary embolism: sensitivity and specificity of ventilation-perfusion scintigraphy in PIOPED II study. Radiology 2008;246(3):941–6.

Computed Tomography Pulmonary Angiography – Enhanced Scan of Pulmonary Arterial System

Remy-Jardin M, Pistolesi M, Goodman LR, et al. Management of suspected acute pulmonary embolism in the era of CT angiography: a statement from the Fleischner Society. Radiology 2007;245(2):315–29.

Schoepf UJ, Costello P. CT angiography for diagnosis of pulmonary embolism: state of the art. Radiology 2004;230(2):329–37.

Stein PD, Fowler SE, Goodman LR, et al. Contrast enhanced multidetector spiral CT of the chest and lower extremities in suspected acute pulmonary embolism: results of the Prospective Investigation of Pulmonary Embolism Diagnosis II (PIOPED II). N Engl J Med 2006;354:2317–27.

Wittram C, Maher MM, Yoo AJ, et al. CT angiography of pulmonary embolism: diagnostic criteria and causes of misdiagnosis. RadioGraphics 2004;24(5):1219–38.

Complications

Kucher N. Catheter embolectomy for acute pulmonary embolism. Chest 2007;132(2):657–63.

Uflacker R. Interventional therapy for pulmonary embolism. J Vasc Interv Radiol 2001;12(2):147–64.

MAGNETIC RESONANCE IMAGING OF THE RESPIRATORY SYSTEM

MRI currently has a limited role in assessing the respiratory system due to the susceptibility artifact from the large volume of air within the lungs. The mediastinum and chest wall are well assessed by MRI due to the ability to image in the coronal and sagittal plane and in particular, malignant invasion of the mediastinum, pericardium and chest wall can be usefully evaluated. MRI is particularly useful in the assessment of superior sulcus and neurogenic tumours as it can give information on the nature and extent of brachial plexus or intraspinal extension. Fast sequences and cardiac gating may be used effectively to minimize motion artifacts. Multidetector CT, however, is quicker, more widely available and can now give excellent multiplanar and three-dimensional reconstruction.

MR of the chest whilst the patient breathes hyperpolarized Helium 3 (^{3}He) allows visualization of the airspaces within the lungs. The technique can detect abnormal distribution of the gas and may develop a clinical role in the assessment of, and subsequent treatment of, airways and parenchymal disease, particularly in asthma, COPD and cystic fibrosis (in the latter allowing regular imaging follow-up without ionizing radiation burden). MR of the lungs, however, is not yet currently used routinely in clinical practice.

Further Reading

Kauczor H-U, Ley-Zaporozhan J, Ley S. Imaging of pulmonary pathologies: Focus on magnetic resonance imaging. Proc Am Thorac Soc 2009;6:458–63.

PET AND PET-CT OF THE RESPIRATORY SYSTEM

In recent years, FDG-PET has become an essential part of lung-cancer imaging, adding metabolic information to the morphological information provided by CT. A PET scan is currently recommended for the investigation of lung cancer where the lesion is greater than 1 cm in size and plays an important role in loco-regional and distant staging of non-small cell lung cancer (NSCLC). The scan can be performed either on a dedicated PET scanner or an integrated PET-CT scanner and should be considered in all patients in whom curative-intent treatment is contemplated. Patient preparation and the technique are fully described in Chapter 11.

In addition to its current primary use in diagnosis and staging of lung cancer, PET and PET-CT has an emerging role in assessment of early metabolic response to therapy which may allow influence subsequent treatment planning and predict eventual prognosis.

Further Reading

De Wever W, Stroobants S, Coolen J, Verschakelen JA. Integrated PET/CT in the staging of non-small cell lung cancer: technical aspects and clinical integration. Eur Respir J 2009;33:201–12.

Erasmus JJ, Rohren E, Swisher SG. Prognosis and reevaluation of lung cancer by positron emission tomography imaging. Proc Am Thorac Soc 2009;6:171–9.

Paul NS, Ley S, Metser U. Optimal imaging protocols for lung cancer staging: CT, PET, MR imaging, and the role of imaging. Radiol Clin North Am 2012;50(5):935–49.

Vansteenkiste JF, Stroobants SS. PET scan in lung cancer: current recommendations and innovation. J Thorac Oncol 2006;1(1):71–3.

Weber WA. Assessing tumor response to therapy. J Nucl Med 2009;50(5):1S–10S.

Heart

Methods of imaging the heart

1. Chest radiography
2. Fluoroscopy and angiocardiography
3. Echocardiography – transthoracic and transoesophageal techniques
4. Computed tomography (CT)
5. Magnetic resonance imaging (MRI).
6. Radionuclide imaging:
   (a) Ventriculography
   (b) Myocardial perfusion imaging.

ANGIOCARDIOGRAPHY

Diagnostic catheterization has largely been replaced by echocardiography (including transoesophageal echocardiography), radionuclide ventriculography and MR imaging.
Angiocardiography is usually used as part of an interventional therapeutic procedure and can be performed simultaneously with cardiac catheterization during which pressures and oximetry are measured in the cardiac chambers and vessels that are under investigation. The right heart, left heart and great vessels are examined together or alone, depending on the clinical problem.

Indications

1. Congenital heart disease and anomalies of the great vessels – mostly in the paediatric population. Either for diagnosis or therapeutic procedures such as transcatheter closure of patent foramen ovale, atrial septal defect (ASD), ventricular septal defect (VSD) and patent ductus arteriosus.
2. Valve disease, myocardial disease and assess ventricular function. Balloon valvuloplasty and, in selected centres, transcatheter aortic valve implantation (TAVI) can be performed to treat stenotic valvular disease.

Contrast medium

Low osmolar contrast material (LOCM) 370 mg I ml^{-1} (see Table 8.1).

Equipment

1. Biplane digital fluoroscopy and cine radiography with C-arms to facilitate axial projections
2. Pressure recording device
3. Electrocardiogram (ECG) monitor
4. Blood oxygen analyser
5. Catheter:
   (a) For pressure measurements and blood sampling: Cournand (Fig. 8.1), 4–7F
   (b) For angiocardiography: National Institutes of Health (NIH) (Fig. 8.2) or pigtail (Fig. 8.3), 4–8F.

Table 8.1 Volumes of contrast media in angiocardiography			
	Injection site		
	Ventricle		**Aorta or pulmonary artery**
Adult	1 ml kg^{-1} at 18–20 ml s^{-1}		0.75 ml kg^{-1} at 18–20 ml s^{-1} (max. 40 ml)
Child First year 2–4 years 5 years	1.5 ml kg^{-1} 1.2 ml kg^{-1} 1.0 ml kg^{-1}	injected over 1–2 s	75% of the ventricular volume

In general, hypoplastic or obstructed chambers require smaller volumes and flow rates and large shunts require greater volumes and flow rates of contrast medium.

Figure 8.1 Cournand catheter. End holes: 1 Side holes: 0.

Figure 8.2 National Institutes of Health (NIH) catheter. End holes: 0 Side holes: 4 or 6.

Figure 8.3 Pigtail catheter. End holes: 1 Side holes: 12.

Technique

1. Right-sided cardiac structures and pulmonary arteries are examined by introducing a catheter into a peripheral vein. In babies the femoral vein may be the only vein large enough to take the catheter. If an atrial septal defect is suspected, the femoral vein approach offers the best chance of passing the catheter into the left atrium across the defect. In adults the right antecubital or basilic vein may be used. The cephalic vein should be avoided as it can be difficult to pass the catheter past the site where the vein pierces the clavipectoral fascia to join the axillary vein. The catheter, or introducer, is introduced using the Seldinger technique. (The NIH catheter must be introduced via an introducer as there is no end hole for a guidewire.)
2. In children it is usually possible to examine the left heart and occasionally the aorta by manipulating a venous catheter through a patent foramen ovale. In adults the aorta and left ventricle are studied via a catheter passed retrogradely from the femoral artery.
3. The catheter is manipulated into the appropriate positions for recording pressures and sampling blood for oxygen saturation. Following this, angiography is performed.

Image acquisition

Using digital angiography at 7.5 frames s^{-1} with alignment to the anatomical axes of the heart, i.e. the X-ray beam is angulated relative to the axial planes of the heart rather the orthogonal planes of the body. The long axis of the heart is usually oblique to the long axis of the patient's body and cardiac angiography suites have movable C-arms which allow correct positioning by movement of the equipment alone without disturbing the patient. Supplementary angulations of the X-ray beam from the cardiac axes are used to profile those areas of the heart under examination. Useful views are:

1. *40° cranial/40° left anterior oblique (LAO) (hepatoclavicular or four-chamber) view* – the beam is perpendicular to the long axis of the heart and aligns the atrial septum and posterior interventricular septum parallel to the beam
2. *Long axial 20° right anterior oblique (RAO) (long axial oblique) view* – the lateral tube and image intensifier are angled 25–30° cranially, to align with the long axis of the heart, and 20° RAO.

CORONARY ARTERIOGRAPHY

Indications

1. Diagnosis of the presence and extent of ischaemic heart disease
2. After revascularization procedures
3. Congenital heart lesions

4. Therapeutic percutaneous coronary intervention – balloon angioplasty and stenting.

Diagnostic arteriography can be supplemented by intravascular ultrasound (US) to determine the nature and extent of plaque within the vessel wall and, in some centres, with angioscopy. Pressure wire studies to determine fractional flow reduction (FFR) across stenoses prior to angioplasty/stenting can be performed; particularly useful in assessment of intermediate lesions.

Contrast medium

LOCM 370 mg I ml^{-1}, 8–10 ml given as a hand injection for each projection.

Equipment

1. Digital angiography with C-arm
2. Pressure recording device and ECG monitor
3. Selective coronary artery catheters:
  (a) Judkins (Fig. 8.4) or Amplatz (Fig. 8.5) catheters – the left and right coronary artery catheters are of different shape. These can be used for both femoral or radial approaches (usually utilizing smaller Judkins for the left coronary artery)
  (b) Tiger II catheter (Fig. 8.6) – specifically designed for right radial approach. Single catheter used for both left and right coronary arteries (reduces procedure time, radiation exposure and less manipulation leading to less radial artery spasm)

| 4 cm: normal aortic arch |
| 5 cm: unfolded aortic arch |

Figure 8.4 Judkins coronary artery catheters. End holes: 1 Side holes: 0.

Figure 8.5 Amplatz coronary artery catheters. End holes: 1 Side holes: 0.

Figure 8.6 Tiger II coronary artery catheter. End holes: 1 Side holes: 0.

(c) For assessment of grafts: Judkins, Simmons and others (for both femoral and radial approaches).

Patient preparation
As for routine arteriography.

Preliminary image
Chest X-ray.

Technique
The catheter is introduced using the Seldinger technique via the radial (most commonly), brachial or femoral artery and advanced until its tip lies in the ostium of the coronary artery.

Image acquisition
Optimum visualization of vessels is obtained with images acquired perpendicular to the vessel under examination so multiple, compound projections using rotation around the patient axis as well as cranio-caudal angulations of the X-ray beam are utilized for each coronary vessel.

Angiography (7.5 frames s⁻¹) is performed in the following projections:

1. Right coronary artery*
   - RAO 30°
   - LAO 30°
   - LAO 30°/cranial 30°

2. Left coronary artery*
   - PA
   - LAO 45°/caudad 30° ('spider view')
   - RAO 45°/caudad 30°
   - RAO 45°/cranial 30°
   - LAO 45°/cranial 30°

(* though each projection will show good visualization of various segments of the other coronary artery).

Complications

In addition to the general complications discussed in Chapter 9, patients undergoing coronary arteriography may be liable to:

1. Arrhythmias – such as non-sustained atrial fibrillation with right heart catheterization or non-sustained ventricular arrhythmia with left ventriculography
2. Ostial dissection by the catheter
3. Access site complications (more commonly seen with femoral approach) – local haematoma, femoral artery pseudoaneurysm or arterio-venous fistula.

Further Reading
Di Mario C, Sutaria N. Coronary angiography in the angioplasty era: projections with a meaning. Heart 2005;91(7):968–76.

CARDIAC CT

The rapid evolution of multi-detector CT scanner technology over the last 5 years has resulted in cardiac CT and coronary CT angiography becoming well-established techniques in the investigation and management of cardiovascular disease. Greater temporal resolution, sophisticated ECG-gating software and post processing algorithms and, very importantly, radiation dose-reducing strategies allow cardiac CT to be used widely. CT has a high accuracy in detecting coronary vessel stenoses and a very high negative predictive value in excluding significant disease.

Indications

1. Patients with known or suspected chronic coronary artery disease
2. Assessment of suspected anomalous coronary artery anatomy
3. As a screening test in symptomatic patients with typical chest pain but a low clinical probability of significant coronary artery disease
4. As a screening test in asymptomatic but high-risk patients or patients with atypical chest pain
5. Assessment of coronary artery grafts, including left internal mammary artery (LIMA) grafts

6. As an alternative to diagnostic coronary angiography when planning percutaneous angiographic intervention or as post-procedure follow-up.
7. Assessment of left atrium and pulmonary vein anatomy prior to electrophysiological studies and ablation.

Contraindications

1. Standard contraindications to iodinated contrast media administration – previous significant contrast reaction, renal insufficiency, etc.
2. Inability to lie still, breath hold or cooperate with scan instructions
3. Clinical instability
   (a) Cardiac failure, acute myocardial infarction, severe hypotension
   (b) Cardiac dysrhythmia: including atrial fibrillation, frequent ventricular extrasystoles and bigeminy
   (c) Elevated heart rate (in presence of contraindication to beta-blockade).

Patient preparation

1. Avoid caffeine – this includes tea, coffee and caffeine-containing soft drinks (including 'decaffeinated' varieties), 'energy' pills and Viagra-type medication.
2. Drugs – patients should take all their normal cardiac medication as usual on the day of the test.
3. Thorough explanation of the procedure to the patient aids compliance, particularly with regard to breath-hold (suggest patient takes a '¾ breath' when instructed – less likely to move during scan and avoids 'Valsalva' manoeuvre affecting contrast bolus entering chest).
4. 18G cannula in right antecubital fossa – siting cannula in right arm reduces artefact as contrast crosses the mediastinum. For graft studies this avoids streak artefact obscuring origin of LIMA grafts.
5. Assess suitability for administration of β-blockers and sublingual nitrates (see below).

Beta-blockers

Optimal imaging quality and radiation dose are significantly influenced by heart rate, which ideally should be between 55–65 bpm. With basic precautions and simple monitoring, safe and dose-titratable heart rate reduction can be achieved in the majority of patients using β-blocker administered within the radiology department. Metoprolol is commonly used and can be given orally or intravenously, or in combination.

- The patient may already be on oral β-blockers (either as regular medication or specifically prescribed by the referrer for the purposes of the examination). In most cases the scan can proceed without further medication.

- If the patient is not on β-blockers, requires heart rate reduction to optimize scan and has no contraindication to β-blocker administration, metoprolol can be given orally or i.v.

(Contraindications to β-blockade include heart failure, significant aortic stenosis, heart block, asthma/COPD, use of other antiarrhythmic medication including calcium channel blockers and digoxin.)

- Metoprolol 100 mg orally 1 h prior to scan. Pulse and blood pressure monitored regularly until heart rate reaches desired level. (If the heart rate does not reach a satisfactory level additional metoprolol can be given intravenously whilst the patient is on the scanner.)
- Metoprolol can be given solely in i.v. form (or to 'top up' oral dose where optimal heart rate has not been achieved with oral administration) just before the start of the scan with the patient on the scanner table. 5–30 mg i.v. given in aliquots of 5 mg titrated against heart rate.

Nitrates

Sublingual glyceryl trinitrate 400–800 μg (1–2 tablets) can be given a few minutes prior to scanning to produce coronary dilatation and improve image quality. Temporary effect of hypotension is unlikely to be an issue with the patient lying on the CT table and transient physiological elevation of heart rate usually resolves by the time of image acquisition. (Contraindications to nitrates include: hypotension, hypovolaemia, severe aortic valve stenosis, hypertrophic cardiomyopathy, recent MI, severe anaemia, recent 'Viagra'-type medication.)

Technique

Cardiac CT remains a high radiation dose procedure and careful attention to dose reduction measures, whilst maintaining image quality, is essential. The use of 'prospective' rather than 'retrospective' scanning and, where possible, single heart beat acquisition reduce radiation dose very significantly.

Scan technique will be determined by the clinical question to be answered and by patient heart rate; the exact protocol will be determined by the manufacturer and model of the CT scanner.

Scan protocol

All scans are ECG-gated (a) to allow retrospective reconstruction of images timed to specific points in the cardiac cycle, (b) where possible, to allow prospective ECG triggering of the scan with X-ray exposure only during specific parts of the cardiac cycle (usually mid-late diastole to derive coronary artery images) or (c) if prospective triggering is not possible, to modulate the tube current – by decreasing X-ray exposure during parts of the cardiac cycle where image quality is not so critical (usually systole and early diastole) to reduce overall radiation dose.

Plain CT heart

Prospective ECG-triggered non-contrast scan acquired during diastole (usually c. 65–80% of R–R interval) over 3–4 cardiac cycles. Used to detect and quantify coronary artery calcification from which the age- and sex-matched *Calcium Score* is calculated. Higher scores are associated with increasing risk of significant atheromatous disease and the technique can be used as a screening tool for subclinical cardiac disease. Absence of coronary artery calcification however does not completely exclude atheroma but is associated with a low risk of adverse coronary event. The plain scan can then be used to plan the range of the subsequent contrast-enhanced scan.

Contrast-enhanced cardiac scan

Contrast administration

The rapidity of the scan acquisition necessitates very accurate timing of contrast bolus to ensure optimal vessel opacification (but also means that generally smaller volumes of contrast medium can be utilized). Biphasic injection of contrast followed by saline 'chaser' (or if desired, diluted contrast) improves geometry of delivery of contrast and 'washes out' the right side of the heart to reduce streak artefact. Typically 90–100 ml LOCM 350 mg I ml^{-1}-given at 5–7 ml s^{-1} followed by 40–50 ml saline at 4–7 ml s^{-1}. Graft studies need higher volume of contrast 100–120 ml LOCM 350 mg I ml^{-1} at 5–6 ml s^{-1}.

Bolus timing can be achieved using:

1. Empirical delay of c. 25 s. Unreliable and not recommended
2. 'Bolus-tracking' – a selected region-of-interest (ROI) – usually ascending aorta – is scanned every second or so following contrast injection and the full acquisition scan is automatically triggered (after a short delay) once the ROI has enhanced to a preset level e.g. 120 HU
3. 'Test bolus' – a small initial injection of contrast (e.g. 20 ml contrast with 40 ml saline 'chaser' bolus) is given and the ROI (ascending aorta) is scanned and time-to-peak enhancement is derived. The full scan is then performed using this timing delay. (Usually add 3 s to allow for maximal coronary vessel enhancement). This method is probably the most reliable and accurate, confirms i.v. line patency and familiarizes the patient ready for the final crucial acquisition scan.

Retrospective scan

Helical acquisition throughout the cardiac cycle. Retrospective reconstruction of images from data acquired during diastole (c 75% of RR) to show coronary and cardiac structures and from entire data set to show functional imaging of entire cardiac cycle. This is a high radiation dose procedure (approximately 14 mSv) and is utilized in patients with higher heart rates, less stable heart rhythms, for graft assessment and in patients where functional data from the whole cardiac cycle is required. Modulation of tube current in systole and early diastole should be used whenever possible to decrease overall radiation dose (by up to 50%) – image quality is reduced during these less critical parts of the cardiac cycle but useful functional data are preserved.

Prospective scan

ECG-gated prospective triggered sequential axial scan X-ray exposure is limited to specific part of cardiac cycle acquiring data over successive heart beats. Usually centred at approximately 75% of R–R interval in mid/late diastole in order to optimally image the coronary arteries. Requires careful patient selection and preparation; low heart rate and regular rhythm and does not acquire any data from other parts of the cardiac cycle, i.e. no functional information is obtained. Dose reduction of up to 90% compared to retrospective acquisition (currently 2–4.5 mSv – comparable to conventional catheter angiogram c. 5 mSv).

Single-beat acquisition

Using advanced CT technology, acquires data from whole heart in a single cardiac cycle using either wide-area detector covering whole volume of heart or dual-source high-pitch helical acquisition. Requires cooperative patient, low heart rate and very stable rhythm but offers potential of low radiation dose approaching 1 mSv and reduced contrast media volume.

Further Reading

Bastarrika G, Lee YS, Huda W, et al. CT of coronary artery disease. Radiology 2009;253(2):317–38.

Boxt LM. Coronary computed tomography angiography: a practical guide to performance and interpretation. Semin Roentgenol 2012;47(3): 204–19.

Mahesh M, Cody DD. AAPM/RSNA physics tutorial for residents: physics of cardiac imaging with multiple-row detector CT. RadioGraphics 2007;27:1495–509.

Pannu HK, Alvarez W, Fishman EK. Review: β-blockers for cardiac CT: a primer for the radiologist. Am J Roentgenol 2006;186:S341–5.

Schoepf UJ, Zwerner PL, Savino G, et al. Coronary CT angiography: how I do it. Radiology 2007;244:48–63.

Sun Z, Ng KH. Prospective versus retrospective ECG-gated multislice CT coronary angiography: a systematic review of radiation dose and diagnostic accuracy. Euro J Radiol 2012;81(2):94–100.

Taylor CM, Blum A, Abbara S. Cardiac CT: Patient preparation and scanning techniques. Radiol Clin North Am 2010;48(4):675–86.

CARDIAC MR

Cardiac MR imaging has a major role in the assessment of cardiac disease. MR is well established in the evaluation of cardiac and major vessel anatomy, ventricular volumes and mass; functional imaging to assess ventricular and valve motion; and flow quantification allowing measurement of blood velocity and volume to assess intracardiac shunts and stenotic and regurgitant, valvular disease. More recently contrast-enhanced MR has evolved as a powerful tool in assessing myocardial viability and perfusion both in the evaluation of acute myocardial ischaemia and also in assessment of myocardial viability and potential reversibility prior to revascularization. Coronary artery MR imaging has yet to be developed to be of routine use and, for the present, has been comprehensively overtaken by recent advances in CT coronary imaging.

Indications

1. Assessment of chamber dimensions, mass and function
2. Assessment of complex congenital heart disease
3. Diagnosis and evaluation of cardiomyopathies – e.g. sarcoid, amyloid, hypertrophic cardiomyopathy, arrhythmogenic right ventricular cardiomyopathy
4. Evaluation of cardiac masses
5. Evaluation of pericardial disease
6. Evaluation of:
   (a) myocardial viability
   (b) extent of myocardial necrosis/fibrosis
   (c) inducible ischaemia to guide revascularization strategies
7. Imaging and quantification of flow:
   (a) to assess valvular disease – stenosis and incompetence
   (b) to assess shunts – ASD/VSD/PDA/PAPVR
   (c) to assess coarctation of the aorta.

Contraindications

1. Non-MRI-compatible pacemaker
2. Other active implant/device
3. Claustrophobia.

Relative contraindications

1. Asthma is a relative contraindication in adenosine stress perfusion imaging.
2. Frequent ectopics, bigeminy or rhythms such as AF with fast ventricular response may render functional imaging non-diagnostic.

Patient preparation

1. Standard MRI safety screening
2. Placement of MRI-compatible ECG electrodes for gating of sequences
3. IV cannulation
4. Patients for adenosine stress imaging must avoid caffeine.

Technique

Technique will be varied depending on indication, but will consist of elements from the following.

Localizer images
fGRE or SSFP.

Thoracic overview, cardiac morphology
HASTE black blood imaging.

Functional imaging
Long-axis and short-axis SSFP multi-phase retrospectively gated imaging in the standard cardiac planes viz. echocardiography (Flash/fGRE may be used at high field strengths) 6–8 mm with 2–4 mm gap (spatial resolution ~1.5 × 1.5 × 8 mm, temporal resolution <50 ms). Post processing of these images produces quantification of chamber volumes, myocardial mass and ventricular ejection fraction.

In patients with arrhythmia or an inability to breath-hold lower-resolution untriggered real-time functional imaging can be helpful. Typically temporal resolution is ~40 ms, spatial resolution 2–3 mm.

Tissue characterization
1. T2tse or STIR imaging of oedema for myocarditis and peri-infarct 'region at risk'
2. $T2^*$ mapping for iron load in haemochromatosis
3. T1tse imaging for fatty infiltration (esp ARVC), pericardial anatomy and accurate two-dimensional analysis of the endovasculature.

Myocardial perfusion
Apical, mid and basal Flash/fGRE images every heartbeat during rapid administration of i.v. gadolinium:
  (a) during infusion of a vasodilator such as adenosine
  (b) at rest.

Dobutamine stress imaging
Functional imaging of ischaemic wall motion abnormalities produced by increasing doses of infused dobutamine.

Early gadolinium enhancement
IRfGRE images immediately following administration of gadolinium chelate to detect/exclude intracardiac thrombus or microvascular obstruction.

Late gadolinium enhancement

Phase sensitive IRfGRE images 10–20 min following administration of gadolinium in the standard cardiac planes. Patterns of enhancement/hyperenhancement are characteristic for myocardial infarction, and for mid-wall fibrosis and infiltration in various cardiomyopathies.

Flow quantification

Phase contrast imaging with velocity encoding ~120% of expected velocity:

1. For assessment of transvalvular velocities and flow volumes in valve disease
2. For derivation of Qp:Qs ratio in intracardiac shunts
3. For demonstration of shunts, including septal defects and conduits.

MR angiography

3D-T1SSFP volumes for coronaries using navigator respiratory gating, or 2D breathhold SSFP.

Contrast-enhanced angiography using isovolumetric 3DT1fGRE sequences for demonstration of aorta, pulmonary artery or pulmonary veins.

Further Reading

Belloni E, De Cobelli F, Esposito A, et al. MRI of cardiomyopathy. Am J Roentgenol 2008;191(6):1702–10.

Ginat DT, Fong MW, Tuttle DJ, et al. Review: cardiac imaging: Part 1, MR pulse sequences, imaging planes, and basic anatomy. Am J Roentgenol 2011;197(4):808–15.

Kramer CM, Barkhausen J, Flamm SD, et al. Standardized cardiovascular magnetic resonance imaging (CMR) protocols, society for cardiovascular magnetic resonance: board of trustees task force on standardized protocols. J Cardiovasc Mag Res 2008;10:35.

O'Donnell DH, Abbara S, Chaithiraphan V, et al. Cardiac tumours: optimal cardiac MR sequences and spectrum of imaging appearances. Am J Roentgenol 2009;193(2):377–87.

Schwitter J, Arai AE. Assessment of cardiac ischaemia and viability: role of cardiovascular magnetic resonance. Euro Heart J 2011;32:799–809.

8

RADIONUCLIDE VENTRICULOGRAPHY

Indications

Gated blood-pool study[1]

1. Evaluation of ventricular function; particularly left ventricular ejection fraction (LVEF)
2. Assessment of myocardial reserve in coronary artery disease
3. Cardiomyopathy, including the effects of cardio-toxic drugs.

(Previous indications of *first pass radionuclide angiography* – for evaluation of right ventricular ejection fraction (RVEF) and detection and quantification of intracardiac shunts are now superseded by echocardiography and MR unless for very specialist indications and will not be described here.)

Contraindications

Significant arrhythmias may make gated blood-pool imaging impossible.

Radiopharmaceuticals

^{99m}Technetium-in-vivo-labelled red blood cells, 800 MBq max (8 mSv ED).

Before radiolabelling with ^{99m}Technetium (^{99m}Tc)-pertechnetate, the red blood cells are 'primed' with an injection of stannous pyrophosphate. The stannous ions reduce the pertechnetate and allow it to bind to the pyrophosphate which adsorbs on to the red blood cells.

Equipment

1. Gamma-camera: equipped with low-energy general purpose collimator
2. Imaging computer: list-mode or multigated acquisition (MUGA)
3. ECG monitor with gating pulse output.

Patient preparation

1. An i.v. injection of 'cold' stannous pyrophosphate (20 µg kg^{-1}) is given directly into a vein 20–30 min before the pertechnetate injection. (Avoid injection via long plastic Teflon-coated cannula which may result in a poor label.)
2. Three ECG electrodes are placed in standard positions to give a gating signal.

Technique

1. Patient supine
2. The ECG trigger signal is connected
3. I.v. injection of ^{99m}Tc pertechnetate
4. One minute is allowed for the bolus to equilibrate before computer acquisition is commenced (see 'Images' below).

List mode is best, where individual events are stored as their x,y coordinates along with timing and gating pulses. This allows maximum flexibility for later manipulation and framing of data. Around 5 million counts should be acquired. However, MUGA mode is adequate, and is still the most commonly used. In this, the start of an acquisition cycle is usually triggered by the R wave of the patient's ECG. A series of 16–32 fast frames are recorded before the next R wave occurs. Each of these has very few counts in from a single cycle, so every time the R wave trigger arrives another set of frames is recorded and summed with the first. The sequence continues until 100–200 kilo-counts per frame have been acquired in about 10 min. Some degree of arrhythmia can be tolerated using the technique of 'buffered bad beat rejection', where cardiac cycles of irregular length are rejected and the data not included in the images. The length of time to acquire an image set increases as the proportion of rejected beats rises.

Images

A number of views may be recorded, depending on the clinical problem:

1. LAO 35–45° with a 15–30° caudal tilt, chosen to give best separation between left and right ventricles. Patient supine. This view is sufficient if only LVEF is required
2. Anterior, patient supine
3. LPO, chosen to give best separation between atria and ventricles. Patient in right lateral decubitus position.

Analysis

1. The LVEF is calculated
2. Systolic, diastolic, phase and amplitude images are generated
3. The frames can be displayed in cine mode to give good visualization of wall motion.

Additional techniques

1. Gated blood-pool imaging can be carried out during controlled exercise with appropriate precautions to assess ventricular functional reserve. Leg exercise using a bed-mounted bicycle ergometer is the method of choice. Shoulder restraints and hand grips help to reduce upper body movement during imaging. For patients unable to exercise effectively, stress with dobutamine infusion is used.[2] Under continuous monitoring, the dose is incrementally increased from 5 to 20 µg kg^{-1} min^{-1}, infusing each dose for 3 min. The infusion is stopped when S-T segment depression of >3 mm, any ventricular arrhythmia, systolic blood pressure >220 mmHg, attainment of maximum heart rate, or any side effects occur.
2. Gated single photon emission computed tomography (SPECT) blood pool acquisition can be used for measurement of left as well as the right ventricular function using special software (Autoquant+) which calculates the left and right ventricular volumes.
3. With gated SPECT using the myocardial perfusion imaging agents ^{99m}Tc-MIBI and ^{99m}Tc-tetrofosmin (see 'Radionuclide myocardial perfusion imaging'), it is possible to combine ventriculography and perfusion scans in a single study.[3,4]

When acquiring gated SPECT studies ventricular parameters are usually measured during rest study only because of the length of the examination (20 min).

Aftercare

1. Monitor recovery from exercise
2. Normal radiation safety precautions (see Chapter 1).

Complications

Complications are related to the exercise test and include induction of angina, cardiac arrhythmias and cardiac arrest.

References
1. Metcalfe MJ. Radionuclide ventriculography. In: Sharp PF, Gemmell HG, Murray AD, editors. Practical Nuclear Medicine. London: Springer; 2005.
2. Konishi T, Koyama T, Aoki T, et al. Radionuclide assessment of left ventricular function during dobutamine infusion in patients with coronary artery disease: comparison with ergometer exercise. Clin Cardiol 1990;13:183–8.
3. Fukuoka S, Maeno M, Nakagawa S, et al. Feasibility of myocardial dual-isotope perfusion imaging combined with gated single photon emission tomography for assessing coronary artery disease. Nucl Med Commun 2002;23(1):19–29.
4. Anagnostopoulos C, Underwood SR. Simultaneous assessment of myocardial perfusion and function: how and when? Eur J Nucl Med 1998;25:555–8.

RADIONUCLIDE MYOCARDIAL PERFUSION IMAGING

Indications

1. Diagnosis and assessment of extent and severity of myocardial ischaemia or infarction
2. Assessment of myocardial viability
3. Evaluation of prognosis
4. Evaluation of effects of angioplasty and bypass surgery on myocardial perfusion with pre- and post-intervention imaging.

Contraindications

1. Unstable angina
2. Frequent ventricular arrhythmias at rest
3. Contraindications to pharmacological stress agent
4. Second-degree heart block
5. Severe valvular disease, especially aortic valve stenosis.

Radiopharmaceuticals[1,2]

1. ^{99m}Tc-methoxyisobutylisonitrile (MIBI or sestamibi), up to 800 MBq (8 mSv ED) for planar imaging, 800 MBq (8 mSv ED) for SPECT

(or 1600 MBq max. for the total of two injections in single day rest/exercise protocols). Cationic complex with myocardial uptake in near proportion to coronary blood flow but minimal redistribution. There is also, normally, liver uptake and biliary excretion, which can cause inferior wall artifacts on SPECT if care is not taken. Separate injections are required for stress/rest studies, but image timing is flexible due to minimal redistribution.

2. ^{99m}Tc-tetrofosmin (Myoview) (activity and radiation dose as for MIBI). Similar uptake characteristics and diagnostic efficacy to MIBI, but with easier preparation.

3. ^{201}Tl-thallous chloride, 80 MBq max. (18 mSv ED). Thallium is a potassium analogue with initial rapid myocardial uptake in near proportion to coronary blood flow, and subsequent washout and redistribution. Hence, unlike the ^{99m}Tc agents, same-day stress/rest redistribution studies can be performed with a single injection. With principal photon energies of 68–72 and 167 keV and $T_{1/2}$ of 73 h, it is not ideal for imaging and gives a higher radiation dose than the newer ^{99m}Tc alternatives. It is increasingly being replaced by ^{99m}Tc agents. However, many still consider ^{201}Tl for assessment of myocardial viability and hibernation, with either re-injection at rest or a separate day rest-redistribution study giving the greatest sensitivity.

4. ^{18}FDG + blood flow PET. The radio-isotope gold standard for viability assessment, but not widely available.[3]

5. Rubidium-82 PET. This study can be used to assess myocardial perfusion. Not widely available.

Equipment

1. SPECT-capable gamma-camera, preferably dual-headed
2. Low-energy, high-resolution, general purpose or specialized cardiac collimators
3. Pharmacological stressing agent (adenosine or dobutamine [dipyridamole now rarely used]) or exercise (bicycle ergometer or treadmill)
4. Nitroglycerin (tablets or sublingual spray) to enhance resting uptake of ischaemic, but viable segments
5. ECG monitor
6. Resuscitation facilities including defibrillator
7. Lidocaine to reverse serious arrhythmias caused by dobutamine infusion.

Patient preparation

1. Nil by mouth or light breakfast 4–6 h prior to test
2. Cessation of cardiac medication on the day of the test if possible. ß-blockers can be continued and adenosine stress used. Avoid caffeine for 24 h if using dipyridamole or adenosine.

Technique

The principle of the technique is to compare myocardial perfusion under conditions of pharmacological stress or physical exercise, with perfusion at rest. Diseased but patent arterial territories will show lower perfusion under stress conditions than healthy arteries, but will show relatively improved perfusion at rest. Infarcted tissue will show no improvement at rest. Hence, prognostic information on the likelihood of adverse cardiac events and the benefits of revascularization can be gained.[4]

Stress regimen

Pharmacological stress has become increasingly widely used instead of physical exercise.[5] The optimal stress technique aims to maximize coronary arterial flow. The preferred pharmacological stressing agent is adenosine infusion (0.14 mg kg^{-1} min^{-1} for 6 min).[6] Adenosine is a potent coronary vasodilator. It reproducibly increases coronary artery flow by more than maximal physical exercise (which often cannot be achieved in this group of patients). It has a short biological half-life of 8–10 s, so most side effects are reversed simply by discontinuing infusion. Stressing with adenosine has now almost completely replaced dipyridamole and will not be discussed here.

There are circumstances where adenosine is contraindicated, e.g. asthma, second-degree heart block or systolic blood pressure <100 mmHg. Dobutamine stress may be employed in these circumstances.[7] Dobutamine acts as a β_1 receptor agonist, increasing contractility and heart rate. Under continuous monitoring, the dose is incrementally increased from 5 to 20 μg kg^{-1} min^{-1}, infusing each dose for 3 min. The infusion is terminated when S-T segment depression of >3 mm, any ventricular arrhythmia, systolic blood pressure >220 mmHg, attainment of maximum heart rate, or any side effects occur. Dobutamine is contraindicated in patients with aortic aneurysm. New, more specific targeted agents such as regadenoson (A_{2A} adenosine receptor agonist) are being developed which could be used in asthmatic patients rather than dobutamine.[8]

^{99m}Tc-MIBI or tetrofosmin rest/stress test

Because MIBI and tetrofosmin have minimal redistribution, separate injections are needed for stress and rest studies. Two-day protocols are optimal, but it is often more convenient to perform both studies on the same day. A number of groups have shown that this is possible without significantly degrading the results, most effectively when the resting study is performed first.[9]

2-Day protocol (stress/rest)

1. Initiate pharmacological stress or exercise
2. Up to 800 MBq MIBI or tetrofosmin is administered i.v. at maximal stress, continuing the stress protocol for 2 min post injection to allow uptake in the myocardium

3. 10–30 min post injection, a milky drink or similar is given to promote biliary clearance; high fluid intake will dilute bowel contents

4. Images are acquired 15–30 min after tetrofosmin or 60–120 min after sestamibi injection. If there is excessive liver uptake or activity in small bowel close to the heart, imaging should be delayed by a further 60 min

5. Depending on the clinical situation, if the stress scan is completely normal the patient may not need to return for the rest scan[10]

6. Preferably 2–7 days later, the patient returns for a resting scan

7. Glyceryl trinitrate (GTN) (two 0.3 mg tablets) or equivalent sublingual spray may be given to improve blood flow to ischaemic, but viable segments[11]

8. Immediately, up to 800 MBq MIBI or tetrofosmin i.v., is administered and proceed as for stress imaging.

1-Day protocol (stress/rest)

1. Initiate pharmacological stress or exercise; up to 400 MBq MIBI or tetrofosmin i.v. is administered at maximum stress

2. Image as per 2-day protocol

3. A minimum of 2 h after first tetrofosmin injection and minimum of 4 h after sestamibi injection, GTN is administered as above, followed by up to 1200 MBq MIBI or tetrofosmin (with longer period between injections, the activity of the second injection may be reduced)

4. Image as per 2-day protocol.

^{201}Tl stress/rest test

Since ^{201}Tl redistributes after injection, stress/rest studies can be performed with a single injection. However, stress image timing is more critical:

1. Initiate pharmacological stress or exercise

2. Administer 80 MBq ^{201}Tl i.v. at maximal stress, continuing the stress protocol for 1 min post injection to allow uptake in the myocardium

3. Image immediately (<5 min)

4. Image at rest 3–4 h after redistribution period, during which time patients should not eat

5. If fixed defects are present in exercise and rest images and assessment of viability and hibernation is required, either:

   (a) administer a second smaller dose of 40 MBq ^{201}Tl, giving GTN pre injection, and image 20–30 min later. If defects still persist, image again at 18–24 h

   OR

   (b) perform a separate day rest-redistribution study with 80 MBq ^{201}Tl after GTN, and image at 20–30 min and 3–4 h.

Images

SPECT

1. Position patient as comfortably as possible with their arms above their head (or at least the left arm) if possible. SPECT images may be severely degraded by patient movement, so attention should be paid to keeping the patient very still.
2. For the ^{99m}Tc agents, check for activity in bowel loops close to the inferior wall of the heart. This can cause artifacts in the reconstructed images, so if significant activity is seen, delay the imaging to give greater time for clearance.
3. 180° orbit from RAO 45° to LPO 45°, elliptical if possible. With modern dual-headed systems, this can be achieved with the heads at 90° to each other to minimize the amount of camera rotation required.
4. Matrix size and zoom to give a pixel size of 6 mm.
5. 60 projections, with a total imaging time of about 30–40 min for single and 15–25 min for dual-head systems.
6. View the projections as a cine before the patient leaves the department. If available, perform software motion correction. If there is significant movement that cannot be corrected, repeat imaging. Beware 'diaphragmatic creep', particularly on ^{201}Tl patients breathless after exercise, where the average position of the diaphragm changes as they recover.

Analysis

1. Short, vertical long and horizontal long axis views are reconstructed, taking care to use the same orientation for stress and rest image data sets (modern systems have automatic alignment software).
2. Two-dimensional circumferential profile or 'bull's-eye' polar maps may be generated.

Additional techniques

1. Gated SPECT is now recommended,[12] and with special software (e.g. Cedars Sinai QGS package, Emory cardiac tool box) can provide additional information on ventricular wall motion, ejection fraction and chamber volume. It can also improve specificity by reducing artifactual defects caused by regional myocardial motion and wall thickening.
2. Bull's-eye maps can be compared to normal databases and displayed quantitatively in terms of severity and extent of relative underperfusion.[13]
3. Attenuation and scatter correction using scanning transmission line sources or CT are now available on most modern dual-headed systems. This technique can improve diagnostic specificity by correcting attenuation artifacts and thereby increasing the

normalcy rate. However, algorithms are still being improved, so at present it is wise to view the attenuation-corrected and uncorrected images together to identify possible introduced artifacts.[14]

4. The combination of rest ^{201}Tl and exercise ^{99m}Tc MIBI or tetrofosmin can be used to assess both ischaemia and viability.[15]

Aftercare

1. Monitoring of patient post-exercise
2. Normal radiation safety precautions (see Chapter 1).

Complications

Complications are related to stress and exercise and include: induction of angina, cardiac arrhythmias, cardiac arrest and bronchospasm after adenosine.

References

1. Reyes E, Loong CY, Harbinson M, et al. A comparison of Tl-201, Tc-99m sestamibi, and Tc-99m tetrofosmin myocardial perfusion scinitgraphy in patients with mild to moderate coronary stenosis. J Nucl Cardiol 2006;13(4):488–94.
2. Kapur A, Latus KA, Davies G, et al. A comparison of three radionuclide myocardial perfusion tracers in clinical practice: the ROBUST study. Eur J Nucl Med Mol Imaging 2002;29(12):1608–16.
3. Nandalur KR, Dwamena BA, Choudhri AF, et al. Diagnostic performance of positron emission tomography in the detection of coronary artery disease: a meta-analysis. Acad Radiol 2008;15(4):444–51.
4. Travin MI, Bergmann SR. Assessment of myocardial viability. Semin Nucl Med 2005;35(1):2–16.
5. Travain MI, Wexler JP. Pharmacological stress testing. Semin Nucl Med 1999;29:298–318.
6. Takeishi Y, Takahashi N, Fujiwara S, et al. Myocardial tomography with technetium-99m-tetrofosmin during intravenous infusion of adenosine triphosphate. J Nucl Med 1998;39:582–6.
7. Verani MS. Dobutamine myocardial perfusion imaging. J Nucl Med 1994;35:737–9.
8. Iskandrian AE, Bateman TM, Belardinelli L, et al. Adenosine versus regadenoson comparative evaluation in myocardial perfusion imaging: results of the ADVANCE phase 3 multicenter international trial. J Nucl Cardiol 2007;14(5):645–58.
9. Tadehara F, Yamamoto H, Tsujiyama S, et al. Feasibility of a rapid protocol of 1-day single-isotope rest/adenosine stress Tc-99m sestamibi ECG-gated myocardial perfusion imaging. J Nucl Cardiol 2008;15(1):35–41.
10. Lavalaye JM, Shroeder-Tanka JM, Tiel-van Buul MM, et al. Implementation of technetium-99m MIBI SPECT imaging guidelines: optimizing the two-day stress-rest protocol. Int J Card Imaging 1997;13:331–5.
11. Thorley PJ, Sheard KL, Wright DJ, et al. The routine use of sublingual GTN with resting ^{99m}Tc-tetrofosmin myocardial perfusion imaging. Nucl Med Commun 1998;19:937–42.

8

12. Travin MI, Heller GV, Johnson LL, et al. The prognostic value of ECG-gated SPECT imaging in patients undergoing stress Tc-99m sestamibi myocardial perfusion imaging. J Nucl Cardiol 2004;11(3):253–62.
13. Schwaiger M, Melin J. Cardiological applications of nuclear medicine. Lancet 1999;354:661–6.
14. Banzo I, Pena FJ, Allende RH, et al. Prospective clinical comparison of non-corrected and attenuation- and scatter-corrected myocardial perfusion SPECT in patients with suspicion of coronary artery disease. Nucl Med Commun 2003;24(9):995–1002.
15. Kim Y, Goto H, Kobayshi K, et al. A new method to evaluate ischemic heart disease: combined use of rest thallium-201 myocardial SPECT and Tc-99m exercise tetrofosmin first pass and myocardial SPECT. Ann Nucl Med 1999;13:147–53.

Arterial system

Methods of imaging the arterial system

1. Catheter angiography
2. Ultrasound (US)
3. Computed tomography (CT)
4. Magnetic resonance imaging (MRI).

Further Reading

Collins R, Cranny G, Burch J, et al. A systematic review of duplex ultrasound, magnetic resonance angiography and computed tomography angiography for the diagnosis and assessment of symptomatic, lower limb peripheral arterial disease. Health Technol Assess 2007;11(20):iii–iv, xi–xiii, 1–184.

Kaufman JA, Lee MJ, editors. Vascular and Interventional Radiology: The Requisites. Philadelphia: Elsevier-Mosby; 2004.

INTRODUCTION TO CATHETER TECHNIQUES

The basic technique of arterial catheterization is also applicable to veins.

Patient preparation

1. The patient will need admission to hospital. Careful preparation before the procedure and observation after are required. With the introduction of smaller-diameter catheters, day-case admission may be appropriate for routine peripheral angiography and some angioplasty cases.
2. If the patient is on anticoagulant treatment, blood clotting should be within an acceptable therapeutic 'window'.
3. The radiologist or a suitably trained person should see the patient, preferably several days prior to the procedure, in order to:
   (a) explain the procedure
   (b) obtain informed consent
   (c) assess the patient, with special reference to renal function, blood pressure and peripheral pulses as a baseline for post-arteriographic problems.

Puncture sites
1. Femoral artery – most frequently used
2. Brachial artery
3. Axillary artery
4. Radial artery.

Equipment for the Seldinger technique

Needles
The technique of catheter insertion via double-wall needle puncture and guidewire is known as the Seldinger technique. The original Seldinger needle consisted of three parts:

1. An outer thin-walled blunt cannula
2. An inner needle
3. A stilette.

Many radiologists now prefer to use modified needles:

1. Double-wall puncture with a two-piece needle consisting of a bevelled central stilette and an outer tube
2. Single-wall puncture with a simple sharp needle (without a stilette) with a bore just wide enough to accommodate the guidewire.

Guidewires
Basic guidewires consist of two central cores of straight wire around which is a tightly wound coiled wire spring (Fig. 9.1). The ends are sealed with solder. One of the central core wires is secured at both ends – a safety feature in case of fracturing. The other is anchored

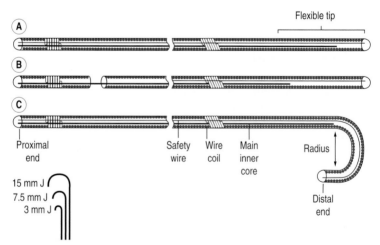

Figure 9.1 Guidewire construction. (a) Fixed core, straight. (b) Movable core, straight. (c) Fixed core, J-curve.

in solder at one end, but terminates 5 cm from the other end, leaving a soft flexible tip. Some guidewires have a movable central core so the tip can be flexible or stiff. Others have a J-shaped tip which is useful for negotiating vessels with irregular walls. The size of the J-curve is denoted by its radius in mm. Guidewires are polyethylene coated but may be coated with a thin film of Teflon to reduce friction. Teflon, however, also increases the thrombogenicity, which can be countered by using heparin-bonded Teflon. The most common sizes are 0.035 and 0.038 inch diameter. More recently hydrophilic guidewires have been developed. These frequently have a metal mandrel as their core. They are very slippery with excellent torque and are useful in negotiating narrow tortuous vessels. They require constant lubrication with saline.

Catheters

Most catheters are manufactured commercially, complete with end hole, side holes, preformed curves and Luer lock connection. They are made of polyurethane or polyethylene. Details of the specific catheter types are given with the appropriate technique.

Some straight catheters may be shaped by immersion in hot sterile water until they become malleable, forming the desired shape and then fixing the shape by cooling in cold sterile water. For the average adult a 100-cm catheter with a 145-cm guidewire is suitable for reaching the thoracic aortic branches from a femoral puncture. If abdominal aortography or peripheral arteriography of the legs is to be performed shorter catheters may be used.

The introduction of a catheter over a guidewire may be facilitated by dilation of the track with a dilator (short length of tapered diameter tubing). If the patient has a large amount of subcutaneous fat in the puncture area, catheter control will be better if it is manipulated through an introducer sheath. This is also indicated where it is anticipated that frequent catheter exchanges may be required.

Taps and connectors

These should have a large internal diameter that will not increase resistance to flow. Taps should be removed during high-pressure injections.

FEMORAL ARTERY PUNCTURE

This is the most frequently used puncture site providing access to the left ventricle, aorta and its branches and has the lowest complication rate of the peripheral sites.

Relative contraindications

1. Blood dyscrasias
2. Femoral artery aneurysm or pseudoaneurysm

3. Local soft-tissue infection
4. Severe hypertension
5. Ehlers–Danlos syndrome (due to the vessel wall being easily torn).

Technique (Fig. 9.2)

1. The patient lies supine on the X-ray table. Both femoral arteries are palpated and if pulsations are of similar strength the side opposite the symptomatic leg may be chosen, which gives the option to proceed to angioplasty by crossing over the aortic bifurcation. If all else is equal, then the right side is technically easier (for right-handed operators).
2. The appropriate catheter and guidewire are selected and their compatibility checked by passing the guidewire through the catheter and needle.
3. The location and point of puncture of the femoral artery must be considered. The external iliac artery arches anteriorly and laterally as it passes under the inguinal ligament and continues as the femoral artery. Attempts to puncture the artery cephalad to the ligament may result in a puncture deep in the pelvis at a point where haemostasis is difficult to achieve by manual compression and where peri-catheter and post-procedure bleeding may be

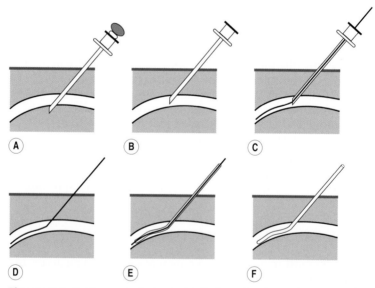

Figure 9.2 Seldinger technique. (a) Both walls of vessel punctured. (b) Stilette removed. Needle withdrawn so that bevel is within the lumen of the vessel and blood flows from the hub. (c) Guidewire inserted through needle. (d) Needle withdrawn, leaving guidewire in situ. (e) Catheter threaded over wire. (f) Guidewire withdrawn.

obscured by preferential passage of blood into the retroperitoneum. Brief preliminary fluoroscopy of the groin can identify the centre of the femoral head with the intention of puncturing the artery at this point. This increases the likelihood of hitting the common femoral artery and facilitates haemostasis post procedure by allowing the artery to be compressed against bone. The inguinal skin fold does not reliably correlate with the position of the inguinal ligament. The entire common femoral artery lies above the skin fold in more than 75% of Western European subjects.[1] Direct US guidance is increasingly routinely used for vascular puncture.

4. Using aseptic technique, local anaesthetic is infiltrated either side of the artery down to the periosteum. A 3–5-mm stab incision is made over the artery to reduce binding of soft tissues on the catheter. In thin patients the artery may be very superficial and the skin may need to be pinched-up or deflected laterally, to avoid cutting the artery.

5. The artery is immobilized by placing the index and middle fingers of the left hand on either side of the artery, and the needle is held in the right hand. The needle is advanced through the soft tissues until transmitted pulsations are felt. Either both walls of the artery are punctured through-and-through or a single wall puncture is performed depending on the needle used. If present, the stilette is removed and the needle hub is depressed so that it runs more parallel to the skin and is then withdrawn until pulsatile blood flow indicates a satisfactory puncture. Poor flow may be due to:

   (a) the end of the needle lying in or against the vessel wall or within plaque
   (b) aorto-iliac stenosis resulting in low femoral artery pressure
   (c) hypotension – due to vasovagal reaction during the puncture
   (d) femoral vein puncture.

6. When good flow is obtained the guidewire is introduced through the needle and advanced gently along the artery using intermittent fluoroscopy to avoid engaging the vessel wall. When the wire is in the descending thoracic aorta the needle is withdrawn over the guidewire, keeping firm pressure on the puncture site to reduce bleeding. The free portion of guidewire is then wiped clean with a wet sponge and the catheter threaded over it. For 5F or greater diameter catheters, particularly those which are curved, a dilator is recommended matched to catheter size. The catheter is advanced up the descending aorta, under fluoroscopic control, and when in a satisfactory position the guidewire is withdrawn.

7. Catheter patency can be maintained by continuous flushing from a pressurized bag of heparinized saline (2500 units in 500 ml of 0.9% saline) attached through a three-way tap, or by intermittent

9

manual flushing throughout the procedure. Flushing should be done rapidly otherwise the more distal catheter holes will remain unflushed.
8. At the end of the procedure the catheter is withdrawn and manual compression of the puncture site should be maintained for 5–10 min.

Aftercare

1. Bed rest – typically for 4 h, but longer at the discretion of the operator. Larger catheters, antiplatelet therapy and anticoagulation require longer observation
2. Careful observation of the puncture site for haemorrhage
3. Pulse and blood pressure observation, e.g. half-hourly for 4 h and then 4-hourly for the remainder of 24 h, if the larger catheter systems are used.

HIGH BRACHIAL ARTERY PUNCTURE

Indications

As for femoral artery puncture, but as this approach is associated with a higher incidence of complications, it should only be used if femoral artery puncture is not possible.

Contraindications

1. Atherosclerosis of the axillary or subclavian arteries
2. Subclavian artery aneurysm.

Technique

1. The patient lies on the X-ray table with his arm in supination. The peripheral pulses are palpated and the brachial artery localized approximately 10 cm above the elbow.
2. A small incision is made in the skin, 1–2 cm distal to the selected point of arterial puncture.
3. A single-wall puncture needle is used, with an acute angle of entry into the artery.
4. A straight, soft-tipped guidewire is introduced when good pulsatile flow is obtained.
5. A 5F pigtail catheter is introduced over the guidewire and its pigtail formed in the aorta.
6. At the end of the procedure the catheter tip is straightened using the guidewire and then removed. This reduces the risk of intimal damage and flap formation during withdrawal of the catheter.

AXILLARY ARTERY PUNCTURE

Indications

As for femoral artery puncture, but this approach is associated with a higher incidence of complications than femoral or high brachial artery puncture and should only be used if these techniques are not possible.

Contraindications

1. Atherosclerosis of the axillary or subclavian arteries
2. Subclavian artery aneurysm.

Technique

1. The patient lies supine on the X-ray table with the arm fully abducted. The puncture point is just distal to the axillary fold. It is infiltrated with local anaesthetic.
2. A small incision is made in the skin 1–2 cm distal to the point of the arterial puncture.
3. The needle is directed more horizontally than the femoral approach and along the line of the humerus.
4. Following satisfactory puncture the remainder of the technique is as for femoral artery catheterization.

Reference

Aftercare

1. Lechner G, Jantsch H, Waneck R, et al. The relationship between the common femoral artery, the inguinal crease, and the inguinal ligament: a guide to accurate angiographic puncture. Cardiovasc Intervent Radiol 1988;11(3):165–9.

GENERAL COMPLICATIONS OF CATHETER TECHNIQUES

Due to the anaesthetic

See Chapter 18.

Due to the contrast medium

See Chapter 2.

Due to the technique

Diagnostic angiography is an invasive procedure and complications are expected. The majority of these are minor, e.g. groin haematoma. Recommended upper limits for complication rates have been produced by the Society of Interventional Radiology (SIR):[1] these rates are included in the following discussion.

Local

The most frequent complications occur at the puncture site. The complication rate is lowest for femoral artery punctures:

1. *Haemorrhage/haematoma* – the commonest complication. Small haematomas occur in up to 20% of examinations and large haematomas in up to 4%. The SCIR threshold for haematomas requiring transfusion, surgery or delayed discharge after diagnostic angiography is 0.5%. Haematoma formation is greater with larger catheters, more frequent catheter exchanges and heparin, antiplatelet or thrombolytic agents. Haematoma formation is also greater when the femoral artery is punctured high because of inadequate compression of the artery following catheter removal.

2. *Arterial thrombus* may be due to:
   (a) stripping of thrombus from the catheter wall as it is withdrawn
   (b) trauma to the vessel wall.
   Factors implicated in increased thrombus formation are:
   (a) large catheters
   (b) excessive time in the artery
   (c) many catheter changes
   (d) inexperience of the radiologist
   (e) polyurethane catheters, because of their rough surface.
   The incidence is decreased by the use of:
   (a) heparin-bonded catheters
   (b) heparin-bonded guidewires
   (c) flushing with heparinized saline.

3. *Infection at the puncture site.*

4. *Damage to local structures;* especially the brachial plexus during axillary artery puncture. Femoral nerve palsy can result from inadvertent infiltration of the nerve with local anaesthetic. It is short-lived but should prompt very cautious subsequent mobilization of the patient in case the leg 'gives way'. More protracted femoral nerve damage can be due to excessive haematoma or pseudoaneurysm formation in the groin.

5. *Pseudoaneurysm.* The SIR threshold for diagnostic angiography is 0.2%. It presents as a pulsatile mass at the puncture site any time after arteriography and is due to communication between the lumen of the artery and a cavity within semi-solid or organized haematoma. Arterial puncture below the common femoral artery bifurcation increases the risk of this complication. Some may require surgical or interventional radiological repair.

6. *Arteriovenous fistula* – rare. SIR threshold is 0.1%. More common when puncture is below the common femoral artery bifurcation, because at this level the vein lies posterior to the

artery and both are punctured in the standard double-wall technique.

Distant

1. *Peripheral embolus* – from stripped catheter thrombus. Emboli to small digital arteries will resolve spontaneously; emboli to large arteries may need aspiration thrombectomy through a catheter or surgical embolectomy. The SCVIR threshold is 0.5%.
2. *Atheroembolism* – more likely in older subjects. J-shaped guidewires are less likely to dislodge atheromatous plaques.
3. *Air embolus.* May be fatal in coronary or cerebral arteries. It is prevented by:
   (a) ensuring that all taps and connectors are tight
   (b) always sucking back when a new syringe is connected
   (c) ensuring that all bubbles are excluded from the syringe before injecting
   (d) keeping the syringe vertical, plunger up, when injecting.
4. *Cotton fibre embolus.* Occurs when syringes are filled from a bowl containing swabs or when a guidewire is wiped with a dry gauze pad. This very bad practice is prevented by:
   (a) separate bowls of saline for flushing and wet swabs
   OR, preferably,
   (b) a closed system of perfusion.
5. *Artery dissection* – due to entry of the catheter, guidewire or contrast medium into the subintimal space. It is recognized by resistance to passage of the guidewire or catheter, poor back-bleeding from the catheter hub, increased resistance to injection of contrast medium or subintimal contrast medium on fluoroscopy. The risk of serious dissection is reduced by:
   (a) using floppy J-shaped guidewires
   (b) using catheters with multiple side holes
   (c) employing a small volume manual test injection prior to a pump injection
   (d) careful and gentle manipulation of catheters.
6. *Catheter knotting* – more likely during the investigation of complex congenital heart disease. Non-surgical reduction of catheter knots is discussed by Thomas and Sievers.[2] Withdrawal of the knotted end to the groin followed by surgical removal may be the only solution in some cases.
7. *Catheter impaction*:
   (a) In a coronary artery produces cardiac ischaemic pain
   (b) In a mesenteric artery produces abdominal pain. There should be rapid wash-out of contrast medium after a selective injection. A sound of sucking air on removing the guidewire and poor back-bleeding from the catheter indicate an impacted (wedged) catheter tip.

9

8. *Guidewire breakage* – less common with modern guidewires and tended to occur 5 cm from the tip, where a single central core terminates.

9. *Bacteraemia* – rarely of clinical significance.

References
1. Singh H, Cardella JF, Cole PE, et al. Quality improvement guidelines for diagnostic arteriography. J Vasc Interv Radiol 2003;14(9 Pt2):S283–8.
2. Thomas HA, Sievers RE. Nonsurgical reduction of arterial catheter knots. Am J Roentgenol 1979;132(6):1018–19.

ASCENDING AORTOGRAPHY

Echocardiography, multislice CT, and MRI are preferable initial imaging modalities for assessment of the ascending aorta.

Indications

1. Aortic aneurysm, trauma or dissection
2. Atheroma at the origin of the major vessels
3. Aortic regurgitation (echocardiography is more sensitive and less invasive if available)
4. Congenital heart disease – particularly the demonstration of congenital or iatrogenic aorto-pulmonary shunts and coarctation
5. As a preliminary to endovascular intervention, e.g. aneurysm repair.

Contrast medium

Low osmolar contrast material (LOCM) 370 mg I ml^{-1}, 0.75 ml kg^{-1} (max. 40 ml). Inject at 18–20 ml s^{-1}.

Equipment

1. Digital fluoroscopy unit with C-arm capable of 20–30 frames s^{-1}
2. Pump injector
3. Catheter:
    (a) Pigtail (Fig. 8.3)
    OR
    (b) Gensini (Fig. 9.3)
    OR
    (c) National Institutes of Health (NIH) (Fig. 8.2).

Figure 9.3 Gensini catheter. Note tapered end. End holes: 1 Side holes: 6.

Technique

1. The catheter is introduced using the Seldinger technique via the femoral artery, and its tip sited 1–3 cm above the aortic valve.
2. The C-arm is positioned 45° left anterior oblique (LAO) to open out the aortic arch, and to show the aortic valve and the left ventricle to best advantage.
3. A test injection is performed to ensure that:
   (a) the catheter is correctly placed in relation to the aortic valve (which is particularly important in the hyperkinetic heart)
   (b) the catheter tip is not in a coronary artery.

Images

2–3 frames s^{-1}.

Additional images

If, on the original run, the right common carotid artery overlies the right innominate artery or an aneurysm is present on the anterior aspect of the ascending aorta, the injection is repeated with C-arm positioned right anterior oblique (RAO).

ARTERIOGRAPHY OF THE LOWER LIMB

Indications

1. Arterial ischaemia
2. Trauma
3. Arteriovenous malformation.

Methods

Both lower limbs

1. Catheter angiography – using a pigtail catheter introduced via the femoral artery and sited proximal to the aortic bifurcation
2. Brachial or axillary puncture.

One lower limb

1. Using a femoral artery catheter:
   (a) Introduced retrogradely and sited in the ipsilateral common iliac artery
   (b) Introduced retrogradely from the contralateral side and sited in the common iliac, external iliac or femoral artery (sidewinder catheter)
   (c) Introduced antegradely.

If thin 4F catheters are used, only day-case admission is necessary.

Contrast medium

All of these techniques can be performed under local anaesthesia with LOCM. 10–20 ml of 300 mg I ml^{-1} concentration is suitable for the examination of one limb. 50 ml of 350 mg I ml^{-1}, at a rate of 12–15 ml s^{-1}, is suitable for a catheter aortogram.

BALLOON ANGIOPLASTY

Also known as percutaneous transluminal angioplasty or balloon dilation.

Indications

1. Dilation of localized vascular stenoses, mainly of the renal, iliac, lower limb and coronary arteries.
2. Recanalization of occluded segments of vessels in selected cases.

Dilation procedures are often combined with preparatory diagnostic angiography in the same session; the majority are done under local anaesthetic. The procedure is often needed after lysis of arterial thrombus: this is outlined below.

Equipment

1. Digital fluoroscopy unit with C-arm capable of angiography and preferably with 'road mapping' facilities
2. Arterial pressure measuring equipment (optional)
3. Catheters:
   (a) Gruntzig double-lumen balloon dilation catheters. Various manufacturers offer a wide range of balloon length and diameter combinations as well as catheter-shaft lengths, depending on the site and size of the vessel to be treated
   (b) van Andel dilation catheter (a tapered, straight Teflon catheter, occasionally useful)
   (c) straight Teflon or polyethylene catheters
4. Guidewires:
   (a) 0.035- or 0.038-inch diameter wires, typically 145 cm long; hydrophilic guidewires may be helpful for crossing tight stenoses
   (b) 250 cm exchange guidewire
5. Thrombolytic agents may be infused into recently thrombosed vessels, prior to angioplasty.

Technique

Principles
1. Adequate angiograms must be obtained before proceeding to angioplasty.

2. Angioplasty is always performed with the guidewire remaining across the stenosis or occlusion until the procedure is completed.
3. Adequate vascular surgical assistance must be readily available before attempting angioplasty.
4. If the history suggests that a thrombosis has occurred within the previous 3 weeks, thrombolysis may be helpful.
5. The patient should be anticoagulated during the procedure, using 3000–5000 units of heparin.
6. The balloon diameter is selected by reference to the measured size of the normal artery on the preceding angiogram, allowing for magnification.

Renal arteries

1. The tip of a suitable guidewire is negotiated through and beyond the stenosis in the renal artery, from either the femoral or high brachial artery approach.
2. A balloon catheter of appropriate diameter is positioned across the stenosis and distended (approx. 7 atmospheres for 1 min) after injecting 3000 units of heparin. A post-dilation angiogram is then taken. If a residual stenosis remains, further dilations or implantation of a metallic stent may be necessary.

Iliac arteries

1. These are preferably dilated from a retrograde femoral puncture on the side of the lesion.
2. If the femoral pulse is absent or difficult to feel, it may be located using US guidance or road mapping from a contralateral femoral approach. Alternatively, a sidewinder catheter can be introduced from the opposite groin and a guidewire directed over the aortic bifurcation and across the lesion.
3. It can be helpful to measure the femoral artery pressure immediately after introducing the catheter, and before a guidewire is passed through the lesion. This is to assess the severity of the pressure gradient before and after angioplasty.
4. A suitable guidewire is then advanced carefully through the stenosis. If the lesion is eccentrically situated, it may be preferable to advance using a pre-shaped catheter, inject contrast medium to position the catheter, and then to advance through the patent lumen, avoiding possible intimal dissection from below. If the lesion is particularly tight, a hydrophilic wire may be useful.
5. A catheter is passed over the guidewire and into the distal aorta.
6. Heparin 3000–5000 units should be administered.
7. The guidewire is removed, to allow a pressure measurement in the aorta. It is then replaced and the catheter exchanged for a balloon catheter. After dilating the lesion, an angiogram is performed to assess the result. Pressure measurements may be checked to ensure that a significant gradient no longer exists. A wire or catheter remains across the stenosis until this is confirmed.

9

Femoral arteries (common, and origins of superficial femoral and profunda femoris arteries)

1. These cannot easily be approached by an antegrade puncture on the side of the lesion since there is little room to manoeuvre and exchange catheters.
2. The contralateral femoral artery is catheterized using a sidewinder catheter. The tip is positioned in the iliac artery ipsilateral to the lesion and a guidewire advanced down through the lesion. The catheter is then exchanged for a balloon catheter and, after injecting heparin 3000 units, the lesion is dilated and a check angiogram performed before the guidewire is withdrawn. A long introducer sheath placed across the bifurcation facilitates smooth tracking of catheters and permits check arteriography throughout the procedure whilst still maintaining the wire across the lesion.

Superficial femoral and popliteal arteries

1. An antegrade puncture is performed (pointing in the direction of arterial flow) aiming to hit the femoral artery as it passes over the femoral head. The skin puncture site is correspondingly higher than a retrograde puncture. US is invaluable in antegrade punctures and most experienced operators use it wherever possible.
2. A 15 mm J-guidewire can be used to select the required branch; usually the superficial femoral artery.
3. The guidewire is advanced almost down to the lesion, and a straight Teflon or polyethylene catheter is inserted over the guidewire to the same point. The wire is then gently passed across the lesion with the catheter following. Digital road mapping guidance is helpful in many instances. A van Andel dilation catheter may be useful once the lesion has been traversed by the guidewire.
4. If gentle injection of contrast medium outlines a channel parallel to the expected lumen, dissection has occurred. The catheter should be withdrawn and attempts made to regain the lumen.
5. When the lesion has been passed the catheter is exchanged for a balloon catheter (usually 5 mm in diameter), 3000 units of heparin are injected and dilation is performed. The distal 'run-off' should be carefully assessed on the post-angioplasty films; success is related to the adequacy of 'run-off' and it is necessary to ensure that there has been no distal embolization of thrombus or atheroma.

Catheter-directed arterial thrombolysis

1. Chemical thrombolysis plays a role in the treatment of acute ischaemia of the leg due to:
   (a) in situ thrombosis of a stenosed vessel
   (b) occluded lower-limb arterial bypass graft
   (c) thrombosed popliteal aneurysm with no demonstrable distal run-off

    (d) infra-inguinal embolus (sometimes iatrogenic post-angioplasty).

2. Thrombolysis should be undertaken in consultation with a vascular surgeon and should not compromise the leg unnecessarily by delaying surgical treatment. An acute episode less than 24 h old is more likely to respond to thrombolysis. After 14 days surgery is preferable to thrombolysis.[1]

3. Irreversible limb ischaemia requires amputation to avoid reperfusion syndrome.

4. Absolute contraindications to thrombolysis include stroke within the preceding 2 months, a recent gastrointestinal bleed and neurosurgery or head trauma. Relative contraindications are major trauma or surgery, severe hypertension, brain tumour and recent eye surgery.

5. Recombinant tissue plasminogen activator (rt-PA) is the most widely used agent in the UK. It can be used as local boluses of, for example, 5 mg at 5–10 min intervals or as a low-dose infusion at 0.5–2 mg h^{-1}.

6. Catheter placement for thrombolysis is typically achieved by passing a guidewire alongside or through the thrombus and advancing a catheter into the proximal end. The catheter is firmly fixed to the skin to prevent dislodgement. A bolus of rt-PA followed by infusion is then administered through the catheter and the patient returned to a high-dependency ward for observation for signs of haemorrhage. Monitoring of clotting factors such as fibrinogen levels does not predict the likelihood of haemorrhagic complications.

7. Depending on the initial progress and discretion of the operator the patient returns after several hours for check angiography through the catheter. If necessary, the catheter is advanced and infusion continued until satisfactory lysis, or the procedure is discontinued if progress is poor. Successful thrombolysis often reveals underlying stenoses as the cause of the occlusion. These are angioplastied at completion.

8. There are catheters manufactured for delivering fibrinolytics as a high-pressure spray through multiple side holes over several centimetres of occluded vessel. These may be used manually or connected to a dedicated pump that measures and times the 'pulse sprays'. This method has an added mechanical lytic effect and allows faster lysis. Other devices used in thrombolysis include hydrolyzing and mechanical thrombectomy catheters.

9. Bleeding complications are frequent, including haemorrhagic stroke in up to 2%.[2]

10. Thrombolysis is used widely wherever arterial and venous thrombosis occurs in the body. Many applications are not universally accepted and are off-license uses of the thrombolytic agent.

It is an important tool in the management of thrombosed haemodialysis access.

Aftercare

1. The pulses distal to the artery that has been dilated and the colour of the toes should be observed half-hourly for 4 h
2. Aspirin 150 mg daily (for life, unless there is a contraindication)
3. Reinforcement of the need to stop smoking.

Complications

Due to technique

1. Perforation of iliac artery leading to retroperitoneal haemorrhage
2. Embolization of clot or atheroma distally down either leg. This may be removed by aspiration thrombo-embolectomy or surgical embolectomy
3. Occlusion of main artery
4. Occlusion of collateral artery
5. Major groin haematoma formation, which may suddenly develop several hours after the procedure is completed
6. False aneurysm formation at the puncture site
7. Cholesterol embolization. Catheter manipulation disrupts atheroma and releases cholesterol crystals into the arterial circulation causing occlusion at arteriolar level. Pulses may be present and arteries patent angiographically, but patients are restless and develop severe tissue ischaemia in the affected vascular territory with skin mottling, limb loss, stroke, bowel infarction and renal failure.

References

1. Ouriel K, Shortell CK, DeWeese JA, et al. A comparison of thrombolytic therapy with operative revascularization in the initial treatment of acute peripheral arterial ischemia. J Vasc Surg 1994;19(6):1021–30.
2. Dawson K, Armon A, Braithwaite BD, et al. Stroke during intra-arterial thrombolysis: a survey of experience in the UK (abstr). Br J Surg 1996;83(S2):5–8.

Further Reading

Working Party on Thrombolysis in the Management of Limb Ischemia. Thrombolysis in the management of lower limb peripheral arterial occlusion a consensus document. J Vasc Interv Radiol 2003;14(9 Pt 2): S337–49.

VASCULAR EMBOLIZATION

Indications

1. To control bleeding – from the gastrointestinal and genitourinary tracts, from the lungs and after trauma
2. To infarct or reduce the blood supply to tumours or organs

3. To reduce or stop blood flow through arteriovenous malformations, aneurysms, fistulae or varicoceles
4. To reduce the blood flow in high-flow priapism
5. As treatment for uterine fibroids.

Equipment

1. Digital fluoroscopy unit with C-arm capable of angiography and preferably with 'road mapping' facilities.
2. Pre-shaped femoro-visceral catheters. These should not have side holes since their presence promotes clumping of particles and fibres at the catheter tip leading to blockage of the lumen. Size and shape will depend on the particular problem. Balloon occlusion catheters and co-axial catheters may also be useful.
3. Embolic materials:
   (a) Liquid – 50% dextrose, alcohol, quick-setting glues and polymers
   (b) Particulate – gel-foam, polyvinyl alcohol, autologous clot
   (c) Solid – metallic embolization coils, detachable balloons.

The material used depends on the lesion, its site and the duration of the occlusion required. Use of materials other than those listed has been reported.

Patient preparation

1. As for arteriography
2. Some procedures are painful and sedo-analgaesia may be needed (see Chapter 18).

Technique

Principles

1. All therapeutic occlusions are potentially dangerous: the expected gain must justify the risk.
2. Adequate knowledge of the vascular anatomy must be available before commencing.
3. The operator must be an experienced angiographer.
4. The lesion must be selectively catheterized. When permanent occlusion is required, the centre of the lesion should be filled with non-absorbable material (e.g. silicone spheres, polyvinyl-alcohol, polymer) before the supplying blood vessels are occluded.
5. Reflux of embolic material is likely to occur as the blood flow slows down; injection of emboli should be done slowly with intermittent gentle injections of contrast medium to assess flow and progress.
6. It is safer to come back another day than to continue for too long.

Aftercare

1. Observation of temperature pulse and blood pressure for signs of sepsis or bleeding

9

2. Observation of the tissues distal to the occluded vessel should be maintained for 24 h
3. Analgesia as required (patient-controlled administration).

Complications

1. Misplacement of embolic material: this may occur without the operator being aware that it has happened.
2. There may be propagation of thrombus, with embolization to the lungs or elsewhere.
3. Post-embolization syndrome results from infarcted tissue releasing toxins into the circulation. It comprises pain, fever, malaise, raised white cell count and inflammatory indices and transient impairment of renal function. Infarcted tissue can cause fever for up to 10 days. However, this tissue can become infected, and antibiotics may be required.

VASCULAR ULTRASOUND

US is a reliable, non-invasive, inexpensive test which is well tolerated by patients and widely used for assessment of the arterial system. Intra-abdominal or pelvic arteries can be examined with US, but it is best suited to relatively superficial vessels such as those of the neck or lower limb. Chest arteries cannot be assessed by US because the sound will not adequately penetrate air or bone. The main disadvantages of US are the marked operator-dependent nature of the technique and lengthy examination times for some studies.

The main components of arterial vascular US studies are:

1. Grey-scale US: gives anatomical information and detailed assessment of vessel wall including areas of intimal thickening or calcification
2. Pulsed-wave Doppler: measures changes in frequency of US waves reflected by moving blood within the vessel (Doppler shift). These data are used to calculate a detailed graph of direction and velocity of flow in the vessel. The normal pattern of flow differs between various arteries and flow patterns change at sites of disease such as narrowing (i.e. increases in velocity)
3. Colour Doppler: uses the same information as pulsed-wave Doppler but displays flow as colour superimposed in the arterial lumen on grey-scale imaging. Colour encoding represents the direction and velocity of flow with red conventionally indicating flow towards the US transducer and blue representing flow away from the transducer. Rapid flow is displayed as white or yellow. This is helpful in selection of regions for detailed assessment with pulsed-wave Doppler or detection of A-V fistulae or pseudo-aneurysm

4. Power Doppler: a modification of colour Doppler which is more sensitive to slow flow or flow in small structures. However, it does not give information on direction or velocity of flow.

Further Reading
Pellerito JS. Current approach to peripheral arterial sonography. Radiol Clin North Am 2001;39(3):553–67.

COMPUTED TOMOGRAPHIC ANGIOGRAPHY

As CT technology has developed during the past few years, particularly with the introduction of multidetector CT (MDCT) scanners with up to 256 (or more) slices, the quality and diagnostic usefulness of CT angiography (CTA) have improved dramatically.

CTA is performed as a block of very thin axial MDCT images obtained during the rapid peripheral intravenous (i.v.) infusion of iodinated contrast. The acquisition is timed to coincide with the peak density of contrast in arteries and the images subsequently re-constructed using post-processing techniques such as multiplanar reconstruction (MPR) or maximum intensity projections (MIP).

Although CTA involves administration of iodinated contrast (see Chapter 2) and significant radiation dose, there are many advantages: imaging is very rapid – usually less than 30 s to acquire the main dataset even for extended scans including lower limbs, scanners are readily available, unstable patients can be monitored with standard equipment, and valuable information is obtained about the blood vessel wall and surrounding structures.

9

PERIPHERAL (LOWER LIMB) COMPUTED TOMOGRAPHIC ANGIOGRAPHY

Descriptions of other specific CTA methods are found in appropriate chapters.

Indications
1. Lower-limb ischaemia
2. Arterio-venous malformation
3. Trauma.

Patient preparation
General precautions for use of ionizing radiation (Chapter 1) and iodinated contrast (Chapter 2). The nature and purpose of the examination is explained to the patient.

Technique

For optimum images a MDCT scanner with at least a 16-slice detector is used:

1. Contrast: 100–150 ml LOCM 300 mg I ml^{-1} (volume determined by scanner and scan protocol)
2. Contrast injection rate: 4 ml s^{-1} via a peripheral vein
3. Range: lower abdominal aorta to heel, or extended as upper abdominal aorta to heel
4. Slice thickness: 3 mm or less
5. Reconstruction increment: 0.6 mm
6. Delay:
   (a) Preset empirical delay, using manufacturer's guidelines for individual scanner
   OR, preferably,
   (b) Bolus tracking technique, choosing a region of interest (ROI) in the aorta just above the upper range of the scan and monitoring contrast density in ROI during injection until it reaches a predetermined value (usually 100–120 Hounsfield units), which triggers the CT acquisition. This is the preferred technique.

Aftercare and complications

For iodinated contrast see Chapter 2.

Further Reading

Chow LC, Rubin GD. CT angiography of the arterial system. Radiol Clin North Am 2002;40(4):729–49.

Duddalwar VA. Multislice CT angiography: a practical guide to CT angiography in vascular imaging and intervention. Br J Radiol 2004;77(Suppl. 1):S27–38.

MAGNETIC RESONANCE ANGIOGRAPHY

Guidelines on MR safety and selection of patients must be followed (see Chapter 1).

MR angiography (MRA) is now in widespread clinical use and is a highly sensitive and specific tool for assessment of the arterial system. For most examinations contrast-enhanced MRA with i.v. gadolinium (see Chapter 2) is now the preferred method. Gadolinium i.v. shortens the T1 relaxation time of blood so blood appears bright when imaged with a very short RT (repetition time) and other structures on the image appear dark. Timing of the contrast injection is critical. Imaging without contrast is used infrequently, but may be either a 'bright blood' cine technique, to demonstrate both anatomical and functional data, or 'black blood' imaging, which gives useful morphological information.

The thoracic and abdominal aorta, carotid arterial system and major branches of the aorta including, subclavian, coeliac, superior mesenteric and renal arteries, are routinely imaged with MRA. The pulmonary arteries are harder to image at MRA. Images are most often obtained as a block of thin coronal images (three-dimensional imaging) with contrast enhancement. Images are post-processed, including maximum-intensity projection (MIP) series.

Previously, the arteries of the pelvis and peripheral arteries of the lower limb were difficult to image due to limited longitudinal field of view in MR scanners. More recent developments including elongated MR coils and 'moving-table' multistation MRA have made high-quality examination of these vessels possible with a single injection of contrast and short imaging time. In some centres peripheral MRA is now routine and has replaced diagnostic catheter angiography.

Further Reading

Earls JP, Edelman RR. Magnetic resonance angiography: body applications. In: Edelman RR, Hesselink JR, Zlatkin MB, editors. Clinical Magnetic Resonance Imaging. Philadelphia: Saunders-Elsevier; 2006.

Ho VB, Corse WR. MR angiography of the abdominal aorta and peripheral vessels. Radiol Clin North Am 2003;41(1):115–44.

9

Venous system

Methods of imaging the venous system

1. Contrast venography
2. Ultrasound (US)
3. Impedance plethysmography
4. Radionuclide imaging
5. Computed tomography (CT)
6. Magnetic resonance imaging (MRI).

Further Reading

Kaufman JA, Lee MJ, editors. Vascular and Interventional Radiology:
   The Requisites. Philadelphia: Elsevier-Mosby; 2004.
Scarvelis D, Wells PS. Diagnosis and treatment of deep-vein thrombosis.
   Can Med Assoc J 2006;175(9):1087–92.

PERIPHERAL VENOGRAPHY

Intravenous (i.v.) peripheral venography is an invasive procedure
requiring i.v. injection of contrast medium and the use of ionizing
radiation. Marked limb swelling can result in failure to cannulate
a vein which precludes use of the technique. False-negative results
do occur. It is still considered the gold standard for diagnosis of
deep venous thrombosis, but is now only very rarely performed.

LOWER LIMB

Method

Intravenous venography.

Indications

1. Deep venous thrombosis
2. To demonstrate incompetent perforating veins (Doppler ultrasound
   is preferable)

3. Oedema of unknown cause
4. Congenital abnormality of the venous system.

Contraindications

Local sepsis.

Contrast medium

Low osmolar contrast material (LOCM) 240.

Equipment

1. Fluoroscopy unit with spot film device
2. Tilting radiography table.

Patient preparation

The leg should be elevated overnight to lessen oedema if leg swelling is severe.

Technique

1. The patient is supine and tilted 40° head up, to delay the transit time of the contrast medium.
2. A tourniquet is applied tightly just above the ankle to occlude the superficial venous system. The compression may also occlude the anterior tibial veins, and so their absence should not automatically be interpreted as due to venous thrombosis.
3. A 19G butterfly needle (smaller if necessary) is inserted into a vein on the dorsum of the foot. If the needle is too near the ankle, the contrast medium may bypass the deep veins and so give the impression of deep venous occlusion.
4. 40 ml of contrast medium is injected by hand. The first series of spot films is then taken.
5. A further 20 ml bolus is injected quickly whilst the patient performs a Valsalva manoeuvre to delay the transit of contrast medium into the upper thigh and pelvic veins. The patient is tilted quickly into a slightly head down position and the Valsalva manoeuvre is relaxed. Alternatively, if the patient is unable to comply, direct manual pressure over the femoral vein whilst the table is being tilted into the head-down position will achieve the same effect. Films are taken 2–3 s after releasing pressure.
6. At the end of the procedure the needle should be flushed with 0.9% saline to lessen the chance of phlebitis due to contrast medium.

Images

Collimated to include all veins:

1. Anterior posterior (AP) of calf
2. Both obliques of calf (foot internally and externally rotated)
3. AP of popliteal, common femoral and iliac veins.

Aftercare

The limb should be exercised.

Complications

Due to the contrast medium

1. As for the general complications of intravascular contrast media (Chapter 2)
2. Thrombophlebitis
3. Tissue necrosis due to extravasation of contrast medium. This is rare, but may occur in patients with peripheral ischaemia
4. Cardiac arrhythmia – more likely if the patient has pulmonary hypertension.

Due to the technique

1. Haematoma
2. Pulmonary embolus – due to dislodged clot or injection of excessive air.

UPPER LIMB

Method

Intravenous venography.

Indications

1. Oedema
2. To demonstrate the site of venous occlusion or stenosis
3. Superior vena cava obstruction.

Contrast medium

LOCM 300 mg I ml^{-1}.

Equipment

Fluoroscopy unit with spot film device.

Patient preparation

None.

Technique

For i.v. venography:

1. The patient is supine
2. An 18G butterfly needle is inserted into the median cubital vein at the elbow. The cephalic vein is not used, as this bypasses the axillary vein
3. Spot films are taken of the region of interest during a hand injection of 30 ml of contrast medium. Alternatively a digital subtraction angiographic run can be performed at 1 frame sec^{-1}.

10

Aftercare

None.

Complications

Due to the contrast medium
See Chapter 2.

CENTRAL VENOGRAPHY

SUPERIOR VENA CAVOGRAPHY

Indications

1. To demonstrate occlusion or stenosis of the central veins
2. As a preliminary examination in transvenous interventional techniques
3. Congenital abnormality of the venous system, e.g. left-sided superior vena cava.

Contrast medium

LOCM 370 mg I ml^{-1}, 60 ml.

Equipment

A C-arm with digital subtraction angiography.

Patient preparation

None.

Technique

1. The patient is supine
2. 18G butterfly needles are inserted into the median antecubital vein of both arms
3. Hand injections of contrast medium 30 ml per side are made simultaneously, as rapidly as possible, by two operators. The injection is recorded by rapid serial radiography (see 'Films' below). The film sequence is commenced after about two-thirds of the contrast medium has been injected.

N.B. If the study is to demonstrate a congenital abnormality, or on the rare occasion that the opacification obtained by the above method is too poor, a 5-F catheter with side holes, introduced by the Seldinger technique, may be used.

Images

Images are obtained at a rate of one frame s^{-1} for 10 s.

Aftercare

None, unless a catheter is used.

Complications

Due to the contrast medium
See Chapter 2.

INFERIOR VENA CAVOGRAPHY

Indications

1. To demonstrate the site of venous obstruction, displacement or infiltration
2. As a preliminary examination in transvenous interventional techniques
3. Congenital abnormality of the venous system.

Contrast medium

LOCM 370 mg I ml^{-1}, 40 ml.

Technique

1. With the patient supine, the catheter is inserted into the femoral vein using the Seldinger technique (see Chapter 9). A Valsalva manoeuvre may facilitate venepuncture by distending the vein. The vein can be punctured blindly by palpating the femoral artery pulsation and aiming to its medial side, but it is preferable to puncture the vein under direct US guidance.
2. Any obstruction to the passage of the catheter may indicate thrombus in the iliac veins or that the catheter and wire have entered an ascending lumbar vein. Fluoroscopy and gentle hand injection of contrast will clarify.
3. An injection of 40 ml of contrast medium is made at 20 ml s^{-1} by a pump injector, and recorded by rapid serial radiography or as a digital subtraction run at 2 frames s^{-1}.

Aftercare

1. Pressure at venepuncture site
2. Routine observations for 2 h.

Complications

Due to the contrast medium
See Chapter 2.

Due to the technique
See Chapter 9 – complications of catheter technique.

10

PORTAL VENOGRAPHY

Methods

1. Late-phase superior mesenteric angiography (see p. 77)
2. Trans-splenic approach (discussed below)
3. Paraumbilical vein catheterization
4. Transjugular transhepatic approach.[1]

Indications

1. To demonstrate prior to operation the anatomy of the portal system in patients with portal hypertension
2. To check the patency of a portosystemic anastomosis.

Contrast medium

LOCM 370 mg I ml^{-1}, 50 ml.

Equipment

1. Rapid serial radiography unit
2. Arterial catheter (SMA approach)
3. 10-cm needle (20G) with stilette and outer plastic sheath, e.g. Longdwell (trans-splenic approach).

Patient preparation

1. Admission to hospital. A surgeon should be informed in case complications of procedure arise (for the trans-splenic approach)
2. Clotting factors are checked
3. Severe ascites is drained
4. Nil orally for 5 h prior to the procedure
5. Premedication, e.g. diazepam 10 mg orally.

Technique

Superior mesenteric angiography
See page 77.

For trans-splenic approach
1. With the patient supine, the position of the spleen is percussed or identified with US. The access point is as low as possible in the midaxillary line, usually at the level of the tenth or eleventh intercostal space.
2. The region is anaesthetized using a sterile procedure.
3. The patient is asked to hold their breath in mid-inspiration, and the needle is then inserted inwards and upwards into the spleen (about three-quarters of the length of the needle is inserted, i.e. 7.5 cm). The needle and stilette are then withdrawn, leaving the

plastic cannula in situ. Blood will flow back easily if the cannula is correctly sited. The patient is then asked to breathe as shallowly as possible to avoid trauma to the spleen from excessive movement of the cannula.

4. A test injection of a small volume of contrast medium under screening control can be made to ensure correct siting of the cannula. If it has transfixed the spleen, simple withdrawal into the body of the spleen is not acceptable, as any contrast medium subsequently injected would follow the track created by the withdrawal. A new puncture is necessary.

5. When the cannula is in a satisfactory position, the splenic pulp pressure may be measured with a sterile manometer (normally 10–15 cmH$_2$O).

6. A hand injection of 50 ml of contrast medium is made over 5 s and recorded by rapid serial radiography/digital subtraction angiography. The cannula should be removed as soon as possible after the injection to minimize trauma to the spleen.

7. Occasionally a patent portal vein will fail to opacify, owing to major portosystemic collaterals causing reversed flow in the portal vein. The final arbiter of portal vein patency is direct mesenteric venography performed at operation. The maximum width of a normal portal vein is said to be 2 cm.

Images
Rapid serial radiography or digital subtraction runs: one image s^{-1} for 10 s.

Aftercare
1. Blood pressure and pulse; initially quarter-hourly, subsequently 4-hourly.
2. The patient must remain in hospital overnight.

Complications
Due to the contrast medium
See Chapter 2.

Due to the technique
1. Haemorrhage
2. Subcapsular injection
3. Perforation of adjacent structures (e.g. pleura, colon)
4. Splenic rupture
5. Infection
6. Pain (especially with an extra-capsular injection).

Due to the catheter
See Chapter 9.

Reference
1. Rösch J, Antonovic R, Dotter CT. Transjugular approach to the liver, biliary system, and portal circulation. Am J Roentgenol 1975;125(3):602–8.

Further Reading
Tamura S, Kodama T, Kihara Y, et al. Right anterior caudocranial oblique projection for portal venography; its indications and advantages. Eur J Radiol 1992;15(3):215–19.

TRANSHEPATIC PORTAL VENOUS CATHETERIZATION

Indications

To localize pancreatic hormone-secreting tumours before operation.

Contraindications

There are none specific to the technique. Ascites and hepatic cirrhosis make the procedure more difficult.

Contrast medium

LOCM 370 mg I ml^{-1}, to demonstrate anatomy and position of catheter.

Technique

1. 5-ml samples of blood are taken at points along the splenic vein, superior mesenteric vein and first part of the portal vein. The samples are numbered sequentially, and the site from which each was taken is marked on a sketch map of the portal drainage system. Simultaneous peripheral blood samples should be obtained at the same time as each portal sample to assess changing blood levels.
2. The accuracy of sampling can be improved by selective catheterization of pancreatic veins using varying shapes of catheter.[1]

Reference
1. Reichardt W, Ingemansson S. Selective vein catheterization for hormone assay in endocrine tumours of the pancreas: technique and results. Acta Radiol Diagn 1980;21(2A):177–87.

ULTRASOUND

Ultrasound is the most widely used imaging method for the venous system; the advantages are that it is low cost and readily available. It can be used to assess the following:

1. Lower limb veins
2. Upper limb veins
3. Abdominal veins including renal veins, hepatic and portal veins, and inferior vena cava
4. Venous anatomy to assist in central venous line placement, e.g. for the internal jugular or subclavian vein.

US is most commonly used for assessment of patients with suspected venous thrombosis, particularly of the lower limb. It is also useful to assess arterio-venous fistulae; both therapeutic fistulae created for haemodialysis and those occurring as a complication of interventional vascular procedures, and for pre-surgical planning in patients with varicose veins. Both duplex and colour Doppler techniques are utilized.

Duplex

Duplex scanning involves a combination of pulsed Doppler and real-time US for direct visualization. Expansion and filling of the normal echo-free lumen can be identified but slow-moving blood may be misinterpreted as thrombus. Valsalva manoeuvre will cause expansion in the normal vein but is not a totally reliable sign. Pulsed Doppler assesses flow. Enhancement of flow due to respiratory excursion or manual calf compression suggests patency. The most reliable sign of patency is compressibility. Direct pressure with the US probe over the vein will cause the normal vein to collapse. If thrombus is present, this will not occur.

Colour Doppler

Colour Doppler examination gives a visual representation of flow over a segment of vein.

10

LOWER LIMB VENOUS ULTRASOUND

Indications

1. Suspected deep vein thrombosis
2. Follow-up of known deep vein thrombosis
3. To guide access for interventional venous procedures.

Equipment

5–7.5-MHz transducer with colour Doppler.

Technique

1. Patient supine with foot-down tilt. The popliteal and calf veins can easily be examined with the patient sitting with legs dependent or lying on a tilted couch with flexed knees and externally rotated

hips. The femoral veins and external iliac veins are examined supine. The popliteal veins may be examined with the patient prone.

2. Longitudinal and transverse scans for external iliac, femoral and popliteal veins. For tibial and peroneal veins, these may be supplemented by oblique coronal scans.

3. Each vein may be identified by real-time scanning and colour Doppler. If in any doubt it may be confirmed as a vein by the spectral Doppler tracing. A normal patent vein should be completely occluded in real time by directly applied transducer pressure (though this is not always possible for the superficial femoral vein at the adductor canal).

4. The normal venous signal is phasic and in the larger veins varies with respiration. Flow can be stopped by a Valsalva manoeuvre and is transiently augmented by distal compression of the foot or calf. Acute thrombus may be non-echogenic but the vein should not be completely compressible nor fill with colour Doppler. Thrombus tends to become echogenic after a few days.

5. Although this technique is less well established for the exclusion of thrombus in the calf vessels, it has been shown to have a sensitivity and specificity close to that of venography. Cannulation of a vein and injection of contrast medium can thus be avoided.

UPPER LIMB VENOUS ULTRASOUND

Indications
As for lower limb US, upper limb US is much less commonly performed.

Equipment
5–7.5-MHz transducer with colour Doppler.

Technique
1. The patient should be recumbent on a couch wide enough to support the upper limb and trunk comfortably.

2. With the arm in a neutral position at the patient's side, the subclavian vein is assessed either from above or below the clavicle. The image plane is parallel to the long axis of the vein. Diagnostic criteria for upper limb thrombosis are the same as those used for the lower limb, but the Doppler waveform in the upper limb venous system is more pulsatile because of proximity to the heart. The upper limb also has a much more extensive network of potential collateral venous pathways and care should be taken to avoid confusion of a patent collateral vein with the potentially occluded deep venous structure under examination.

3. The arm is then abducted and the axillary and brachial veins examined. The transducer should be placed high in the axilla to identify the proximal axillary vein and the Doppler characteristics of the axillary and brachial veins followed to assess for spontaneous and phasic flow, and appropriate response to augmentation and Valsalva manoeuvre. Both transverse and longitudinal imaging planes should be used, including assessment of response to compression.

The examination can be extended to include the cephalic, basilic and forearm veins.

Further Reading

Hamper UM, DeJong MR, Scoutt LM. Ultrasound evaluation of the lower extremity veins. Radiol Clin North Am 2007;45(3):525–47.

Weber TM, Lockhart ME, Robbin ML. Upper extremity venous Doppler ultrasound. Radiol Clin North Am 2007;45(3):513–24.

IMPEDANCE PLETHYSMOGRAPHY

This technique depends on the principle of the capacity of the veins to fill and empty in response to temporary obstruction to venous outflow by occlusion of the thigh veins with a pneumatic cuff. Changes in calf volume produce changes in impedance measured by electrodes applied to the calf. The technique is demanding and requires skilled personnel. Clinical states that impair venous return, such as cardiac failure and pelvic pathology and also arterial insufficiency, produce abnormal results. Many centres use impedance plethysmography in conjunction with clinical pretest probability scoring and/or plasma D-dimer assay to identify patients who do not need to proceed to US or venography.[1]

Reference

1. Ginsberg JS, Kearon C, Douketis J, et al. The use of D-dimer testing and impedance plethysmographic examination in patients with clinical indications of deep vein thrombosis. Arch Intern Med 1997;157:1077–81.

RADIOISOTOPES

Thrombus may be imaged with ^{111}In- or ^{99m}Tc-in vitro-labelled platelets. These are of limited routine clinical application.

COMPUTED TOMOGRAPHY

Multidetector CT (MDCT) with standard i.v. contrast and scan delay protocols for the chest or abdomen/pelvis (see Chapter 1) is very effective for detection of compression or thrombosis of major veins including the superior and inferior vena cavae, iliac and renal veins.

Although it would be possible to perform direct lower-limb CT venography after infusion of contrast via a foot vein, this technique has found little application and is not used in clinical practice.

In a group of selected patients with suspected pulmonary embolus (PE), MDCT of the lower limbs from iliac crest to popliteal fossa, 2 min after completion of CT pulmonary angiography (indirect CT venography), may be used as an alternative to US for detection of lower limb deep venous thrombosis. However, there is a significant associated radiation dose and there is no diagnostic advantage over US.[1] Indirect CT venography is not recommended in patients with suspected deep vein thrombosis, but without suspected PE. It should only be used as an alternative to US in patients undergoing CT for suspected PE for whom identification of DVT is considered necessary[2] or those with a high probability of PE, including patients with history of previous venous thrombo-embolism and possible malignancy.[3]

References

1. Goodman LR, Stein PD, Matta F, et al. CT venography and compression sonography are diagnostically equivalent: data from PIOPED II. Am J Roentgenol 2007;189(5):1071–6.
2. Thomas SM, Goodacre SW, Sampson FC, et al. Diagnostic value of CT for deep vein thrombosis; results of a systematic review and meta-analysis. Clin Radiol 2008;63(3):299–304.
3. Hunsaker AR, Zou KH, Poh AC, et al. Routine pelvic and lower extremity CT venography in patients undergoing pulmonary CT angiography. Am J Roentgenol 2008;190(2):322–6.

MAGNETIC RESONANCE

Standard guidance applies on selection of patients suitable for MRI examination (see Chapter 1).

MRI is well suited to imaging the venous system, but because of cost and limited availability it is used infrequently. Peripheral MR venography (MRV)[1] is currently used in selected cases of venous thrombosis in pregnant subjects and where fractured limbs are immobilized in casts. It is useful in evaluation of congenital abnormalities of peripheral venous anatomy and venous malformations.

The multi-planar imaging capabilities allow demonstration of complex venous anatomy and cine sequences, including velocity-encoded phase mapping, can provide functional information regarding direction and velocity of venous blood flow. MRI can be used to 'age' thrombus and differentiate acute from chronic clot. MRV does not involve ionizing radiation and i.v. gadolinium has a wider safety profile than iodinated contrast used for CT. Imaging can be performed using slice-by-slice (two-dimensional) or volume (three-dimensional) acquisition. Post-processing techniques, including maximum-intensity projection (MIP) images, are used.

MRV sequences can be performed without i.v. contrast, e.g. time-of-flight imaging or phase contrast imaging sequences. However, these techniques are susceptible to signal loss due to slow flow or turbulence, and have largely been replaced by faster and more accurate i.v. gadolinium contrast-enhanced MRV studies.

MR venography offers unique diagnostic possibilities for abdominal, pelvic and thoracic veins,[2] and development of blood pool contrast agents (see Chapter 2) will further improve clinical usefulness of these procedures.[3]

References

1. Sampson FC, Goodacre SW, Thomas SM, et al. The accuracy of MRI in diagnosis of suspected deep vein thrombosis: systematic review and meta-analysis. Eur Radiol 2007;17(1):175–81.
2. Butty S, Hagspiel KD, Leung DA, et al. Body MR venography. Radiol Clin North Am 2002;40(4):899–919.
3. Prince MR, Sostman HD. MR venography: unsung and underutilized. Radiology 2003;226(3):630–2.

10

Radionuclide imaging in oncology and infection

POSITRON EMISSION TOMOGRAPHY IMAGING

Positron emission tomography (PET) imaging is a technique used to detect and accurately stage malignant disease, to differentiate benign and malignant tissue, and to assess response to treatment. Until recently, PET imaging availability was restricted due to high capital cost and logistics of radiopharmaceutical supply. It uses short-lived cyclotron-produced radionuclides such as [18]Fluorine, [11]Carbon, [13]Nitrogen and [15]Oxygen with half-lives of 110, 20, 10 and 2 min respectively. [18]Fluorine is the only one of these that has a half-life long enough to allow it to be produced off-site. This does permit 2-[^{18}F]fluoro-2-deoxy-d-glucose (^{18}F-FDG), the single most important PET radiopharmaceutical, to be used by sites without their own cyclotron.

The widespread acceptance of PET as a major advance is due to two major factors:

1. There is increased recognition in the literature of the role of the main PET tracer ^{18}F-FDG, a glucose analogue that is taken up in tissue in proportion to cellular glucose metabolism. This is particularly useful for tumour imaging, since most tumours have increased glucose metabolism and will concentrate FDG. Malignant cells are characterized by increased glucose transporter molecules at the cell surface. FDG is phosphorylated by the enzyme hexokinase to a polar intermediate which does not cross cell membranes well and is, therefore, trapped in the cell. Hexokinase levels and activity are increased in malignant cells. The reverse reaction (glucose-6-phosphatase) is slow and the enzyme is commonly deficient in cancer cells.
2. Integrated PET CT scanners are now widely available and are the standard of care. These units have separate PET and CT scanners installed in the same gantry. The patient undergoes a conventional

CT scan (usually performed with low exposure factors to reduce radiation dose) immediately followed by a PET scan without moving, on the same table-top. This allows fusion of the anatomical information from CT with the functional data from the PET scan, and hence accurate anatomical localization of metabolically active disease and recognition of normal anatomical and physiological uptake. The density data from the CT scan are also used to correct the PET data for differential attenuation of the emitted photons within the patient.

Normal physiological uptake is seen in organs that are hyper-metabolic and big glucose users, especially the brain and the heart, or active or recently active skeletal muscle. Variable uptake is seen in the gut and there is normal excreted urinary activity in the urinary tract. One confounding factor for interpretation may be normal physiological uptake in brown fat – particularly in the neck and paraspinal regions. Differentiation of this normal activity from pathology is greatly aided by the image registration afforded by combined PET CT scanners.

However, FDG is not specific for cancer cells as any hypermetabolic cell will show increased uptake of FDG such as those in sites of inflammation or infection, so interpretation with reference to full clinical details and other imaging is important to avoid false-positive scans.

As the only PET pharmaceutical currently widely available and widely used, this section is restricted to FDG imaging. Other pharmaceuticals tagged with carbon-11 or other short-lived isotopes are restricted to sites with a dedicated cyclotron. Other fluorine-labelled pharmaceuticals such as ^{18}F-choline are, however, being produced and have a role in imaging of prostate cancer metastases for example.

2-[^{18}F]FLUORO-2-DEOXY-D-GLUCOSE (^{18}F-FDG) PET SCANNING

Indications (oncology)

General

1. Distinguishing benign from malignant disease, e.g. lung nodules, brain lesions, etc.
2. Establishing the grade of malignancy, e.g. brain tumours, soft-tissue masses
3. Establishing the stage of disease, e.g. lung cancer, lymphoma, etc.
4. Establishing whether there is recurrent or residual disease, e.g. lymphoma, teratoma, seminoma, etc.
5. Establishing the site of disease in the face of rising tumour markers, e.g. colorectal, germ cell tumours, etc.

6. Establishing the response to therapy – pre, during and post therapy imaging
7. Identifying occult malignancy, e.g. paraneoplastic syndrome or the unknown primary in the setting of proven metastatic disease.

Specific

The following tumours are commonly imaged for staging and follow-up purposes and in cases of diagnostic difficulty:

1. Lung cancer
2. Lymphoma
3. Colorectal cancer
4. Oesophageal cancer
5. Melanoma
6. Thyroid cancer
7. Seminoma/teratoma
8. Sarcoma
9. Gynaecological cancer.

A full list of tumour-specific indications can be found in the 2012 guidance document produced by the Royal Colleges of Physicians and Radiologists listed under further reading.

Contraindications

1. Recent chemotherapy – minimum interval of 2–3 weeks recommended
2. Recent radiotherapy – minimum interval of 8–12 weeks recommended
3. Poorly controlled diabetes, i.e. serum glucose >8.5 mmol l^{-1} at time of scanning.

Patient preparation

1. Fasting for 4–6 h, with plenty of non-sugary fluids. Even a small snack or sweet can alter the pattern of ^{18}FDG uptake.
2. Measure blood glucose before injection to ensure it is not elevated. Elevated blood glucose levels result in diversion of glucose to muscle. Consider rescheduling patient if blood glucose elevated. Administration of insulin is counter-productive as this diverts glucose uptake to muscle.
3. A mild sedative such as diazepam may be given to reduce physiological muscle and brown fat uptake.
4. Oral contrast may be administered to aid interpretation of the CT. Previous concerns about attenuation correction artifact on the PET images secondary to the high-density contrast has been shown not to be clinically significant.

Technique

1. Up to the UK limit of 400 MBq ^{18}FDG intravenously (i.v.) (10 mSv effective dose (ED)) is administered.

11

2. To reduce muscle uptake of FDG, patients should remain in a relaxed environment such as lying in a darkened room (without talking if head and neck area are being imaged) between injection and scan.

3. Image at 1 h post injection.

4. Imaging is preferred with the arms above the head to reduce beam hardening artifact on the CT.

5. CT:
   (a) Low dose (example exposure factors 120 kv, 80 mAs)
   (b) No i.v. contrast medium
   (c) Positive or negative oral contrast agents according to local protocol may be used, but care should be taken with image interpretation as there may be bowel movement between the short initial CT scan and the 15–30 minutes taken for the PET acquisition.

6. PET:
   (a) From the base of skull to upper thighs (occasionally extended if melanoma or limb or head and neck tumours)
   (b) 3–4 min for each of 5–6 bed positions for the PET.

7. In some instances a diagnostic standard dose CT with i.v. contrast may be acquired as well, but in routine practice a diagnostic scan will usually be already available. A scan performed with i.v. contrast may result in attenuation artefacts on the reconstructed PET images if used for attenuation correction.

Other applications

Coronary artery disease (Chapter 8)
Assessment of myocardial viability.

Neurology (Chapter 13)
1. Location of epileptic foci
2. Assessment of dementia.

Imaging of infection and inflammation
See last section of this chapter.

Further reading
Cook GJ, Wegner EA, Fogelman I. Pitfalls and artifacts in ^{18}FDG PET and PET/CT oncologic imaging. Semin Nucl Med 2004;34(2):122–33.

Kapoor V, McCook BM, Torok FS. An introduction to PET CT imaging. RadioGraphics 2004;24(2):523–43.

Rohren EM, Turkington TG, Coleman RE. Clinical applications of PET in oncology. Radiology 2004;231(2):305–32.

The Royal College of Physicians and the Royal College of Radiologists. Evidence based guidelines for the use of PET CT in the United Kingdom 2012. London: The Royal College of Physicians and the Royal College of Radiologists; 2012.

von Schulthess GK, Steinert HC, Hany TF. Integrated PET/CT: current applications and future directions. Radiology 2006;238(2):405–22.

GALLIUM RADIONUCLIDE TUMOUR IMAGING

This is rarely used, having almost entirely been superseded by cross-sectional techniques and PET scanning.[1] The main disadvantages are the high radiation dose, the extended nature of the investigation, its non-specific nature, and difficulties in interpretation in the abdomen due to normal bowel activity.

Indications

1. Hodgkin's and non-Hodgkin's lymphoma: assessment of residual masses after therapy and early diagnosis of recurrence[1]
2. Gallium imaging has been used with variable success in a variety of other tumours, e.g. hepatoma, bronchial carcinoma, multiple myeloma and sarcoma
3. It has also been used in benign conditions such as sarcoidosis and for localization of infection or in suspected orthopaedic infection.

Contraindications

None.

Radiopharmaceutical

^{67}Ga-Gallium citrate, 150 MBq maximum (17 mSv ED).

Normal accumulation is seen in the liver, bone marrow and nasal sinuses, and variably in the spleen, salivary and lacrimal glands. There is significant excretion via the gut and some via the kidneys. ^{67}Ga has a half-life of 78 h and principal γ-emissions at 93, 185 and 300 keV, so image quality is fairly poor.

Equipment

1. Gamma camera, preferably with whole-body and single-photon emission computed tomography (SPECT) facilities
2. Medium- or high-energy collimator.

Patient preparation

If the abdomen is being investigated, laxatives may be given (if not contraindicated) for 2 days after injection of ^{67}Ga-citrate to clear bowel activity. Additionally, an enema or suppository may be given on the day of imaging.

Technique

1. ^{67}Ga-citrate is administered i.v.
2. Delayed images are acquired as below with energy windows about the lower two or all three of the main photopeaks.

11

Images

1. 48 and 72 h. Whole-body, spot views and single photon emission computed tomography (SPECT) as appropriate. SPECT can increase the sensitivity and specificity of the investigation
2. Non-specific bowel activity can be discriminated by imaging on two separate occasions. Activity in bowel contents should move between scans and abnormal areas of accumulation will be stationary. If there is still any doubt at 72 h, later images at up to 7 days may prove helpful.

Additional techniques

1. A radionuclide bone scan may be performed prior to gallium imaging
2. A radiocolloid scan may help to discriminate between lesions in the region of the liver or spleen and normal uptake in these organs. Image subtraction techniques may be used.

Aftercare

Normal radiation safety precautions.

Complications

None.

Reference

1. Seam P, Juweid ME, Cheson BD. The role of FDG-PET scans in patients with lymphoma. Blood 2007;110(10):3507–16.

Further Reading

Bombardieri E, Aktolun C, Baum RP, et al. ^{67}Ga scintigraphy: procedure guidelines for tumour imaging. Eur J Nucl Med Mol Imaging 2003;30(12):BP125–31.

Front D, Bar-Shalom R, Israel O. The continuing clinical role of gallium 67 scintigraphy in the age of receptor imaging. Semin Nucl Med 1997;27(1):68–74.

Palestro CJ, Love C, Tronco GG, et al. Role of radionuclide imaging in the diagnosis of postoperative infection. RadioGraphics 2000;20:1649–60.

RADIOIODINE METAIODOBENZYLGUANIDINE SCAN

Metaiodobenzylguanidine (MIBG) is a noradrenaline (norepinephrine) analogue. It is taken up actively across cell membranes of sympathetic and adrenal medullary tissue into intracellular storage vesicles. There is no further metabolism, and it remains sequestered and localized in the storage vesicles of catecholamine-secreting tumours and tumours of neuroendocrine origin.[1]

Indications

Localization and staging of the following tumours of neuroendocrine origin:

1. Neuroblastoma
2. Phaeochromocytoma
3. Carcinoid tumours
4. Medullary thyroid carcinoma
5. Other neuroendocrine tumours.

Contraindications

None.

Radiopharmaceuticals

1. ^{123}Iodine(I)-metaiodobenzylguanidine (MIBG), 250 MBq typical, 400 MBq max (6 mSv ED with thyroid blockade). The 13-h half-life of ^{123}I allows imaging up to 48 h
2. ^{131}I-labelled MIBG is also available, and is still in common use outside Europe where ^{123}I-MIBG is not made commercially. However, the higher photon energy of the emitted gamma rays renders it an inferior imaging agent and results in a higher radiation dose to the patient. It should only be considered where ^{123}I-MIBG cannot be obtained.

Equipment

1. Gamma-camera, preferably with whole-body imaging and SPECT capabilities. Many centres are now using hybrid CT-SPECT cameras for improved anatomical localization and consequently improved specificity
2. Low-energy general purpose collimator for ^{123}I.

Patient preparation

1. Where possible, stop medications that interfere with MIBG uptake.[2] These include tricyclic antidepressants, antihypertensives, cocaine, sympathomimetics, decongestants containing pseudoephedrine, phenylpropanolamine and phenylephrine (many available over the counter) and others.
2. Thyroid blockade, to reduce radiation dose to the thyroid continuing for 24 h after ^{123}I-MIBG injection:
   (a) Adults – either oral potassium perchlorate (400 mg, 1 h before MIBG injection, then 200 mg every 6 h) or oral potassium iodate (85 mg twice daily starting 24 h before MIBG injection)
   (b) Children – Lugol's iodine 0.1–0.2 ml diluted with water or milk three times a day starting 48 h before MIBG injection. Potassium iodate is more palatable – the tablets need splitting for paediatric dosage.

11

Technique

1. MIBG is administered slowly i.v. over 1–2 min (a fast injection may cause adrenergic side-effects)
2. Imaging at 24 h (sometimes additionally at 4 or 48 h), emptying bladder before pelvic views.

Images

1. Anterior and posterior abdomen, 10–20 min per view
2. Whole-body imaging for comprehensive search for metastases
3. SPECT may help to localize lesions, particularly in thorax and abdomen. Hybrid CT-SPECT scanners will help anatomical localization.

Additional techniques

1. If therapy with ^{131}I-MIBG is being considered, quantitative assessment can be performed using geometric mean and attenuation correction to calculate percentage of administered dose residing in tumour at 24 h
2. ^{111}In-octreotide, which binds to somatostatin receptors frequently expressed in neuroendocrine and other tumours, is an alternative imaging agent to MIBG. It appears to be more sensitive for carcinoids, and may be useful in cases where the MIBG scan is negative. It also has therapeutic analogues under development
3. PET imaging with novel radiopharmaceuticals such as 18-F fluorodopamine and 18-F fluorodopa is available in only a few centres but has been reported to offer additional value over MIBG.[3,4] Conventional 18-F FDG PET imaging is also of value in assessing metastatic disease.

Aftercare

Normal radiation safety precautions (see Chapter 1).

Complications

None.

References

1. Ilias I, Divgi C, Pacak K. Current role of metaiodobenzylguanidine in the diagnosis of pheochromocytoma and medullary thyroid cancer. Semin Nucl Med 2011;41:364–8.
2. Solanki KK, Bomanji J, Moyes J, et al. A pharmacological guide to medicines which interfere with the biodistribution of radiolabelled meta-iodobenzylguanidine (MIBG). Nucl Med Commun 1992;13(7):513–21.
3. Chrisoulidou1 A, Kaltsas G, Ilias I, et al. The diagnosis and management of malignant phaeochromocytoma and paragangliomas. Endocrine-Related Cancer 2007;14:569–85.
4. Timmers H, Chen C, Jorge A, et al. Comparison of 18f-fluoro-l-dopa, 18f-fluoro-deoxyglucose, and 18f-fluorodopamine pet and 123i-mibg scintigraphy in the localization of pheochromocytoma and paragangliomas. J Clin Endocrinol Metab 2009;94:4757–67.

SOMATOSTATIN RECEPTOR IMAGING

Somatostatin is a physiological neuropeptide which has biological effects including inhibition of growth hormone release, and suppression of insulin and glucagon excretion. Octreotide (a long-acting analogue of the human hormone, somatostatin) can be used therapeutically to inhibit hormone production by carcinoids, gastrinomas and insulinoma, etc. A number of tumours, particularly those of neuroendocrine origin, express neuroendocrine receptors. Imaging after the administration of radionuclide-labelled somatostatin analogues such as octreotide, therefore, allows their localization.[1,2]

Indications

Localization and staging of the following tumours of neuroendocrine origin:

1. Carcinoid
2. Gastrinoma
3. Phaeochromocytoma
4. Medullary cell cancer thyroid
5. Small cell lung cancer
6. Pituitary.

Although sometimes used for the assessment of insulinomas, these latter tumours are more variably visible with octreotide (approx. 50%) than carcinoids, gastrinomas and phaeochromocytomas, which are seen in 80–100% of cases.

Contraindications

None.

Radiopharmaceuticals

[111]Indium (In) pentetreotide (a DTPA conjugate of octreotide) 220 MBq i.v. (ED 17 mSv).

Equipment

1. Gamma-camera, preferably with whole-body imaging and SPECT capabilities
2. Medium energy for [111]In.

Patient preparation

1. Some centres use bowel preparation
2. Oral hydration to help with renal clearance. There is usually high renal uptake.

11

3. In patients with possible insulinoma i.v. glucose should be available because of a small risk of inducing hypoglycaemia

4. Discontinue oral somatostatin to avoid competitive inhibition.

Technique

Image at 24 h and 48 h if necessary:

1. Anterior and posterior abdomen, 10–20 min per view

2. Whole-body imaging for comprehensive search for metastases

3. SPECT and now hybrid CT-SPECT scanners are increasingly available and will help anatomical localization, and improve specificity by differentiating tumour uptake from bowel uptake for example.

Additional techniques

MIBG may be positive in octreotide-negative tumours and vice versa.

Other novel agents for conventional isotope and PET imaging have been investigated.[2]

Aftercare

Normal radiation safety precautions (see Chapter 1).

Complications

None.

References

1. Krenning EP, Kwekkeboom DJ, Bakker WH, et al. Somatostatin receptor scintigraphy with [^{111}In-DTPA-D-Phe1] and [^{123}I-Tyr3]-octreotide: the Rotterdam experience with more than 1000 patients. Eur J Nucl Med 1993;20(8):716–31.
2. Rufini V, Calcagni M, Baum R. Imaging of neuroendocrine tumors. Sem Nucl Med 2006;36:228–47.

LYMPH NODE AND LYMPHATIC CHANNEL IMAGING

RADIOGRAPHY

On plain films lymph nodes may show:

1. Directly:
   (a) as a soft tissue mass, e.g. hilar lymph glands on a chest X-ray
   (b) calcified nodes, e.g. following tuberculosis or treatment of malignancy.

2. Indirect evidence from displacement of normal structures, e.g. displacement of ureters seen during excretion urography.

ULTRASOUND

Advantages

1. Non-invasive and without risk to the patient
2. Helpful in the neck and axilla in particular, especially with morphological and Doppler analysis and US-guided fine-needle aspiration or core biopsy.

Disadvantages

Intestinal gas is a major factor in poor visualization of abdominal nodes. Unsuitable for the mediastinum.

COMPUTED TOMOGRAPHY

Technique is dealt with in other chapters.

Advantages

1. Can image all nodes
2. Technically easy to perform.

Disadvantages

1. Internal nodal structure is not seen
2. Gives no indication of nature, apart from on the basis of size, and possibly on basis of enhancement characteristics.

11

MAGNETIC RESONANCE IMAGING

Technique is dealt with in other chapters.

Advantages

1. Can image all nodes
2. Technically easy to perform.

Disadvantages

1. Internal structure is not seen
2. Gives no indication of nature, apart from on the basis of size.

RADIOGRAPHIC LYMPHANGIOGRAPHY

This is a technically difficult and invasive examination requiring limited operative exposure of lymphatic vessels for cannulation, usually in the feet. Lipiodol, the usual contrast material, is no longer available and operator expertise is also largely no longer available. It has been superseded by cross-sectional imaging techniques such as US, CT and MRI, and functional assessment with FDG PET and some other radionuclide imaging procedures.

RADIONUCLIDE LYMPHOSCINTIGRAPHY

Lymphoscintigraphy provides a less invasive alternative to conventional lymphography. High-resolution anatomical detail is not possible (see MR lymphangiography under further techniques below).

Indications

1. Localization of the 'sentinel' node in breast carcinoma[2,3] and malignant melanoma[4] using a hand-held probe. In recent years, this has become the major indication for lymphoscintigraphy. The technique in itself does not diagnose nodes affected by malignancy; rather it identifies the node most likely to be involved and, therefore, to allow histological sampling. Although still awaiting completion of long-term clinical trials, the early indications are that if the first or 'sentinel' node in the lymphatic drainage chain from the primary site is shown to have negative histology (approx. 60% of cases in breast cancer), then more extensive nodal clearance and associated morbidity can be avoided. SPECT CT can improve anatomical localization[4]
2. Differentiation of lymphoedema from venous oedema
3. Assessment of lymphatic flow in lymphoedema.[5]

Contraindications

Hypersensitivity to human albumin products.

Radiopharmaceuticals

1. [99m]Technetium (Tc)-nanocolloidal albumin (particle size <80 nm), 40 MBq maximum (0.4 mSv ED) total for all injections. The colloid

is injected intradermally and cleared from the interstitial space by lymphatic drainage.

2. A number of other colloids are used around the world for sentinel node imaging, and other radiopharmaceuticals have been used for lymphoscintigraphy.

Equipment

1. Gamma-camera
2. High-resolution general purpose collimator.

Patient preparation

Clean injection sites.

Technique

1. Sentinel node imaging:
   Example protocols are:
   (a) breast carcinoma: inject ^{99m}Tc-colloid in approximately 5 ml volume intradermally for palpable lesions and around the tumour under US guidance for non-palpable lesions
   (b) melanoma: inject ^{99m}Tc-colloid intradermally in a ring of locations around the melanoma site, with a volume of about 0.1 ml for each injection.

   Static images are taken at intervals until the first node is seen. For breast cancer, take anterior and left or right lateral images with the arm raised as for surgery. Mark the skin over the node in both axes to guide surgical incision and intraoperative location with a gamma-detecting probe.

   With effectively no background activity in the body, anatomical localization on the images is needed. A ^{57}Cobalt flood source (usually available for routine camera quality assurance) can be placed for a short period under the imaging couch to produce a body outline on the image.

2. Other anatomical sites of investigation or for investigation of lymphatic drainage/lymphoedema:
   (a) 99mTc-colloid in 0.1–0.3 ml volume is injected intradermally at sites depending upon the area to be studied, e.g. for nodes below diaphragm and lower limb drainage – injections in each foot in the first and second web spaces for drainage or over the lateral dorsum of the foot for lymphatics or for axillary nodes and upper limb drainage injections in each hand in the second and third web spaces
   (b) Static images are taken of the injection site(s) immediately, followed by injection site, drainage route and liver images at intervals, e.g. 15, 30, 60 and 180 min, continuing up to 24 h

11

or until the liver is seen. Visualization of the liver indicates patency of at least one lymphatic channel (except early liver activity within 15 min, which implies some colloid entry into blood vessels).

Analysis

If more frequent imaging or a long dynamic study is performed, time–activity curves for regions along the drainage route can be plotted and used to quantify flow impairment.

Aftercare

Normal radiation safety precautions.

Complications

Anaphylactic reaction – rare.

Other techniques – MR lymphangiography[6]

Although this technique has not yet been widely taken up, this is equivalent to radionuclide lymphoscintigraphy in principle but provides high-resolution anatomical imaging and direct visualization of draining lymph vessels. Instead of radionuclide agents, small volumes of gadolinium-based MR contrast agents are injected intracutaneously into the webspaces of the feet or other relevant anatomical area. T2 weighted imaging is used to demonstrate the lymphoedema, and post contrast a 3D spoiled gradient-echo sequence (volumetric interpolated breath-hold examination [VIBE]) at multiple time intervals up to an hour is used to demonstrate the lymph channels directly.

References

1. Harisinghani MG, Barentsz J, Hahn PF, et al. Noninvasive detection of clinically occult lymph-node metastases in prostate cancer. New Engl J Med 2003;348(25):2491–9.
2. Krynyckyi BR, Kim CK, Goyenechea MR, et al. Clinical breast lymphoscintigraphy: optimal techniques for performing studies, image atlas, and analysis of images. RadioGraphics 2004;24(1):121–45.
3. Husarik DB, Steinert HC. Single-photon emission computed tomography/computed tomography for sentinel node mapping in breast cancer. Semin Nucl Med 2007;37(1):29–33.
4. Intenzo CM, Truluck CA, Kushen MC, et al. Lymphoscintigraphy in cutaneous melanoma: an updated total body atlas of sentinel node mapping. RadioGraphics 2009;29(4):1125–35.
5. Witte CL, Witte MH, Unger EC, et al. Advances in imaging of lymph flow disorders. RadioGraphics 2000;20(6):1697–719.
6. Lohrmann C, Foeldi E, Speck O, et al. High-resolution MR lymphangiography in patients with primary and secondary lymphedema. Am J Roentgenol 2006;187(2):556–61.

RADIONUCLIDE IMAGING OF INFECTION AND INFLAMMATION

A number of radionuclide techniques exist for this, the most commonly used of which is radionuclide-labelled leucocyte imaging.[1,2] The ready availability and sensitivity for collections and inflammation of anatomical imaging techniques such as US and CT has, however, reduced the demand for radionuclide procedures.

Indications

1. Diagnosis and localization of obscure infection and inflammation in soft tissue and bone
2. Assessment of inflammatory activity in disorders such as inflammatory bowel disease, e.g. Crohn's.

Contraindications

None.

Radiopharmaceuticals

1. ^{111}In-labelled leucocytes, 20 MBq maximum (9 mSv ED). ^{111}In-oxine, tropolonate and acetylacetonate are highly lipophilic complexes that will label leucocytes, erythrocytes and platelets. The leucocytes have to be labelled in vitro and the labelled cell suspension reinjected. ABO/Rh-matched donor leucocytes can be used with neutropenic patients or to reduce infection hazard in HIV-positive patients.[111]In has a half-life of 67 h and principal gamma emissions at 171 and 245 keV. There is no confounding uptake in bowel and this technique may be more suitable for chronic or more low-grade infections because of the longer imaging window (4–48 h).
2. ^{99m}Tc-hexamethylpropyleneamineoxime (HMPAO)-labelled leucocytes, 200 MBq max (3 mSv ED). HMPAO is also a highly lipophilic complex which preferentially labels granulocytes. The cell-labelling technique is similar to that for ^{111}In, but HMPAO has the advantage that kits can be stocked and used at short notice. There is more bowel uptake as a result of biliary excretion than with ^{111}In-labelled leucocytes, so images must be taken earlier than 4 h post injection for diagnosis of abdominal infection. The ^{99m}Tc label delivers a lower radiation dose than ^{111}In-labelled leucocytes and has better imaging resolution, which can, for example, help to identify inflammation in small bowel.
3. ^{67}Ga-gallium citrate, 150 MBq max (17 mSv ED). This localizes in inflammatory sites. Formerly the most commonly used agent, it has now largely been replaced by labelled leucocyte imaging.

11

There is significant bowel activity up to 72 h, so delayed imaging may be necessary for suspected abdominal infection, and accuracy in the abdomen is less than elsewhere. ^{67}Ga, with a T1/2 of 78 h and principal γ-emissions at 93, 185 and 300 keV, delivers a significantly higher radiation dose than ^{99m}Tc-HMPAO- and 111In-labelled leucocytes, but it has the advantage of requiring no special preparation.

4. ^{99m}Tc- or ^{111}In-human immunoglobulin (HIG). This is an agent for which a commercial kit is available for ^{99m}Tc labelling. It has the advantage of not requiring a complex preparation procedure, but its place relative to labelled leucocytes is still a matter of debate.

5. ^{99m}Tc-sulesomab (Leukoscan). This is another commercial agent comprising a labelled antigranulocyte monoclonal antibody fragment. It also has a simple preparation procedure, and is finding a role in the diagnosis of orthopaedic infections.

6. ^{18}F-FDG PET has been used to evaluate obscure infection or suspected infection of orthopaedic hardware.

Equipment

1. Gamma camera, preferably with whole body imaging facility
2. Low-energy high-resolution collimator for ^{99m}Tc, medium-energy for ^{111}In, medium- or high-energy for ^{67}Ga.

Patient preparation

None.

Technique

1. The radiopharmaceutical is administered intravenously
2. Image timing depends upon the radiopharmaceutical used and the suspected source of infection. Whole-body imaging may be employed for all of the radiopharmaceuticals:
    (a) ^{111}In-labelled white cells. Static images are acquired at 3 and 24 h post injection. Further imaging at 48 h may prove helpful
    (b) ^{99m}Tc-HMPAO-labelled white cells. For suspected abdominal infections, image at 0.5 and 2 h, i.e. before significant normal bowel activity is seen. For other sites, image at 1, 2 and 4 h. Additional 24-h images may be useful
    (c) ^{67}Ga-citrate. Images are acquired at 48 and 72 h for regions where normal bowel, urinary and blood pool activity may obscure abnormal collection sites. Later images may prove helpful in non-urgent cases. Extremities and urgent cases may be imaged from as early as 6 h. If not contraindicated, laxatives given for 48 h post injection will help to clear bowel activity.

Additional techniques

1. The diagnosis of bone infection may be improved by combination with three-phase radioisotope bone scanning or bone marrow imaging
2. Comparison with a radiocolloid scan may help to discriminate between infection in the region of the liver or spleen and normal uptake in these organs.

Aftercare

Normal radiation safety precautions (see Chapter 1).

Complications

None.

References
1. Peters AM, Lavender JP. Editorial. Imaging inflammation with radiolabelled white cells; ^{99m}Tc-HMPAO or ^{111}In. Nucl Med Commun 1991;12:923–5.
2. Love C, Palestro CJ. Radionuclide imaging of infection. J Nucl Med Technol 2004;32(2):47–57.

11

Bones and joints

Imaging modalities

1. **Plain films**. These are cheap, widely available and valuable screening tools in the preliminary assessment of osteoarticular symptoms. Standard views require a minimum of two views perpendicular to each other, e.g. antero-posterior and lateral projections. The pathological processes underlying osteolysis and osteosclerosis, e.g. infection, tumours, articular erosions, etc., are well advanced before they become radiographically visible and radiographs may appear normal despite the presence of significant bone and joint disease. Although there are limitations, plain films are very useful in the characterization and differential diagnosis of disease, e.g. trauma, bone tumours, arthritis. Despite the recent advances in imaging techniques, the radiograph remains the single most important investigation in the characterization of bone tumours.

2. **Arthrography**. The injection of radiographically positive (iodinated) and negative (air) contrast medium directly into the joint allows radiographic assessment of articular structures in conventional arthrography. The examination can then be supplemented with CT (CT arthrography) which provides more detailed assessment of intra-articular status and structures using bone and soft-tissue window settings. For optimal evaluation, reformatted CT images in three planes with MDCT are obtained. Arthrography using a dilute gadolinium-DTPA solution and imaging with MRI (MR arthrography) is increasingly used in the study of large joint disease, e.g. shoulder, hip and, to a lesser extent, wrist, elbow and ankle.

3. **Radionuclide imaging**. Bone scintigraphy enjoys a high sensitivity but a low specificity. It is widely used in the detection and follow-up of metastatic disease, characterization of lesions shown by other imaging modalities, and as a sensitive test for the detection of pathology such as infection.

4. **Ultrasound (US)**. Advances in US technology have increasingly been applied to musculoskeletal disorders in both adult and paediatric age groups. Peri-articular structures (capsule, ligaments, and tendons) are optimally imaged. Under US-guidance, therapy to soft-tissue disease can be accurately targeted, joint fluid aspirated and arthrographic agents instilled into joints.

5. **Computed tomography (CT)**. This is very useful in complex bone trauma for accurate surgical planning and also in many applications in assessment of bone tumours and infection. Joint anatomy and pathology in joints which are difficult to image in two perpendicular planes and in which there is bone overlap, e.g. shoulder, hip, sternoclavicular, sacroiliac joints are best depicted using CT. When employed in CT arthrography, the intra-articular status of joints can be optimally assessed.

6. **Magnetic resonance imaging (MRI)**. MRI is the best imaging modality for joint assessment. In many joints, e.g. knee, it can be employed as the first and only means of imaging. In other joints, e.g. shoulder, MRI alone is used to image the rotator cuff, but MR arthrography is required for optimal imaging of the ligaments, capsule and labrum in post-traumatic instability. Direct MR arthrography using intra-articular injection of dilute gadolinium solution is also employed, in the hip primarily to image the labrum and in the wrist to assess the interosseous ligaments of the proximal carpal row and the triangular fibrocartilage. Indirect MR arthrography following intravenous (i.v.) injection of gadolinium-DTPA, which quickly diffuses into the joint via the synovium, is used in the detection and quantification of active synovitis, e.g. rheumatoid arthritis. This is particularly of value in small joints and in the post-operative assessment of large joints. MRI is widely used in the assessment of bone pathology such as tumour or infection.

MUSCULOSKELETAL MAGNETIC RESONANCE IMAGING – GENERAL POINTS

1. The large variety of MR sequences provides an opportunity to tailor the sequences to the tissues that need to be optimally imaged. See Table 12.1.
2. I.v. gadolinium-DTPA is used in musculoskeletal imaging for:
   (a) infections – to differentiate abscess from phlegmon
   (b) tumours – to differentiate viable tumour from necrosis – to differentiate solid from cystic components
   (c) post-operative spine – to differentiate recurrent disc herniation from scar tissue
   (d) synovial disease, e.g. rheumatoid arthritis – to determine activity/response to treatment

Table 12.1 Optimizing magnetic resonance imaging sequences for musculoskeletal tissues

Tissue type	Optimal magnetic resonance (MR) imaging sequences		
Bone	T1	STIR	T2 fat sat
Cartilage	GRE + fat sat	T2 fat sat	PD fat sat
Labrum	T1 fat sat (MR arthrogram)	T1 spin echo (MR arthrogram)	GRE T2*
Meniscus	T1	GRE T2*	PD fat sat
Tendons/ligaments	T2 fat sat	GRE T2*	T1
Muscle	T1	STIR	T1 fat sat
Marrow	T1	STIR	PD fat sat
Synovium	T1 fat sat (i.v. gadolinium)	T1 spin echo (i.v. gadolinium)	T1

STIR = short tau inversion recovery; GRE = gradient echo; PD = proton density.

   (e) avascular necrosis, e.g. Perthes' disease, scaphoid fracture – to show viable tissue

   (f) indirect MR arthrography – to delineate articular cartilage status, meniscal repair.

3. MR arthrography. Direct MR arthrography involves joint puncture and the intra-articular injection of a dilute gadolinium solution (saline and local anaesthetic can also be used). The amount of gadolinium needed to produce contrast by shortening the T1 effect of fluid is very small and too much gadolinium-DTPA results in signal loss of the fluid ('black out'). Gadolinium-DTPA is, therefore, diluted in a ratio of 1:100 with sterile saline solution before use. The joint is distended and the recesses filled, delineating the intra-articular structures and separating them from adjacent tissues. In the lower limb, it allows accurate visualization of the labrum of the hip, the operated meniscus in the knee, and the impingement ankle syndromes, demonstrating associated osteochondral defects, loose bodies and synovial pathology more reliably than conventional MRI. In the upper limb, it is mostly utilized in the unstable shoulder to assess the damaged osteoarticular structures, the elbow and wrist joints. T1 spin echo and T1 fat-saturated sequences are used routinely in MR arthrography along with a T2 sequence in at least one plane to detect cysts, bone and soft-tissue oedema. Traction applied to joints at MR arthrography improves visualization of certain structures, e.g. long head of biceps origin in the shoulder, articular

12

cartilage in the hip. MR arthrography avoids the requirement for diagnostic arthroscopy and aids in the therapeutic plan.

Further reading

Bergin D, Schweitzer ME. Indirect MR arthrography. Skeletal Radiol 2003;32:551–8.

Peh WC, Cassar-Pullicino VN. Magnetic resonance arthrography: current status. Clin Radiol 1999;54:575–87.

ARTHROGRAPHY – GENERAL POINTS

1. The conventional radiographs should always be reviewed prior to the procedure.
2. Aspiration of an effusion should always be performed before contrast medium is injected. The aspirate should be sent, where appropriate, for microscopy, culture (aerobic and anaerobic) and sensitivity, crystal analysis, cytology and biochemistry.
3. Conventional arthrography has largely been replaced by MRI, e.g. knee. It is still the mainstay for diagnosing adhesive capsulitis, and in demonstrating the exact site of abnormal articular communications, e.g. wrist and foot. Most arthrograms are currently carried out as a prelude to either CT or MR arthrography.
4. If a needle is correctly sited within a joint space, a test injection of a small volume of contrast medium will stream away from the needle tip around the joint. However, if it is incorrectly sited, the contrast medium will remain in a diffuse cloud around the tip of the needle. For this reason, it is important that the fluoroscopy-guided needle approach should aim to visualize the needle tip at all times during its trajectory. In the knee, fluoroscopy in the AP plane is used as the needle is advanced from a lateral approach; fluoroscopy of the ankle in the lateral projection allows needle-tip visualization as it is advanced via an anterior approach.
5. Needle placement may be 'blind' or under image guidance, e.g. fluoroscopy, CT, CT fluoroscopy or US. Measured effective doses given by an experienced radiologist show significant differences; in shoulder arthrography – fluoroscopy (0.0015 mSv), single slice CT (0.18 mSv) and CT fluoroscopy (0.22 mSv).[1]
6. The positive contrast medium is absorbed from the joint and excreted from the body in a few hours. However, intra-articular air may take up to 4 days to be completely absorbed from the joint space. Every effort should be made to eliminate air bubbles at injection for MR arthrography as they create artifacts.
7. Arthrography is well tolerated by patients with discomfort rated less severe than general MRI-related patient discomfort.[2]
8. Arthrography is a very safe procedure with low complication rates. In a major study there were 3.8% minor complications (vasovagal reaction, pain, synovitis) and 0.02% major complications

(anaphylactic reaction, infection, vascular).[3] This included
13 300 MR arthrograms with only a 0.03% complication rate, all of
which were minor.

9. In the scheduling of CT and MR arthrography it is important to
   ensure that the examination is carried out within 30 min of
   fluoroscopy-guided contrast medium intra-articular instillation.
   After this time contrast medium absorption will result in a
   suboptimal examination with resultant difficulties in interpretation.

ARTHROGRAPHY

Indications

1. **Intra-articular structures**, e.g. cartilage, labrum and tendons. The
   exact status of cartilage overlying osteochondritis dissecans (knee,
   ankle), labral tears (shoulder and hip) and anchor point of the long
   head of biceps requires CT or MR arthrography for accurate
   diagnosis.

2. **Capsular, ligamentous and tendon injuries**. Information regarding
   the presence, type, extent, gap and edges of torn capsular and
   peri-capsular structures (glenohumeral ligaments, rotator cuff
   tendons, lateral ankle ligaments) requires CT/MR arthrography.

3. **Loose body**. Loose bodies can be solitary or multiple, radiolucent
   or radio-opaque. CT arthrography using dilute contrast medium
   solution best depicts radiolucent bodies. Double-contrast CT
   arthrography using only a small amount of positive contrast
   medium is best to delineate radio-opaque loose bodies, determine
   true size and assess articular status of the joint.

4. **Para-articular cyst**. Synovial cysts and ganglia within para-articular
   soft tissues and bones can present with space-occupying lesions,
   which may migrate some distance away from the joint source of
   origin (popliteal cysts, iliopsoas bursa). Arthrography can
   demonstrate the articular communication either immediately or on
   delayed imaging.

5. **Prosthesis assessment**, e.g. loosening, infection. Arthrography
   demonstrates abnormal interposition of contrast medium indicating
   loosening at the cement/bone or metal/bone interface depending
   on the type of arthroplasty procedure carried out, while joint
   irrigation and aspiration fluid specimens are needed to confirm
   associated infection. Subtraction radiographic techniques are
   employed to facilitate interpretation, as the metal prosthesis and the
   barium-impregnated cement are subtracted out of the final image.

6. **Pain block**, e.g. bupivacaine ± steroid therapy. For difficult
   therapeutic decisions, diagnostic tests to confirm the pain source
   origin are increasingly being employed by instilling 0.5%
   bupivacaine intra-articularly. The addition of a steroid preparation
   can also aid in a longer period of pain control. If required, the

12

injectate may act as the arthrographic agent for MRI done immediately after the pain block.

7. **Confirm location of calcified para-articular soft-tissue masses**. Calcified or ossified soft-tissue lesions in a para-articular location may or may not be intra-articular (e.g. synovial osteochondromatosis, myositis ossificans) requiring CT arthrography to help in their accurate localization.

8. **Diagnosis and distension therapy in adhesive capsulitis**. Usually employed in the shoulder in the treatment of frozen shoulder, the combination of anaesthetic, steroid and saline can be used to distend and rupture the joint after arthrographic confirmation of the diagnosis.

9. **Intra-articular chemical therapy**, e.g. hyaluronic acid, fibrinolysis, radioactive synovectomy. The intra-articular injection of hyaluronic acid in joints suffering from mild to moderate osteoarthritis produces viscosupplementation of joint fluid, reducing pain and increasing the articular cartilage thickness. In fibrin-laden effusions due to chronic rheumatoid arthritis, injected intra-articular fibrinolytic agents aid in the aspiration of the joint fluid.

Contraindications

1. Local sepsis
2. Allergy to iodine or gadolinium
3. Contraindication to MRI (see Chapter 2); consider CT arthrography.

Contrast medium

Conventional/CT arthrography

Low osmolar contrast material (LOCM) is used, the most common of which are iohexol and iopamidol. A higher concentration is needed in larger joints but for the purposes of CT arthrography, especially in tight joints, a dilute solution (100–150 mg iodine/100 ml) has distinct advantages. Volume of contrast medium needed is directly proportional to the capacity of the joint in question, e.g. 15 ml in the shoulder, 6 ml in the elbow and 3 ml in the wrist. Double-contrast examination of the knee for a CT arthrogram to assess the patellofemoral joint requires 4 ml iodinated contrast medium with 40 ml of air.

Magnetic resonance arthrography

The contrast used contains both dilute gadolinium-DTPA and iodinated contrast (which is needed to confirm correct needle placement during injection), e.g. a combination of:

1. 0.1 ml gadolinium-DTPA
2. 10 ml sterile saline solution, and
3. 2 ml LOCM 200 mg I ml^{-1}.

The volume required varies according to the joint being assessed.

Equipment
1. Fluoroscopy unit with spot film device and fine focal spot (0.3 mm^2)
2. Overcouch tube.

Patient preparation
None.

Preliminary images
Routine acquisition and evaluation of joint radiographs is recommended.

Radiographic views
1. AP and lateral views are routinely obtained after arthrography.
2. Additional axial (e.g. shoulder) and oblique (e.g. ankle) views may be helpful.
3. Dynamic assessment under fluoroscopic imaging with stress views may be useful, e.g. inversion/eversion in the ankle; abduction/adduction, weight-bearing views of the shoulder.
4. Erect posture with external and internal rotation views in double-contrast shoulder studies.
5. Radial and ulnar deviation views in radio-carpal, midcarpal and inferior radio-ulnar joints.

Aftercare
Driving after the procedure is not advisable. The patient is warned that there may be some discomfort in the joint for 1–2 days after the procedure. It is also necessary to refrain from strenuous exercise during this time. The injected air for a double-contrast procedure precludes air travel.

Complications
Due to the contrast medium
1. Allergic reactions
2. Chemical synovitis.

Due to the technique
1. Pain
2. Infection
3. Capsular rupture
4. Trauma to adjacent structures, e.g. neural/vascular structures
5. Air embolus (rare).

Other
Vasovagal reaction.

12

References

1. Binkert CA, Verdun FR, Zanetti M, et al. CT arthrography of the glenohumeral joint: CT fluoroscopy versus conventional CT and fluoroscopy – comparison of image guidance techniques. Radiology 2003;229:153–8.
2. Binkert CA, Zanetti M, Hodler J. Patient's assessment of discomfort during MR arthrography of the shoulder. Radiology 2001;221:775–8.
3. Hugo PC, Newberg AH, Newman JS, et al. Complications of arthrography. Sem Musculoskelet Radiol 1998;2(4):345–8.

Further reading

Andreisek G, Duc SR, Froehlich JM, et al. MR arthrography of the shoulder, hip, and wrist: evaluation of contrast dynamics and image quality with increasing injection-to-imaging time. Am J Roentgenol 2007;188(4):1081–8.

Tehranzadeh J, Mossop EP, Golshan-Momeni M. Therapeutic arthrography and bursography. Orthop Clin North Am 2006;37(3):393–408.

ARTHROGRAPHY – SITE-SPECIFIC ISSUES

There are various needle approaches using image guidance and the most commonly used ones are described.

KNEE

Technique

1. The patient lies supine; either a medial or a lateral approach can be used and it is as well to be familiar with both.
2. Using a sterile technique, the skin and underlying soft tissue are anaesthetized at a point 1–2 cm posterior to the mid-point of the patella.
3. A 21G needle is advanced into the joint space from this point by angling it slightly anteriorly so the tip comes to lie against the posterior surface of the patella. By virtue of the anatomy, the tip of the needle must be within the joint space (Fig. 12.1). A more horizontal approach may result in the needle penetrating the infra-patellar fat pad, resulting in an extra-articular injection of contrast.
4. Any effusion is aspirated. A test injection of a small volume of contrast medium can be made under fluoroscopic control to ensure the needle is correctly positioned and, if so, the contrast medium should be seen to flow rapidly away from the needle tip. If a satisfactory position is demonstrated, then the full volume of contrast medium (4 ml) and air (40 ml) may be injected for a double-contrast arthrogram.
5. The needle is then removed and the knee is manipulated to ensure even distribution of contrast medium within the joint; this is easily

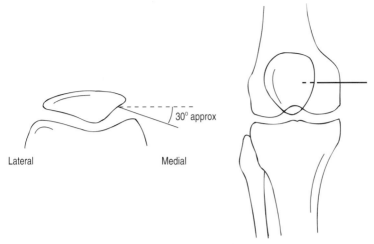

Lateral   Medial

30° approx

Figure 12.1 Technique of knee arthrography.

facilitated by asking the patient to walk around the room several times whilst bending the knee through as full a movement as possible.

6. The arthrogram is usually followed by CT to assess the patellofemoral articular status and its articular geometric relationship. Patellar tracking in different degrees of knee flexion can be done if needed. MDCT also assesses the medial and lateral articular and meniscal status optimally.

HIP

Technique

1. The patient lies supine on the X-ray table, the leg is extended and internally rotated, and the position maintained with sandbags so that the entire length of the femoral neck is visualized.
2. The position of the femoral vessels is marked to avoid inadvertent puncture.
3. The skin is prepared in a standard aseptic manner.
4. A metal marker (sterile needle) or a point on the skin is made to show the position of entry (Fig. 12.2) which should correspond to the midpoint of the inter-trochanteric line. After local anaesthetic infiltration a spinal needle (7.5 cm, 20 or 22G, short bevel) is then advanced vertically with mild forward angulation. The needle tip advances forward towards the femoral neck target under

Figure 12.2 Technique of hip arthrography. x = site of entry into joint.

fluoroscopic control, aiming supero-laterally onto the femoral neck immediately below the junction of the femoral head with the neck laterally. The capsule may be thick and a definite 'give' felt when the needle enters the joint.

5. A test injection of contrast medium will demonstrate correct placement of the needle as it flows away from the needle tip. Any fluid in the joint should be aspirated at this stage and sent for analysis.

6. Approximately 6–8 ml (1–2 ml in children) of contrast medium is injected. The exact amount depends on the capacity of the joint capsule. In MR arthrography, dilute gadolinium solution is used for contrast. Alternatively in a pain block procedure, 6–8 ml of 0.5% bupivacaine is injected intra-articularly and this can also act as the contrast medium for a limited MR arthrogram relying on T2 sequences. If examining a prosthetic joint, larger volumes of contrast medium may be required (15–20 ml). By adding a radioactive tracer to the infusate (^{99m}Tc-colloid) and subsequent imaging with a gamma-camera, a more accurate assessment of loosening can be made, perhaps because the tracer is less viscous than the contrast medium and extends to a greater extent along the prosthesis.

7. After injection of the contrast medium, the needle is removed and the joint is passively exercised to distribute the contrast medium evenly. Radiographic views are taken immediately and the patient sent to CT or MR scanning suites accordingly.

Radiographic views in the paediatric hip arthrogram

In children under the age of 10 years the procedure is usually performed under general anaesthesia. A fuller conventional radiographic series is needed to assess the joint dynamics to help in the evaluation of treatment options particularly in developmental dysplasia of the hip:

1. AP hip
2. Frog lateral
3. Abduction and internal rotation
4. Maximum abduction
5. Maximum adduction
6. Push/pull views to demonstrate instability.

SHOULDER

Technique

1. There are various approaches to needle placement, e.g. anterior (superior or inferior), modified anterior, and posterior to the glenohumeral joint. In the commonly used anterior approach the patient lies supine, with the arm of the side under investigation close to the body and in external rotation. This is to rotate the long head of the biceps out of the path of the needle. The articular surface of the glenoid will face slightly forwards, which is important as it allows a vertically placed needle to enter the joint space without damaging the glenoid labrum.
2. The coracoid process is an important landmark. Using a sterile technique, the skin and soft tissues are anaesthetized at a point 1 cm inferior and 1 cm lateral to the coracoid process. Position of needle entry point is optimized by fluoroscopy which also helps to ensure that the chosen needle trajectory is not impeded by an elongated coracoid process.
3. A spinal needle 21G needle is inserted vertically down into the joint space (Fig. 12.3). The vertical direction should intersect the junction of the middle and lower thirds of the cranio-caudal plane of the glenohumeral joint. This also allows precise control of the medio-lateral course of the needle. The position of the needle should be checked by intermittent screening. When it meets the resistance of the articular surface of the humeral head, it is withdrawn by 1–2 mm to free the tip. In the modified anterior approach where the needle traverses the rotator cuff interval, the needle is aimed towards the upper medial quadrant of the humeral head close to the articular joint line.

12

Figure 12.3 Technique of shoulder arthrography. x = site of entry into joint.

4. The intra-articular position of the needle is then confirmed by the injection of a small amount of the contrast medium under fluoroscopic control.
5. Then either the remainder of the iodinated contrast medium (15 ml in total) is injected for a single contrast examination, or sufficient air to distend the synovial sac (12 ml) is injected for a double-contrast examination. CT arthrography can be done after either type. In MR arthrography a dilute solution of gadolinium needs to be injected into the joint and this can be done by combining 1 ml of lidocaine, 2 ml of iodinated contrast medium (200 mg ml^{-1}) and 12 ml of dilute gadolinium solution (2–2.5 mmol l^{-1}). Sterile, premixed gadolinium-DTPA solutions are available for use in MR arthrography. Patients with an adhesive capsulitis may experience pain after much smaller amounts. If this is severe, then injection should be stopped. Resistance to injection is common, unlike injection into the knee, and more force is often required.
6. The needle is removed and the joint is gently manipulated to distribute the contrast medium.
7. CT arthrography examination is performed with the patient supine and positioned slightly eccentrically within the scanner to ensure that the shoulder is as close to the centre of the scanner as possible. The contralateral arm can be elevated above the head to minimize image artifacts. Scanning should be undertaken during arrested respiration to minimize motion artifact.
8. The area of interest in both CT/MR arthrography should include the acromion to the axillary recess. MDCT provides high-quality reformatted images in the three planes and MR images should also examine the joint in three planes. In addition when the arm is placed in the ABER position (abduction and external rotation), elegant MR views of the inferior capsule-labral complex and supraspinatus optimally study these structures.

ELBOW

Technique

Single contrast
1. The patient sits next to the table with the elbow flexed and resting on the table, the lateral aspect uppermost.
2. The radial head is located by palpation during gentle pronation and supination of the forearm. Using a sterile technique the skin and soft tissues are anaesthetized at a point just proximal to the radial head.
3. A 23G needle is then inserted vertically down into the joint space between the radial head and the capitellum (Fig. 12.4).
4. An injection of a small volume of local anaesthetic will flow easily if the needle is correctly sited. This can be confirmed by the injection of a few drops of contrast medium under fluoroscopic control.
5. The remainder of the contrast medium (6–8 ml) is injected and the joint gently manipulated to distribute it evenly.

Double contrast
1. Position the patient as for single contrast technique and follow steps 1–4 above.
2. Inject 0.5 ml of contrast medium followed by 6–12 ml of air until the olecranon fossa is distended.

12

Figure 12.4 Technique of elbow arthrography. x = site of entry into joint.

WRIST

Technique

Radiocarpal joint

1. The patient is seated next to the screening table with the forearm resting in a neutral prone position. The wrist should be supported over a wedge with about 10–15° of flexion.
2. Using a sterile technique, the skin and soft tissues are anaesthetized at a point over the midpoint of the scapho-capitate joint (Fig. 12.5).
3. A 23G needle is inserted into the joint by advancing it downwards and at an angle of about 15° proximally.
4. Contrast medium (2–4 ml) is injected under fluoroscopic control; if any leakage occurs into the midcarpal joint or distal radio-ulnar joints, then spot views should be taken. If this is not done, it is possible to miss small tears that later become obscured by the anterior and posterior extensions of the radiocarpal joint.

Midcarpal joint

1. The wrist is positioned as for radiocarpal injection, but with ulnar deviation, as this widens the joint space.
2. The skin and soft tissues are anaesthetized at a point over the mid-point of the scapho-capitate joint (Fig. 12.5).
3. A 23G needle is inserted vertically into the joint space under fluoroscopic control.
4. Contrast medium (2 ml) is injected under fluoroscopic control, ideally with video-recording facility, until the joint space is full. Without continuous monitoring it may not be possible to tell which of the ligaments separating the midcarpal from the radiocarpal joint are torn allowing interarticular communication.

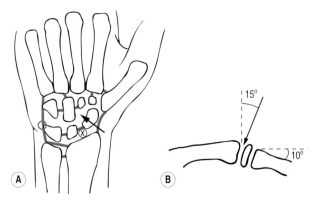

Figure 12.5 Technique of wrist arthrography. (a) AP view, x = point of entry to radiocarpal joint, arrow = point of entry to midcarpal joint. (b) Lateral view, arrow indicates cranial angulation required for needle with dorsal approach to radiocarpal joint.

ANKLE

Technique

1. The patient lies in the lateral decubitus position with the ankle plantar-flexed. An anterior approach is used with fluoroscopic guidance of the needle with the ankle in the true lateral projection (Fig. 12.6).
2. Using a sterile technique, the skin is anaesthetized at a point midway to the bimalleolar distance which places the needle lateral to the dorsalis pedis artery.
3. A 21G needle is inserted and advanced into the anterior joint space and contrast medium injected to confirm correct needle position, and then to distend the joint (4–6 ml).
4. The availability of volume acquisition with MDCT allows reformatted images in the three planes, which can detect small cartilage defects.
5. If MDCT is not available the CT scanner gantry is tilted to obtain, as closely as is possible, true coronal sections through the ankle.

Further Reading

Technique

Coumas JM, Palmer WE. Knee arthrography. Evolution and current status. Radiol Clin North Am 1998;36(4):703–28.

De Filippo M, Bertellini A, Pogliacomi F, et al. Multidetector CT arthrography of the knee: diagnostic accuracy and indications. Eur J Radiol 2008;70(2):342–51.

Mutschler C, Vande Berg BC, Lecouvet FE, et al. Postoperative meniscus: assessment at dual detector row spiral CT arthrography of the knee. Radiology 2003;228(3):635–41.

Radiographic Views in the Paediatric Hip Arthrogram

Aliabadi P, Baker ND, Jaramillo D. Hip arthrography, aspiration, block, and bursography. Radiol Clin North Am 1998;36(4):673–90.

12

Figure 12.6 Technique of ankle arthrography. Arrow = site of entry into joint.

Devalia KL, Wright D, Sathyamurthy P, et al. Role of preoperative arthrography in early Perthes disease as a decision making tool. Is it really necessary? J Pediatr Orthop B 2007;16:196–200.

Grissom L, Harcke HT, Thacker M. Imaging in the surgical management of developmental dislocation of the hip. Clin Orthop Relat Res 2008;466:791–801.

Llopis E, Cerezal L. Direct MR arthrography of the hip with leg traction: feasibility for assessing articular cartilage. Am J Roentgenol 2008;190(4):1124–8.

Temmerman OP, Raijmakers PG, Deville WL, et al. The use of plain radiography, subtraction arthrography, nuclear arthrography, and bone scintigraphy in the diagnosis of a loose acetabular component of a total hip prosthesis: a systematic review. J Arthroplasty 2007;22:818–27.

Technique

Chung CB, Dwek JR, Feng S, et al. MR arthrography of the glenohumeral joint: a tailored approach. Am J Roentgenol 2001;177(1):217–19.

Dépelteau H, Bureau NJ, Cardinal E, et al. Arthrography of the shoulder: a simple fluoroscopically guided approach for targeting the rotator cuff interval. Am J Roentgenol 2004;182(2):329–32.

Farmer KD, Hughes PM. MR arthrography of the shoulder: fluoroscopically guided technique using a posterior approach. Am J Roentgenol 2002;178(2):433–4.

Schneider R, Ghelman B, Kaye JJ. A simplified injection technique for shoulder arthrography. Radiology 1975;114(3):738–9.

Double Contrast

Dubberley JH, Faber KJ, Patterson SD, et al. The detection of loose bodies in the elbow: the value of MRI and CT arthrography. J Bone Joint Surg Br 2005;87:684–6.

Steinbach LS, Schwartz M. Elbow arthrography. Radiol Clin North Am 1998;36(4):635–49.

Waldt S, Bruegel M. Comparison of multislice CT arthrography and MR arthrography for the detection of articular cartilage lesions of the elbow. Eur Radiol 2005;15:784–91.

Midcarpal Joint

Joshy S, Ghosh S, Lee K, et al. Accuracy of direct MR arthrography in the diagnosis of triangular fibrocartilage complex tears of the wrist. Int Orthop 2008;32:251–3.

Linkous MD, Gilula LA. Wrist arthrography today. Radiol Clin North Am 1998;36(4):651–72.

Moser T, Dosch JC, Moussaoui A, et al. Wrist ligament tears: evaluation with MRI and combined MDCT and MR arthrography. Am J Roentgenol 2007;188:1278–86.

Ruegger C, Schmid MR, Pfirrmann CW, et al. Peripheral tear of the triangular fibrocartilage: depiction with MR arthrography of the distal radioulnar joint. Am J Roentgenol 2007;188:187–92.

Tirman RM, Weber ER, Snyder LL, et al. Midcarpal wrist arthrography for the detection of tears of the scapholunate and lunotriquetral ligaments. Am J Roentgenol 1985;144:107–8.

Technique

Cerezal L, Abascal F, García-Valtuille R, et al. Ankle MR arthrography: how, why and when? Radiol Clin North Am 2005;43:693–707.

Davies AM, Cassar-Pullicino VN. Demonstration of osteochondritis dissecans of the talus by coronal computed tomographic arthrography. Br J Radiol 1989;62(744):1050–5.

Schmid MR, Pfirrmann CW, Hodler J, et al. Cartilage lesions in the ankle joint: comparison of MR arthrography and CT arthrography. Skeletal Radiol 2003;32:259–65.

TENDON IMAGING

Methods of imaging tendons

1. Tenography
2. US
3. CT
4. MRI.

GENERAL POINTS

With the advent of CT, US and MRI, the indications for tenography (direct injection of contrast into the tendon sheath) are exceptionally rare. Although CT does show tendons and their relationship to joints and peri-articular structures, US and MRI also show the intrinsic tendon structure and differentiate fluid within the sheath from the tendon. The higher resolution of US enables better depiction of internal architecture of superficial tendons. In addition, dynamic assessment to exclude subluxing tendons can be done sonographically.

ULTRASOUND OF THE PAEDIATRIC HIP

Indications

1. Developmental dysplasia of the hip
2. Hip effusion
3. Slipped femoral capital epiphysis.

Technique

Developmental dysplasia of the hip

With US the unossified elements of the hip – femoral head, greater trochanter, labrum, triradiate cartilage – as well as the bony acetabular roof, can be identified in the first 6 months of life.[1] After 9–12 months, the degree of ossification precludes adequate imaging by US and plain film radiography becomes

12

superior. There are two main methods, static and dynamic, and both may be used during one examination.

Static (Graf) method
This assesses the morphology and geometry of the acetabulum. Although independent of the position of the infant, it is recommended that the infant be placed in the decubitus position. A single longitudinal image is obtained with the transducer placed over the greater trochanter and held at right angles to all the anatomical planes. The following landmarks are identified in the following sequence: chondro-osseous boundary between femoral shaft and head, joint capsule, labrum, cartilaginous roof and superior bony rim of acetabulum. Although most images can be subjectively evaluated, angles can be measured from the image and form the basis for the Graf classification.

Dynamic method
This assesses the stability of the hip when stressed. The hip is studied in the coronal and axial planes with the infant supine. With the hip flexed and adducted, the femur is pushed and pulled with a piston-like action.[2]

Hip-joint effusion
Approximately 50% of children with acute hip pain have intra-articular fluid and the sensitivity of US for detecting effusion approaches 100%.[3] With the child supine, the hip is scanned anteriorly with the transducer parallel to the femoral neck. Bulging of the anterior portion of the joint capsule can be readily identified.[4] The normal distance between the bony femoral neck and the joint capsule is always less than 3 mm, and the difference between the affected and unaffected sides should not be greater than 2 mm.

Slipped femoral capital epiphysis
Although plain radiographs constitute the usual means of diagnosis, a mild posterior slip can be identified in the acute situation by longitudinal scanning along the femoral neck.

References
1. Yousefzadeh DK, Ramilo JL. Normal hip in children: correlation of US with anatomic and cryomicrotome sections. Radiology 1987;165:647–55.
2. Clarke NM, Harcke HT, McHugh P, et al. Real time ultrasound in the diagnosis of congenital dislocation and dysplasia of the hip. J Bone Joint Surg Br 1985;67:406–12.
3. Dörr U, Zieger M, Hauke H. Ultrasonography of the painful hip. Prospective studies in 204 patients. Pediatr Radiol 1988;19:36–40.
4. Miralles M, Gonzalez G, Pulpeiro JR, et al. Sonography of the painful hip in children: 500 consecutive cases. Am J Roentgenol 1989;152: 579–82.

THERMOABLATION OF MUSCULOSKELETAL TUMOURS

Introduction

Image-guided interventional techniques are increasingly being employed in treating bone and soft tissue musculoskeletal tumours. Small painful lesions such as osteoid osteoma can prove difficult to locate at surgery. Using laser and radiofrequency (RF) probes, benign bone tumours are preferentially being treated by thermoablation instead of surgery with a limited role also in managing malignant bone disease. RF ablation is more commonly in use as it does not require the additional safety measures that need to be in place for laser ablation. In this brief section RF treatment is primarily focused in the treatment of osteoid osteomas.

Thermocoagulation

In radiofrequency thermal ablation an alternating current of high-frequency radio waves (>10KHz) is emitted from an electrode tip and this dissipates its energy as heat within the surrounding tissues. It is the tissue around the electrode which is therefore the primary source of heat and not the electrode itself. In response to the RF stimulus ions within local biological tissues vibrate leading to ionic agitation. As a direct result of the ions' attempt to change direction with the alternating electrical current, friction is created around the electrode tip creating heat which desiccates the soft tissues – 'thermal ablation'.[1] The amount of biological tissue that can be ablated is referred to as the 'treatment zone'. Using an electrode tip length of 5 mm, a spherical thermoablation treatment zone of 1 cm is generated. Effective ablation in living bone is achieved with a temperature of 90°C at the active tip for 4–6 min.[2]

Indications

1. Osteoid osteoma
2. Osteoblastoma
3. Chondroblastoma
4. Metastasis.

Rationale

Using CT guidance the target is accurately localized and its dimensions determined. Using a coaxial needle system and drill, a biopsy can be taken and the tip of a thermoablation probe optimally placed in the centre of the lesion. The heat generated causes tumour necrosis over a diameter of 1 cm.[3] Multiple RF

12

probe placements via multiple skin entry points are needed if the lesion is larger than 1 cm to provide the 1 cm wide ablated margin required to cover the entire lesion needed for successful treatment.[4]

Contraindications

1. Cardiac pacemakers are an absolute contraindication as they can be affected by the radiofrequency current.
2. Relative contraindications include lesions that are close to (less than 1 cm) neighbouring peripheral nerves, spinal nerves and spinal cord, although measures can be employed to reduce the risk of damage in treating such lesions. Lesions in the hands and feet also have an additional increased risk of skin damage if they lack an adequate soft tissue cover.

Equipment

1. The Bonopty system is used which incorporates a penetration outer cannula, an inner stylet, a coaxial drill and a coaxial biopsy needle.
2. A radiofrequency generator is the source of the electric current that passes to the electrode tip into the patient, and out through a grounding pad back to the generator.
3. A non-insulated single electrode tip between 0.5 mm and 10 mm in length. A multi-tined electrode system can also be used in larger lesions.

Procedure

Once the lesion is localized by CT, radiopaque markers are placed on the skin. In planning the percutaneous needle route the most direct path to the lesion with the needle angled perpendicular to the cortex is chosen avoiding regional neurovascular structures. If this is not possible a safer but longer route is chosen via the opposite normal cortex.

As the procedure is painful it is carried out under a general anaesthetic. Grounding pads are placed away from the area of interest, e.g. around the thigh to inhibit the transmission of current through the patient.

Using CT guidance the cannula with its inner stylet is guided through the soft tissues to the cortical bone surface. The inner stylet is then replaced by the drill and this is advanced sequentially through the cortex ensuring an optimal intraosseous trajectory which is followed by CT spot images, until the tip of the drill reaches the cortical edge of the tumour. The cannula is then advanced over the drill to maintain the position of the drilled intraosseous path and the drill removed.

Biopsy

Although the imaging characteristics of osteoid osteoma, osteoblastoma and chondroblastoma may be regarded as typical prior to RF ablation, it is important to obtain a biopsy to confirm the diagnosis. This is obtained at the time of the procedure and does not usually require a separate procedure before the RF treatment. It is important to establish the correct diagnosis in case there is a recurrence of the lesion which requires a second thermoablation. Brodie's abscess, intracortical chondroma and stress fracture can mimic the radiological features of osteoid osteoma.

The specially designed biopsy needle is placed in the cannula and slowly advanced through the lesion taking a biopsy after confirming that it has negotiated the tumour tissue by CT images.[5]

Thermoablation

The RF electrode is passed into the cannula and its tip placed in the centre of the lesion. The active business end of the electrode is usually 0.7 cm long. The tip of the electrode should not be more than 0.5 cm away from the peripheral edge of the lesion to ensure successful and complete tumour ablation coverage. It is essential to partially withdraw the cannula (so that it lies more than 1 cm from the electrode tip) over the electrode to avoid the risk of heating adjacent tissue through contact with the metal cannula. These parameters are double-checked by further CT spot images. Both the RF electrode and ground pad dispersive electrode cord are connected to the generator.

Thermal ablation is applied through the RF electrode at a set temperature target of 90°C for a total of 5 min for lesions within a diameter of 1 cm.

Post RF ablation care

1. Introduce local anaesthetic via the cannula after ablation
2. Sterile dressing
3. Oral analgesia
4. Discharge usually within 24 hours
5. Avoid strenuous activities if lesion is in the lower limb for 3 months
6. No imaging required in follow-up unless symptoms recur.

Complications

1. Failed treatment can be due to residual or recurrent tumour. The clinical success rate is close to 90% and is defined as the absence of pain for 2 years. A second RF ablation can be carried out if necessary[5,6]
2. Neural damage
3. Soft tissue necrosis
4. Osteonecrosis

12

5. Skin burns

6. Infection.

References

1. Organ LW. Electrophysiologic principles of radiofrequency lesion making. Appl Neurophysiol 1976;39(2):69–76.
2. Tillotson CL, Rosenberg AE, Rosenthal DI. Controlled thermal injury of bone: report of a percutaneous technique using radiofrequency electrode and generator. Invest Radiol 1989;24(11):888–92.
3. Rosenthal DI, Hornicek FJ, Wolfe MW, et al. Percutaneous radiofrequency coagulation of osteoid osteoma compared with operative treatment. J Bone Joint Surg. American Volume 1998;80(6):815–21.
4. Pinto CH, Taminiau AH, Vanderschueren GM, et al. Technical considerations in CT guided radiofrequency thermal ablation of osteoid osteoma: Tricks of the trade. Am J Roentgenol 2002;179(6):1633–42.
5. Cribb GL, Goude WH, Cool P, et al. Percutaneous radiofrequency thermocoagulation of osteoid osteomas: factors affecting therapeutic outcome. Skeletal Radiol 2005;34(11):702–6.
6. Rimondi E, Mavrogenis AF, Rossi G, et al. Radiofrequency ablation for non-spinal osteoid osteomas in 557 patients. Eur Radiol 2012;22(1): 181–8.

RADIONUCLIDE BONE SCAN

Indications

1. Staging of cancer and response to therapy, especially breast and prostate
2. Assessment and staging of primary bone tumours
3. Painful orthopaedic prostheses to differentiate infection from loosening
4. Bone or joint infection
5. Trauma not obvious on X-ray, e.g. stress fractures
6. Bone pain
7. Avascular necrosis and bone infarction
8. Assessment of non-accidental injury in children
9. Metabolic bone disease for complications such as fractures
10. Arthropathies, e.g. rheumatoid
11. Reflex sympathetic dystrophy
12. Assessment of extent multifocal disorders such as Paget's disease and fibrous dysplasia.

Contraindications

None.

Radiopharmaceuticals

^{99m}Tc-methylene diphosphonate (MDP) or other ^{99m}Tc-labelled diphosphonate, 500 MBq typical, 600 MBq max (3 mSv ED).

For single photon emission computed tomography (SPECT) 800 MBq (5 mSv ED).

These compounds are phosphate analogues which are stable in vivo and rapidly excreted by the kidneys, providing a good contrast between bone and soft tissue.

Equipment

1. Gamma-camera, preferably with SPECT and whole body imaging
2. Low-energy high-resolution collimator.

Patient preparation

The patient must be well hydrated.

Technique

1. ^{99m}Tc-diphosphonate is injected i.v. When infection is suspected or blood flow to bone or primary bone tumour is to be assessed, a bolus injection is given with the patient in position on the camera. A three-phase study is then performed with arterial, blood-pool and delayed static imaging.
2. The patient should be encouraged to drink plenty and empty the bladder frequently to minimize radiation dose.
3. The bladder is emptied immediately prior to imaging to prevent obscuring the sacrum and bony pelvis.
4. Delayed static imaging is performed ≥2 h after injection: up to 4 h for imaging of extremities and up to 6 h for those patients on dialysis or in renal failure.

Images

Standard

High-resolution images are acquired with a pixel size of 1–2 mm:

1. The whole skeleton. The number of views will depend upon the field of view of the camera and whether a whole-body imaging facility is available. A point to consider is that whole-body images will have lower resolution than spot views over parts of the skeleton where the camera is some distance from the patient (unless a body-contour tracking facility is available), since resolution falls off with distance. Spot views should be overlapping.
2. Anterior oblique views of the thorax are useful to separate sternum and spine uptake.
3. For examination of the posterior ribs, scapula or shoulder, an extra posterior thorax view with arms above the head should be taken to move the scapula away from the ribs.
4. For imaging small bones and joints, magnified views should be taken, with a pinhole collimator if necessary.

12

5. SPECT can be useful for lesion localization, e.g. in vertebrae and joints, and to detect avascular necrosis.[1] CT-SPECT fusion is likely to be even more helpful, analogous to the improved specificity and diagnostic confidence seen with PET-CT as opposed to PET alone.[2]

Three-phase

1. *Arterial phase 1*: 1–2 s frames of the area of interest for 1 min post-injection
2. *Blood pool phase 2*: 3-min image of the same area 5 min post injection
3. *Delayed phase 3*: views ≥2 h post injection, as for standard imaging.

Analysis

1. For the arterial phase, time–activity curves are created for regions of interest symmetrical about the mid-line.
2. For SPECT, reconstruction of transaxial, coronal, sagittal and, possibly, oblique slices to demonstrate the lesion.

Additional techniques

SPECT and CT-SPECT can be useful for improved lesion detection and localization in complex bony structures, e.g. spine and knees.[1,2]

Aftercare

Normal radiation safety precautions (see Chapter 1).

Complications

None.

Competing modalities

FDG-PET (see Chapter 11) and whole body MRI (e.g. with diffusion-weighted techniques) may be competitive for oncological purposes. MRI is often preferred for localized orthopaedic applications, but has limited applicability in the presence of a prosthesis.

References
1. Murray IP, Dixon J. The role of single photon emission computed tomography in bone scintigraphy. Skeletal Radiol 1989;18:493–505.
2. Utsunomiya D, Shiraishi S, Imuta M, et al. Added value of SPECT/CT fusion in assessing suspected bone metastasis: comparison with scintigraphy alone and nonfused scintigraphy and CT. Radiology 2006;238:264–71.

Further Reading
Brooks M. The skeletal system. In: Sharp PF, Gemmell HG, Murray AD, editors. Practical Nuclear Medicine. 3rd ed. London: Springer-Verlag; 2005, p. 143–61.
Love C, Din AS, Tomas MB, et al. Radionuclide bone imaging: an illustrative review. RadioGraphics 2003;23:341–58.

Brain

Methods of imaging the brain

Imaging the brain's structure and examining its physiology, both in the acute and elective setting, are now the domain of multiplanar, computer-assisted imaging. The imaging modalities in use today include the following:

1. **Computed tomography (CT).** This is the technique of choice for the investigation of serious head injury; for suspected intracranial haemorrhage, stroke, infection and other acute neurological emergencies. CT is quick, efficient and safer to use in the emergency situation than MRI.
2. **Magnetic resonance imaging (MRI).** This is the best and most versatile imaging modality for the brain, constrained only by availability, patient acceptability, and the logistics and safety of patient handling in emergency situations. New protocols and higher field strength magnets have raised the sensitivity of MRI in epilepsy imaging, acute stroke, aneurysm detection and follow-up post treatment of neoplastic and vascular disorders. It is the only effective way of diagnosing multiple sclerosis.
3. **Angiography.** This is very important in intracranial haemorrhage (ICH), especially subarachnoid haemorrhage (SAH) and, increasingly, in intra-arterial management of ischaemic stroke. However, with the widespread availability of multi-detector CT scanners, CT angiography (CTA) is now preferentially used in ischaemic stroke, SAH and ICH. Angiography is still requested for pre-operative assessment of tumours, vascular malformations and angiographic expertise is vital for the performance of many neurointerventional procedures.
4. **Radionuclide imaging.** There are two principal methods. The first is regional cerebral blood flow scanning, still more used in research than in clinical management, especially in the dementias and in movement disorders such as Parkinsonism; second is positron emission tomography (PET). By this method focal

hyper-metabolism may be shown using ^{18}F fluorodeoxyglucose (^{18}FDG), for example in epilepsy, and cell turnover may be shown using ^{11}C-methionine, for example in tumour studies.

5. **Ultrasound (US)**. This is particularly helpful in neonates and during the first year of life to image haemorrhagic and ischaemic syndromes, developmental malformations, and hydrocephalus using the fontanelles as acoustic windows. In adults, transcranial Doppler may be used for intracerebral arterial velocity studies to assess the severity of vasospasm.

6. **Plain films of the skull**. These are of little value except in head injury.

COMPUTED TOMOGRAPHY OF THE BRAIN

Indications

CT is the imaging modality most commonly used in triaging acute neurological disease. For non-emergency indications CT is second best to MR, but is still widely used, often because it is more broadly available and simpler to interpret. The indications include the following:

1. Following major head injury (if the patient has lost consciousness, has impaired consciousness, or has a neurological deficit). The presence of a skull fracture also justifies the use of CT. NICE (National Institute for Health and Care Excellence) guidance has been issued on the use of imaging for head injuries for adults and children, specifically CT, listing the criteria for assessment based on best relevant data and consensus recommendations.

2. In suspected intracranial infection (the use of contrast enhancement is recommended).

3. For suspected intracranial haemorrhage and cases of ischaemic and haemorrhagic stroke.

4. In suspected raised intracranial pressure, and as a precaution before lumbar puncture once certain criteria are fulfilled. These would include reduced consciousness (a Glasgow coma score of less than 15), definite papilloedema, focal neurological deficit, immune suppression and bleeding dyscrasias.

5. In other situations, such as epilepsy, migraine, suspected tumour, demyelination, dementia and psychosis, CT is a poorer-quality tool. If imaging can be justified, MRI is greatly preferable and is recommended by NICE in these situations except for the first episode of psychosis.

Technique

1. Most clinical indications are adequately covered by 3-mm sections parallel to the floor of the anterior cranial fossa, from the foramen

magnum to the midbrain, with 7-mm sections to the vertex (or contigious 3-mm slices throughout). In all trauma cases, window width and level should be adjusted to examine bone and any haemorrhagic, space-occupying lesions. Review of all trauma studies should be done on brain windows, bone and 'blood windows' (i.e. W175 L75).

2. In suspected infection, tumours, vascular malformations and subacute infarctions, the sections should be repeated following intravenous (i.v.) contrast enhancement, if MR is not available. Standard precautions with regard to possible adverse reactions to contrast medium should be taken.

3. Dynamic studies using iodinated contrast are increasingly being used as a routine in high-velocity head trauma, the assessment of intracerebral bleeding in young patients, aneurysmal SAH, ruptured arteriovenous shunts and dural venous sinus thrombosis. CT angiography (CTA) on a typical 64-slice multidetector scanner is performed using 70–100 ml of contrast and 50 ml saline chaser, injected at 4 ml s^{-1} with a delay of 15 s or triggered by bolus tracking with ROI in the aortic arch. Overlapping slices of 0.75–1.25 mm are reconstructed. CT venography (CTV) involves injecting 90–100 ml of contrast with a delay of 40 s. Images are usually reviewed both as three-dimensional rendered data and multiplanar reformats (MPRs).

Further Reading

Yates D, Aktar R, Hill J. Assessment, investigation, and early management of head injury: summary of NICE guidance. BMJ 2007;335: 719–20.

MAGNETIC RESONANCE IMAGING OF THE BRAIN

Indications

MRI is indicated in all cases of suspected intracranial pathology. Techniques in use change with the development of new sequences and higher field strength magnets. The techniques described below are, therefore, only basic indications as to sequences in use. The greatest advantages in the use of MRI are the improved contrast resolution between grey and white matter, brain and cerebrospinal fluid (CSF); the removal of artifact due to bone close to the skull base and in the posterior fossa; and in obtaining multiplanar images for lesion localization.

13

Technique

1. **Long TR sequences**. The whole brain can be examined with 4-mm sections with 1-mm interspaces using T2-weighted turbo

spin echo imaging. Proton density sequences, long TR and short TE, are used mostly for the assessment of demyelination and intra-articular disc changes in the temporomandibular joints.

2. **Short TR sequences**. T1-weighted sequences are used for the demonstration of detailed anatomy but gadolinium chelate contrast agents are required to view pathology. Common practice is to obtain a sagittal or coronal T1-weighted sequence as part of a standard brain study. Volumetric sequences pre and post contrast are used for image guidance software interfaces for epilepsy imaging, insertion of deep brain stimulators for movement disorders and the removal of intra- and extra-axial tumours.

3. **Gradient-echo T2-weighted sequences and susceptibility weighted imaging**. Although suffering from various artifacts, the sensitivity of these sequences to susceptibility effects makes them very sensitive to the presence of blood products, as in cases of previous head injury, SAH and cavernomas. Haemosiderin produces marked focal loss of signal in such cases, and all patients with a history of head injury or other causes of haemorrhage should be imaged with this sequence. These sequences identify abnormal mineral deposition and can be used in deposition disorders.

4. **FLAIR sequences (*FL*uid *A*ttenuated *I*nversion *R*ecovery)** provide very good contrast resolution in the detection of demyelinating plaques and infarcts, and have the advantage that juxta-ventricular pathology contrasts with dark CSF, and is not lost by proximity to the intense brightness of the ventricular CSF, as in spin-echo T2-weighted studies. There are usually obtained in the sagittal or coronal plane.

5. **Angiographic sequences**. There are many methods, of which 'time-of flight' is one of the more commonly used. This is a very short TR, T1-weighted gradient echo three-dimensional sequence, with sequential presaturation of each partition so that only non-presaturated inflowing blood gives a high signal. Image display is by so-called 'MIP' or maximum intensity projection, giving a three-dimensional model of the intracranial vessels. As it uses the T1 properties, high signal from blood products in the subarachnoid space may reduce the sensitivity to aneurysms. Phase contrast MR angiography uses velocity encoding flow and is useful to detect flow in small and tortuous vessels. Contrast-enhanced MR angiography requires a pump injector and is less susceptible to flow artifacts. Timing of image acquisition is crucial and it is very useful in neck vessel imaging.

6. **Echoplanar or diffusion weighted imaging (DWI)**. This sequence is becoming widely available on scanners. Most units perform DWI on all patients with suspected stroke, vasculitis, encephalitis, abscesses and in the workup of intracranial tumours. DWI examines the free movement, or Brownian motion, of water molecules at a cellular level. In acute infarcts cytotoxic oedema

prevents free movement of water, whereas in tumours there is no restriction. All DWI should be reviewed together with conventional sequences and apparent diffusion coefficient (ADC) maps. Acute infarcts are hyperintense on DWI and hypointense on ADC. DWI is a useful technique in assessment of cholesteatoma both in detecting cholesteatoma if CT is equivocal and is ideal in evaluation of recurrent disease.

Further Reading

Atlas SW. Magnetic resonance imaging of brain and spine. 4th ed. Philadelphia, PA: Lippincott Williams & Wilkins; 2009.

Schwartz KM, Lane JI, Bolster BD, et al. The utility of diffusion-weighted imaging for cholesteatoma evaluation. Am J Neuroradiol 2011;32:430–6.

IMAGING OF INTRACRANIAL HAEMORRHAGE

Imaging of suspected intracranial haemorrhage is one of the most common requests, usually in the emergency setting. Follow-up of haematomas and formulating a differential diagnosis can sometimes be quite challenging. In the acute setting, CT and the neurophysiological information available as a result of multidetector technology, is often the first and only modality used to assess these patients. MRI is more often used in situations where the initial workup has been negative and a more sensitive modality is required.

COMPUTED TOMOGRAPHY

A conventional study consists of 3-mm sections through the brainstem and posterior fossa, and 7-mm sections through the cerebrum. This is the basic multi-detector CT protocol for brain imaging. This is performed without contrast to avoid diagnostic uncertainty in deciding whether a parenchymal lesion is due to enhancement or blood. Acute blood is typically hyperdense on CT. An exhaustive differential diagnosis for bleeding in different compartments of the brain can be sourced elsewhere but, in general, bleeding can be extra-axial (i.e. epidural, subdural, subarachnoid, intraventricular) or intra-axial. Intra-axial bleeding can be due to head trauma, ruptured aneurysms or arteriovenous malformations, bleeding tumours (either primary disease or secondaries), hypertensive haemorrhages (cortical or striatal) or haemorrhagic transformation of venous or arterial infarcts. In the assessment of subarachnoid haemorrhage and ischaemic stroke CTA is becoming increasingly used as the screening modality for deciding further intervention. Neurosurgeons are increasingly using CTA as the sole modality for planning microsurgical clipping, particularly in the cases where haematoma exerting mass

13

effect needs to be evacuated immediately adjacent to a freshly ruptured intracranial aneurysm. In ischaemic stroke CTA can localize an acute embolus and its source. CT perfusion imaging can demonstrate the ischaemic core (irreversibly damaged brain) by calculating the relative cerebral blood volume and the ischaemic penumbra (recoverable brain parenchyma) by evaluating the relative cerebral blood flow (rCBF).

MAGNETIC RESONANCE IMAGING

MRI is predominantly used to exclude the presence of an underlying tumour or a cavernoma at an interval after the initial haemorrhage when there would be less perilesional brain swelling and obscuration of the anatomy due to blood degradation products. It is also used in the setting of subarachnoid bleeding where no aneurysm or arteriovenous malformation is found on CTA or catheter angiography. In these cases the entire neuraxis must be examined to exclude an 'occult' source of the haemorrhage. Diffuse axonal shear injuries, in patients with depressed coma scores post head injury, in light of a normal-appearing CT scan, are best demonstrated on MRI with gradient echo imaging or susceptibility weighted imaging looking for susceptibility artifact due to 'microbleeds'. Where resources are optimal, and MRI is used as part of the initial imaging pathway in ischaemic stroke, MR will help to determine the volumes of brain that can be recovered as well as the presence of early haemorrhage that is not visible on CT which would contraindicate thrombolysis.

Further Reading

Haacke EM, Mittal S, Wu Z, et al. Susceptibility-weighted imaging: technical aspects and clinical applications, part 1. Am J Neuroradiol 2009;30(1):19–30.

Mittal S, Wu Z, Neelavalli J, et al. Susceptibility-weighted imaging: technical aspects and clinical applications, part 2. Am J Neuroradiol 2009;30(2):232–52.

Wada R, Aviv RI, Fox AJ, et al. CT angiography 'spot sign' predicts hematoma expansion in acute intracerebral hemorrhage. Stroke 2007;38(4):1257–62.

Westerlaan HE, Gravendeel J, Fiore D, et al. Multislice CT angiography in the selection of patients with ruptured intracranial aneurysms suitable for clipping or coiling. Neuroradiology 2007;49(12):997–1007.

IMAGING OF GLIOMAS

This is an all-encompassing term for a diverse group of primary brain tumours. This includes astrocytomas, oligodendrogliomas, choroid plexus tumours and ependymomas, amongst others. The most commonly presenting tumour, however, is the WHO grade

IV astrocytoma or glioblastoma multiforme. Other brain tumours are derived from neuronal cell lines, mixed glial-neuronal cell lines, the pineal gland and embryonal cell lines, peripheral cranial nerves (such as the vestibular schwannoma), meningeal tumours and lymphoma. Appropriate differential diagnoses can be derived from noting the age of the patient, the tumour location (i.e. supra- or infratentorial, cortex or white matter, basal ganglia or brainstem, intra- or extra-axial), its consistency (i.e. cyst formation, mural nodule) and its enhancement characteristics.

COMPUTED TOMOGRAPHY

CT is often the first modality to demonstrate the presence of a brain tumour. The indications for scanning can include unrelenting morning headaches, drowsiness, stroke-like presentation and seizures. In addition to making the initial diagnosis, multidetector CT can be used for obtaining high-resolution datasets for image guidance for brain biopsies, with and without stereotactic frames. In the absence of advanced MR neuroimaging software and for patients who are unable to undergo MR, imaging multidetector CT can be used to obtain rCBF data for tumour matrix as well as the normal brain. Studies have been performed to correlate ratios of rCBF with tumour grade, assessment of radiation necrosis or dedifferentiation when following-up tumours.

MAGNETIC RESONANCE IMAGING

MRI is the preferred modality for detailed assessment of brain tumours. In addition to using conventional imaging parameters to assess volume, location and tumour substance in multiple planes, advanced imaging techniques or 'multi-modality' imaging can reveal information about tumour grade and biology. Conventional T1 and T2 images are obtained. Diffusion-weighted imaging and diffusion tractography reveals information about tumour substance and effect on white matter tracts in the brainstem and the cerebrum. Multiple lesions, if present, can be better seen on post-contrast MRI, in which case metastatic disease becomes a consideration in the differential diagnosis. As grade IV gliomas can have a similar appearance, a search for a primary epithelial neoplasm elsewhere (for example breast and lung) would be indicated. MR spectroscopy is a technique whereby relative amounts of cell metabolites are detected to reflect the biochemical environment in a tumour. N-acetylaspartate, choline, creatine, lactate and myo-inositol are a few of the major metabolites assessed. Single voxel techniques are preferable using STEAM

13

(stimulated echo acquisition mode) or point resolved spectroscopy (PRESS). Perfusion-weighted imaging can provide information about tumour grade and help to differentiate between tumour recurrence and radiation necrosis. Susceptibility perfusion imaging is most often used where gradient echo images are obtained of the entire brain during the first pass of gadolinium chelate and analysis of the collated data using small regions of interest is carried out looking at normal brain and the tumour. MPRAGE (magnetization-prepared rapid-acquisition gradient echo) volumetric data can also be used post contrast for image guidance for biopsy or tumour debulking.

Further Reading

Computed Tomography

Jain R. Perfusion CT imaging of brain tumours: an overview. Am J Neuroradiol 2011;32(9):1570–7.

Magnetic Resonance Imaging

Al-Okaili RN, Krejza J, Wang S, et al. Advanced MR imaging techniques in the diagnosis of intraaxial brain tumors in adults. RadioGraphics 2006;26:S173–89.

Osborn AG. Osborn's Brain: Imaging, pathology, anatomy. Salt Lake City: Amirsys, Inc; 2012.

Stadlbauer A, Gruber S, Nimsky C, et al. Preoperative grading of gliomas by using metabolite quantification with high-spatial-resolution proton MR spectroscopic imaging. Radiology 2006;238(3):958–69.

IMAGING OF ACOUSTIC NEUROMAS

MRI is the definitive diagnostic method. The neurophysiological methods, although quite sensitive, produce a large number of false-positive studies.

COMPUTED TOMOGRAPHY

Some departments use 2-mm section i.v. contrast-enhanced CT with bone and soft-tissue windowed images for suspected acoustic neuroma to relieve pressure on their MRI services. This approach is usually reserved for elderly patients, mostly to exclude the presence of large lesions that may require debulking or excision. Intracanalicular tumours cannot be shown by this method but surgically these will not be addressed.

MAGNETIC RESONANCE IMAGING

Most imaging departments will have a 1.5-T scanner where MR cisternography sequences are available, nulling the CSF pulsation artifact and highlighting the appearances of cranial nerves, arteries and veins which may also be contributing to sensorineural deafness and tinnitus. Nulling the pulsation artifact from CSF provides the contrast required and images as thin as 0.8 mm, with no gap, can be obtained. From this kind of data multiplanar, reformatted images can be reviewed. Post-contrast studies are obtained when a change in the contour of the nerve is observed or a filling defect is seen in the labyrinthine structures.

Further Reading

Rupa V, Job A, George M, et al. Cost-effective initial screening for vestibular schwannoma: auditory brainstem response or magnetic resonance imaging. Otolaryngology – Head Neck Surg 2003;128(6):823–8.

RADIONUCLIDE IMAGING OF THE BRAIN

There are currently two main modalities: regional cerebral blood flow imaging and PET imaging. Thallium imaging is also used in specialist centres for brain tumour assessment and there are niche agents in clinical practice used, for example in the diagnosis of Parkinson's disease. Conventional radionuclide brain scanning (blood–brain barrier imaging) is rarely used in modern clinical practice.

CONVENTIONAL RADIONUCLIDE BRAIN SCANNING (BLOOD–BRAIN BARRIER IMAGING)

This technique is not indicated if CT and/or MRI are available. It was a technique that used i.v. injection of the radiopharmaceuticals ^{99m}Tc-DTPA and ^{99m}Tc-pertechnetate to detect areas of blood–brain barrier breakdown and demonstrate cerebral metastases, meningioma and high-grade glioma.

REGIONAL CEREBRAL BLOOD FLOW IMAGING

Indications

1. Localization of epileptic foci
2. Mapping of cerebrovascular disease
3. Investigation of dementias including Huntington and Alzheimer disease
4. Assessment of effects of treatment regimens
5. Confirmation of brain death.

Contraindications

None.

13

Radiopharmaceuticals

1. ^{99m}Tc-hexamethylpropyleneamineoxime (HMPAO or exametazime), 500 MBq (5 mSv ED). The most commonly used agent, HMPAO is a lipophilic complex that crosses the blood–brain barrier and localizes roughly in proportion to cerebral blood flow. It is rapidly extracted by the brain, reaching a peak of 5–6% of injected activity within a minute or so, with minimal redistribution (about 86% remains in the brain at 24 h).
2. ^{99m}Tc-ethyl cysteinate dimer (ECD), 500 MBq (5 mSv ED). This localizes rapidly in proportion to cellular metabolism rather than blood flow, and the distribution has some differences to that of HMPAO, which may need to be taken into consideration for clinical diagnosis.[1,2] It currently has the advantage of greater stability than HMPAO and can be used for up to 6 h after reconstitution, which is of particular benefit for ictal epilepsy studies where an injection is only given once a seizure occurs.

Equipment

1. Single photon emission computed tomography (SPECT) gamma camera, preferably dual-headed
2. SPECT imaging couch with head extension
3. Low-energy high-resolution collimator (or more specialized slant-hole or fan-beam collimator).

Patient preparation

Since cerebral blood flow is continuously varying with motor activity, sensory stimulation, emotional arousal, etc., it is important to standardize the conditions under which the tracer is administered, especially if serial studies are to be undertaken in the same individual. Familiarization with the procedure to reduce anxiety and injection in a relaxing environment through a previously positioned i.v. cannula should be considered.

For localization of epileptic foci, ictal studies are much more sensitive than interictal, and if feasible the patient should be admitted under constant monitoring, with injection as soon as a seizure starts.

Technique

1. Administer 500 MBq of tracer
2. SPECT imaging is performed any time from 5 min to 2 h after injection with the patient supine.

Images

The acquisition protocol will depend upon the system available. Suitable parameters for a modern single-headed gamma-camera might be:

1. 360° circular orbit
2. 60–90° projections or continuous rotation over a 30-min acquisition
3. Combination of matrix size and zoom to give a pixel size of 3–4 mm.

Analysis

A cine film of the projections is reviewed before the patient leaves to detect if any significant movement degradation is present. If movement that cannot be rectified by computer motion correction algorithms has occurred the patient must be re-scanned. SPECT reconstructions are made in three planes.

Additional techniques

1. If blood flow in the carotid and major cerebral arteries is of interest, a dynamic study during injection is performed.
2. Three-dimensional mapping of activity distributions onto standard brain atlases and image registration with MRI, CT and quantitative analysis are areas of increasing interest, particularly with the development of SPECT-CT scanners.

Aftercare

Radiation dose may be reduced by administration of a mild laxative on the day after the study and maintenance of good hydration to promote urine output.

Complications

None.

POSITRON EMISSION TOMOGRAPHY

Indications

1. Localization of epileptic foci
2. Investigation of dementias
3. Grading of brain tumours.

Contraindications

1. Recent chemotherapy – minimum interval of 2–3 weeks recommended
2. Recent radiotherapy – minimum interval of 8–12 weeks recommended
3. Poorly controlled diabetes, i.e. serum glucose >8.5 mmol l^{-1} at time of scanning.

13

Radiopharmaceuticals

Fluorine-18 fluorodeoxyglucose (^{18}FDG) is a glucose analogue which is the most commonly used agent for oncological work and is also used for the investigation of dementias. There are other radiopharmaceuticals, e.g. L-[methyl-^{11}C]methionine ([^{11}C] MET) or 3'-deoxy-3'-[^{18}F] fluorothymidine ([^{18}F] FLT) which have the advantage of little normal cerebral uptake.

Patient preparation

Fasting for 4–6 h, with plenty of non-sugary fluids.

Technique

1. ^{18}FDG -up to the UK limit of 400 MBq i.v. (10 mSv ED) is administered.
2. To reduce muscle uptake of ^{18}FDG, patients should remain in a relaxed environment such as lying in a darkened room, without talking if head and neck area are being imaged, between injection and scan.
3. Image at 1 h post injection. Later imaging has been reported to enhance tumour conspicuity due to a higher tumour to background ratio.
4. If combined with CT scanning:
   (a) Low-dose CT technique
   (b) No i.v. contrast medium.
5. PET imaging of:
   (a) Brain
   (b) Whole body if indicated.

Alternative techniques

1. L-[methyl-^{11}C]methionine ([^{11}C] MET) or 3'-deoxy-3'-[^{18}F] fluorothymidine ([^{18}F] FLT) PET
2. ^{201}Thallium
3. MR spectroscopy.

^{201}THALLIUM BRAIN SCANNING

Indications

1. CNS (and other) tumours:
   (a) Grading
   (b) Differentiation of post surgical or radiotherapy change from residual or recurrent tumours.

This radionuclide procedure has largely been superseded by PET.

Contraindications

None.

Radiopharmaceutical

^{201}Thallium 100 MBq (25 mSv ED).

Equipment

1. SPECT gamma camera
2. VerteX High Resolution (VXHR) gamma camera.

Technique

I.v. injection of radiopharmaceutical.

Analysis

SPECT.

Aftercare

None.

DOPAMINE TRANSPORTER LIGANDS

Indications

Ioflupane, 123-I FP-CIT (DatSCAN, GE Healthcare) contains a
dopamine transporter radioligand and can be used to assess
striatal uptake in possible Parkinson's disease, and differentiate
from other movement disorders.

Contraindications

None.

Radiopharmaceuticals

^{123}I DatSCAN 185 MBq (4.5 mSv ED).

Equipment

1. SPECT gamma camera
2. VXHR.

Patient preparation

Thyroid blockade (400 mg potassium perchlorate orally 1 h before
scan, 200 mg every 6 h for four doses).

13

Technique

I.v. injection of radiopharmaceutical.

Images

Image with SPECT at 3–6 h.

Analysis

Diagnosis depends on an assessment of relative uptake in the caudate and putamen.

Aftercare

None.

References

Complications
1. Asenbaum S, Brücke T, Pirker W, et al. Imaging of cerebral blood flow with technetium-99m-HMPAO and technetium-99m-ECD: a comparison. J Nucl Med 1998;39(4):613–18.
2. Koyama M, Kawashima R, Ito H, et al. SPECT imaging of normal subjects with technetium-99m-HMPAO and technetium-99m-ECD. J Nucl Med 1997;38(4):587–92.

Further Reading

Radionuclide Imaging of the Brain
Freeman LM, Blaufox MD. Functional brain imaging (Part 1). Semin Nucl Med 2003;33(1):1–85.

Complications
Murray AD. The brain, salivary and lacrimal glands. In: Sharp PF, Gemmell HG, Murray AD, editors. Practical Nuclear Medicine. 3rd ed. London: Springer-Verlag; 2005.

Aftercare
Hammoud DA, Hoffman JM, Pomper MG, et al. Molecular neuroimaging: from conventional to emerging techniques. Radiology 2007;245(1):21–42.

ULTRASOUND OF THE INFANT BRAIN

Indications

Any suspected intracranial pathology, particularly suspected germinal matrix haemorrhage, extra-axial haematomas and hydrocephalus.

Equipment

4–7-MHz, sector transducer. A 7.5- or 10-MHz transducer to visualize superficial structures.

Patient preparation

None is required, though a recently fed infant is more likely to tolerate the examination without protest. An agitated child should be calmed by the mother or carer by any appropriate method.

Methods

1. Via the anterior fontanelle
2. Through the squamosal portion of the temporal bone to visualize extracerebral collections and the region of the circle of Willis
3. Via the posterior fontanelle, for the posterior fossa.

Technique

Six coronal and six sagittal images are obtained and supplemented with other images of specific areas of interest. The base of the skull must be perfectly symmetrical on coronal scans. The first image is obtained with the transducer angled forward and subsequent images obtained by angling progressively more posteriorly. The anatomical landmarks that define each view are given below.

Coronal

1. The orbital roofs and cribriform plate (these combine to produce a 'steer's head' appearance); anterior interhemispheric fissure; frontal lobes
2. Greater wings, lesser wings and body of sphenoid (these produce a 'mask' appearance); the cingulate sulcus; frontal horns of lateral ventricles
3. Pentagon view: five-sided star formed by the internal carotid, middle cerebral and anterior cerebral arteries
4. Frontal horns of lateral ventricles; cavum septum pellucidum; basal ganglia. Bilateral C-shaped echoes from the parahippocampal gyri; thalami
5. Trigones of lateral ventricles containing choroid plexus; echogenic inverted V from the tentorium cerebelli; cerebellum
6. Occipital horns of lateral ventricles; parietal and occipital cortex; cerebellum.

Sagittal

For the sagittal images, the reference plane should be a mid-line image with the third ventricle, septum pellucidum and fourth ventricle all on the same image. The more lateral parasagittal images are obtained with the transducer angled laterally and slightly oblique because the occipital horn of the lateral ventricle is more lateral than the frontal horn:

1. Two views of the mid-line
2. Parasagittal scans of the lateral ventricles. These are angled approximately 15° from the mid-line, to show the caudothalamic grooves
3. Steep parasagittal scans, approximately 30° from the mid-line, of the frontal, temporal and parietal cortices.

13

CEREBRAL ANGIOGRAPHY

Indications

1. Intracerebral and subarachnoid haemorrhage
2. Aneurysms presenting as space-occupying lesions
3. Brain arteriovenous shunts, carotico-cavernous fistulas (direct and indirect)
4. Cerebral ischaemia both of extracranial and intracranial origin
5. Pre-operative assessment of intracranial tumours.

Contraindications

1. Patients with unstable neurology (usually following subarachnoid haemorrhage or stroke)
2. Patients unsuitable for surgery
3. Patients in whom vascular access would be impossible or relatively risky
4. Iodine allergy. Relative contraindication as angiography could be performed with gadolinium chelates.

Equipment

A single or biplane digital subtraction angiography apparatus is required, with a C-arm allowing unlimited imaging planes, high-quality fluoroscopy and road-mapping facility.

Three-dimensional rotational angiography is now increasingly available and forms an important part of the analysis of aneurysms during treatment. There should be access to the patient for both the radiologist and the anaesthetist, with appropriate head immobilization.

Preparation

When the patient is able to understand what is proposed, a clear explanation should be given, together with presentation of the risks and benefits. Most patients do not require sedation for diagnostic procedures and this would be contraindicated in acute neurological presentations. Children, patients who are excessively anxious, those who cannot cooperate because of confusion, or those who would be managed better during the procedure with full ventilation control are examined under general anaesthesia. Neurointerventional studies are done under general anaesthesia. Groin shaving is now regarded as unnecessary. Patients should not be starved unless general anaesthesia is to be used, but should, nevertheless, be restricted to fluid intake and only a light meal.

Technique

Catheter flushing solutions should consist of heparinized saline (2500 IU l^{-1} normal saline). Using standard percutaneous catheter introduction techniques, the femoral artery is catheterized. It is a common practice to deliver an access sheath through which catheters are introduced and exchanged if necessary. There is a wide range of catheters available and there are proponents of many types. In patients up to middle age without major hypertension, there will be little difficulty with any standard catheter and a simple 4F polythene catheter with a slightly curved tip or 45° bend will suffice in the majority. Older patients and those with atherosclerotic disease may need catheters offering greater torque control such as the JB2 or Simmons (Figs 13.1, 13.2) as appropriate. Catheter control will be better if passed through an introducer set, and this is also indicated where it is anticipated that catheter exchange may be required. Selective

Figure 13.1 (a) Vertebrale or Berenstein, (b) JB2, (c) Mani. End holes: 1 Side holes: 0.

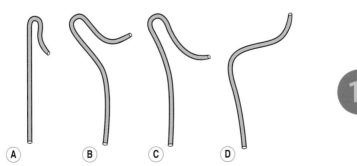

13

Figure 13.2 Simmons (sidewinder) catheters. (a) For narrow aorta. (b) For moderately narrow aorta. (c) For wide aorta. (d) For elongated aorta. End holes: 1 Side holes: 0.

studies of the common carotids and the vertebrals are preferable to super-selective studies of the internal and external carotids unless absolutely necessary. The following points should be noted:

1. The hazards of cerebral angiography are largely avoidable; they consist of the complications common to all forms of angiography (see Chapter 9) and those which are particularly related to cerebral angiography.
2. Any on-table ischaemic event has an explanation. Cerebral angiography does not possess an inherently unavoidable complication rate as has been suggested in the past. If an ischaemic event occurs there has been a complication, and its cause must be identified.
3. The most significant complications are embolic in origin, and the most important emboli are particulate. Air bubbles should be avoided as part of good angiographic practice, but are unlikely to cause a severe neurological complication.
4. Emboli may come from the injected solutions. Avoid contamination from glove powder, and dried blood or clot on gloves. Take care to avoid blood contamination of the saline or of the contrast medium, which is always dangerous. Avoid exposure of solutions to air. Contrast medium or heparin/saline in an open bowl is bad practice.
5. Emboli may arise from dislodgement of plaque or thrombus. Never pass a catheter or guidewire through a vessel that has not been visualized by preliminary injection of contrast medium. Use appropriate angled, hydrophilic guidewires. Do not try to negotiate excessively acute bends in vessels. The splinting effect of the catheter will cause spasm and arrest the flow in the artery. Dissections could occur which may lead to occlusion. Newer catheter designs tend to be softer and allow further distal access for more complex procedures. Sharp curves can otherwise be safely negotiated with microcatheters.
6. Emboli may arise from the formation of thrombus within a catheterized vessel. Always ensure that there is free blood flow past the catheter, and avoid forceful passage of a guidewire or catheter in such a way as may damage the intima of the vessel and cause thrombus formation.
7. Emboli may arise within the catheter. Do not allow blood to flow back into the catheter, or if it does occur then flush regularly or by continuous infusion. Never allow a guidewire to remain within a catheter for more than 1 min without withdrawal and flushing, and never introduce a guidewire into a contrast-filled catheter, but fill the catheter with heparinized saline first.
8. Keep study time to a minimum, but not at the expense of the diagnostic usefulness of the study.

Contrast medium

Non-ionic monomer, e.g. iohexol, iopamidol. The iodine concentration required is equipment-dependent, but with modern DSA, 150 mg I ml^{-1} will be suitable.

Contrast medium volume

1. Common carotid – 10 ml by hand in about 1.5–2 s
2. Internal carotid – 7 ml by hand in about 1.5 s
3. Vertebral artery – 7 ml by hand in about 1.5 s, but this volume can be diluted by 2 ml of saline to opacify the contralateral vertebral on the same injection.

Projections

As required, but basically 20° anterior-posterior (AP), Townes, lateral, occipitomental and oblique views as indicated. Multiple projections are especially needed for aneurysm studies to open loops and profile aneurysms; however, with three-dimensional rotational angiography, contrast runs can now be cut down to a minimum, and computer models of aneurysms and vessels can be analysed instead.

Films

From early arterial to late venous, about 8 s in total in most cases, system acquisitions will be at 2–4 frames s^{-1} depending on the study. With digital fluoroscopy acquisitions typically will be 2 frames s^{-1} for 4 s, and then 1 frame every 2 s for 4 s.

Aftercare

1. Standard nursing care for the arterial puncture site
2. Most departments adopt the practice of maintaining neurological observation for a period of 4 h or so after the procedure
3. Good hydration should be maintained.

13

Spine

Methods of imaging the spine

Many of the earlier imaging methods are now only of historical interest (e.g. conventional tomography, epidurography, epidural venography):

1. **Plain films**. These are widely available, but with low sensitivity. They are of questionable value in chronic back pain because of the prevalence of degenerative changes in both symptomatic and asymptomatic individuals of all ages beyond the second decade. They are, however, useful in suspected spinal injury, spinal deformity and postoperative assessment.
2. **Myelography/radiculography**. This is used when MRI is contraindicated or unacceptable to the patient. It is usually followed by CT for detailed assessment of abnormalities (CT myelography).
3. **Discography**. Advocates still regard it as the only technique able to verify the presence and source of discogenic pain.
4. **Facet joint arthrography**. Facet joint pain origin can be confirmed if it is abolished after diagnostic injection of local anaesthetic, and treated by steroid instillation. The radiological appearances of the arthrogram are not helpful for the most part except in showing a communication with a synovial cyst. Vertical and contralateral facet joint communications can arise in the presence of pars interarticularis defects.
5. **Arteriography**. This is used for further study of vascular malformations shown by other methods, usually MRI, and for assessment for potential embolotherapy. It is not appropriate for the primary diagnosis of spinal vascular malformations. It may be used for pre-operative embolization of vascular vertebral tumours (e.g. renal metastasis).
6. **Radionuclide imaging**. This is largely performed for suspected vertebral metastases and to exclude an occult painful bone lesion (e.g. osteoid osteoma) using a technetium scintigraphic agent, for which it is a sensitive and cost-effective technique.

7. **Computed tomography (CT)**. CT provides optimal detail of vertebral structures and is particularly useful in spinal trauma, spondylolysis, vertebral tumours, spinal deformity and postoperative states, especially if multidetector CT (MDCT) is available.
8. **Magnetic resonance imaging (MRI)**. This is the preferred technique for virtually all spinal pathology. It is the only technique that directly images the spinal cord and nerve roots. MRI with intravenous (i.v.) gadolinium-DTPA is indicated in spinal infection, tumours and postoperative assessment.
9. **Ultrasound (US)**. This is of use as an intra-operative method, and has uses in the infant spine.

IMAGING APPROACH TO BACK PAIN AND SCIATICA

There are a variety of ways to image the spine, many of which are expensive. The role of the radiologist is to ensure that diagnostic algorithms are selected for diagnostic accuracy, clinical relevance and cost-effectiveness. Each diagnostic imaging procedure has a different degree of sensitivity and specificity when applied to a particular diagnostic problem. A combination of imaging techniques can be used in a complementary way to enhance diagnostic accuracy. The appropriate use of the available methods of investigating the spine is essential, requiring a sensible sequence and timing of the procedures to ensure cost-effectiveness, maximal diagnostic accuracy and clinical effectiveness with minimum discomfort to the patient.

The philosophy underlying the management of low back pain and sciatica encompasses the following fundamental points:

1. Radiological investigation is essential if surgery is proposed.
2. Radiological findings should be compatible with the clinical picture before surgery can be advised.
3. It is vital for the surgeon and radiologist to identify those patients who will and who will not benefit from surgery.
4. In those patients judged to be in need of surgical intervention, success is very dependent on precise identification of the site, nature and extent of disease by the radiologist.
5. The demonstration of degenerative disease of the spine by non-invasive methods cannot be assumed to be the cause of the patient's symptoms, as similar changes are often seen in asymptomatic individuals.

The need for radiological investigation of the lumbosacral spine is based on the results of a thorough clinical examination. A useful and basic preliminary step, which will avoid unnecessary investigations, is to determine whether the predominant symptom is back pain or leg pain. Leg pain extending to the foot is indicative of nerve root compression and imaging needs to be directed towards the demonstration of a compressive lesion, typically disc prolapse. This is most commonly seen at the L4/5 or L5/S1 levels (90–95%), and MRI should be employed as the primary mode of imaging. If the predominant symptom is back pain, with or without proximal lower limb radiation, then invasive techniques may be required, including discography and facet joint arthrography. The presence of degenerative disc and facet disease demonstrated by plain films, CT or MRI has no direct correlation with the incidence of clinical symptomatology. The annulus fibrosus of the intervertebral disc and the facet joints are richly innervated, and only direct injection can assess them as a potential pain source. However, unless there are therapeutic implications, there is no indication to go to these lengths, as many patients can be managed by physiotherapy and mild analgesics.

CONVENTIONAL RADIOGRAPHY

Routine radiographic evaluation at the initial assessment of a patient with acute low back pain does not usually provide clinically useful information. Eighty-five per cent of such patients will return to work within 2 months having received only conservative therapy, indicating the potential for non-contributory imaging. Despite the known limitations of radiographs, it is often helpful to obtain routine radiographs of the lumbar spine before another investigation is requested. The role of conventional radiographs can be summarized in the following points:

1. They assist in the diagnosis of conditions that can mimic mechanical or discogenic pain, e.g. infection, spondylolysis, ankylosing spondylitis and bone tumours, though in most circumstances ^{99m}Tc scintigraphy, CT and MRI are more sensitive.
2. They serve as a technical aid to survey the vertebral column and spinal canal prior to myelography, CT or MRI, particularly in the sense of providing basic anatomical data regarding segmentation. Failure to do this may lead to errors in interpreting correctly the vertebral level of abnormalities prior to surgery.
3. Correlation of CT or MRI data with radiographic appearances is often helpful in interpretation.

14

COMPUTED TOMOGRAPHY AND MAGNETIC RESONANCE IMAGING OF THE SPINE

CT and MRI have replaced myelography as the primary method for investigating suspected disc prolapse. High-quality axial imaging by CT is an accurate means of demonstrating disc herniation but, in practice, many studies are less than optimal due to obesity, scoliosis and beam-hardening effects due to dense bone sclerosis. For these reasons, and because of better contrast resolution, MRI is the preferred technique and CT is only employed when MRI cannot be used. MRI alone has the capacity to show the morphology of the intervertebral disc, and can show ageing changes, typically dehydration, in the nucleus pulposus. It provides sagittal sections, which have major advantages for the demonstration of the spinal cord and cauda equina, vertebral alignment, stenosis of the spinal canal, and for showing the neural foramina. Far lateral disc herniation cannot be shown by myelography, but is readily demonstrated by CT or MRI. CT may be preferred to MRI where there is a suspected spinal injury, in the assessment of primary spinal tumours of bony origin, and in the study of spondylolysis and Paget's disease. MRI in spinal stenosis provides all the required information showing all the relevant levels on a single image, the degree of narrowing at each level and the secondary effects such as the distension of the vertebral venous plexus. The relative contributions of bone, osteophyte, ligament or disc, while better evaluated by CT, are relatively unimportant in the management decisions. Furthermore, MRI will show conditions which may mimic spinal stenosis such as prolapsed thoracic disc, ependymoma of the conus medullaris and dural arteriovenous fistula.

In addition to the diagnosis of prolapsed intervertebral disc, CT and MRI differentiate the contained disc, where the herniated portion remains in continuity with the main body of the disc, from the sequestrated disc, where there is a free migratory disc fragment. This distinction may be crucial in the choice of conservative or surgical therapy, and of percutaneous rather than open surgical techniques. MRI studies have shown that even massive *extruded* disc lesions can resolve naturally with time, without intervention. Despite the presence of nerve root compression, a disc prolapse can be entirely asymptomatic. Gadolinium enhancement of compressed lumbar nerve roots is seen in *symptomatic* disc prolapse with a specificity of 95.9%.[1]

Finally, in the decision as to whether to choose CT or MRI it should be remembered that lumbar spine CT delivers a substantial radiation dose, which is important, particularly in younger patients.

The main remaining uses of myelography are in patients with claustrophobia or who are otherwise not suitable for MRI. There are advocates for the use of CT myelography in the investigation of MRI-negative cervical radiculopathy. Myelography also allows a dynamic assessment of the spinal canal in instances of spinal stenosis and instability. The use of a special MR-compatible spinal harness that provides axial loading, and the availability of open and upright MR scanners also provide non-invasive dynamic MR imaging capability.

The problems of the 'post-laminectomy' patient or 'failed back surgery syndrome' are well known. Accurate pre-operative assessment should limit the number of cases resulting from inappropriate surgery and surgery at the wrong level. The investigation of the postoperative lumbar spine is difficult and re-operation has a poor outcome in many cases. Although the investigation of the postoperative lumbar spine is difficult, it is vital to make the distinction between residual or recurrent disc prolapse at the operated level and epidural fibrosis in order to minimize the risk of a negative re-exploration. The best available technique is gadolinium-enhanced MRI.

Arachnoiditis is a cause of postoperative symptoms and its features are shown on myelography, CT myelography and MRI. In the past, many cases were caused by the use of myodil (Pantopaque) as a myelographic contrast medium. It is likely that the use of myodil as an intrathecal contrast agent caused arachnoiditis in most cases, but this became symptomatic in only a minority. The potentiating effects of blood in the CSF, particularly as a result of surgery, have been evident in many cases. New cases of arachnoiditis are now rarely seen, but there is residue of chronic disease still presenting from time to time.

Conclusions

MRI has revolutionized the imaging of spinal disease. Advantages include non-invasiveness, multiple imaging planes and lack of radiation exposure. Its superior soft tissue contrast enables the distinction of nucleus pulposus from annulus fibrosus of the healthy disc and enables the early diagnosis of degenerative changes. However, up to 35% of asymptomatic individuals less than 40 years of age have significant intervertebral disc disease at one or more levels on MRI images. Correlation with the clinical evidence is, therefore, essential before any relevance is attached to their presence and surgery is undertaken. As MRI is, at present, not as accurate as discography in the diagnosis and delineation of annular disease, and in diagnosing the pain source, there has been a resurgence of interest in discography. MRI should be used as a predictor of the causative levels contributing to the back pain

14

with discography having a significant role in the investigation of discogenic pain prior to surgical fusion.[2]

References

1. Tyrrell PN, Cassar-Pullicino VN, McCall IW. Gadolinium-DTPA enhancement of symptomatic nerve roots in MRI of the lumbar spine. Eur Radiol 1998;8(1):116–22.
2. Cassar-Pullicino VN. MRI of the ageing and herniating intervertebral disc. Eur J Radiol 1998;27(3):214–28.

Further Reading

Boden SD, Davis DO, Dina TS, et al. Abnormal magnetic resonance scans of the lumbar spine in asymptomatic subjects. J Bone Joint Surg Am 1990;72(3):403–8.

Butt WP. Radiology for back pain. Clin Radiol 1989;40(1):6–10.

Cribb GL, Jaffray DC, Cassar-Pullicino VN. Observations on the natural history of massive lumbar disc herniation. J Bone Joint Surg Br 2007;89(6):782–4.

du Boulay GH, Hawkes S, Lee CC, et al. Comparing the cost of spinal MR with conventional myelography and radiculography. Neuroradiology 1990;32(2):124–36.

Horton WC, Daftari TK. Which disc as visualized by magnetic resonance imaging is actually a source of pain? A correlation between magnetic resonance imaging and discography. Spine 1992;17(Suppl 6):S164–71.

Hueftle MG, Modic MT, Ross JS, et al. Lumbar spine: post-operative MR imaging with gadolinium-DTPA. Radiology 1988;167(3):817–24.

MYELOGRAPHY AND RADICULOGRAPHY

CONTRAST MEDIA

Historically, the contrast media that have been used for myelography include gas (CO_2, air), lipiodol, abrodil, myodil (Pantopaque, iodophenylate), meglumine iothalamate (Conray), meglumine iocarmate (Dimer X), metrizamide (Amipaque), iopamidol (Niopam), iohexol (Omnipaque) and iotrolan (Isovist). The early oil-based media were diagnostically poor and led to arachnoiditis. The early water-soluble media were very toxic and also led to arachnoiditis, and the first intrathecal contrast medium with acceptably low toxicity was metrizamide, a non-ionic dimer. Iohexol and iopamidol are non-ionic monomers licensed for intrathecal use and the ones most commonly used currently.

CERVICAL MYELOGRAPHY

This may be performed by introduction of contrast medium into the thecal sac by lumbar puncture and then run up to the cervical spine, or by direct cervical puncture at C1/2.

Indications

Suspected spinal cord pathology or root compression in patients unable or unwilling to undergo MRI imaging.

Lateral cervical or C1/2 puncture v lumbar injection

Cervical puncture is quick, safe and reliable but is contraindicated in patients with suspected high cervical or cranio-cervical pathology, and where the normal bony anatomy and landmarks are distorted or lost by anomalous development or rheumatoid disease. Complications are rare but include vertebral artery damage and inadvertent cord puncture. Cervical puncture is particularly indicated where there is severe lumbar disease, which may restrict the flow of contrast medium and may make lumbar puncture difficult, and when there is thoracic spinal canal stenosis. It is also required for the demonstration of the upper end of a spinal block. It is not a good technique for whole-spine myelography; after completion of a cervical myelogram, the contrast medium is too dilute for effective use in the remainder of the spinal canal. When lumbar injection is used, a good lumbar study is possible without dilution, following which a cervical and thoracic study is entirely feasible. Lumbar injection for cervical myelography is as effective as cervical injection when nothing restricts the upward flow of contrast medium. The post-procedural morbidity, mainly consisting of headache, is rather less after cervical puncture.

Contrast medium

Non-ionic contrast medium is used (see above). The total dose should not exceed 3 g of iodine, i.e. 10 ml of contrast medium with a concentration of 300 mg ml^{-1}. Adequate filling for cervical myelography usually only requires 7–8 ml, or even less when the canal is narrow.

Equipment

Tilting X-ray table with a C-arm fluoroscopic facility for screening and radiography in multiple planes.

Patient preparation

Mild sedation with oral diazepam is appropriate in anxious patients, but is not essential. The skin puncture point is outside the hair line and no hair removal is generally needed, though the hair should be gathered into a paper cap.

Technique

1. The patient lies prone with arms at the sides and chin resting on a soft pad so that the neck is in a neutral position or in slight

14

extension. Marked hyperextension is undesirable as it accentuates patient discomfort, particularly in those with spondylosis, who comprise the majority of patients referred for this procedure. In such cases it will further compromise a narrowed canal and may produce symptoms of cord compression. The patient must be comfortable and able to breathe easily.

2. Using lateral fluoroscopy the C1/2 space is identified. The beam should be centred at this level to minimize errors due to parallax. Head and neck adjustments may be needed to ensure a true lateral position. The aim is to puncture the subarachnoid space between the laminae of C1 and C2, at the junction of the middle and posterior thirds of the spinal canal, i.e. posterior to the spinal cord. A 20G spinal needle is used. There is better control with the relatively stiff 20G needle, and the requirement for a small needle size to minimize CSF loss does not apply in the cervical region, where CSF pressure is very low.

3. Using aseptic technique, the skin and subcutaneous tissues are anaesthetized with 1% lidocaine. The spinal needle is introduced with the stilette bevel parallel to the long axis of the spine, i.e. to split rather than cut the fibres of the interlaminar ligaments. Lateral fluoroscopy is used to adjust the direction of the needle, and ensure the maintenance of a perfect lateral position as the needle is advanced. It is very helpful if a nurse steadies the patient's head.

4. The sensation of the needle penetrating the dura is similar to that experienced during a lumbar puncture and the patient may experience slight discomfort at this stage. A feature that indicates that the needle tip is close to the dura is the appearance of venous blood at the needle hub as the epidural space is traversed. If the needle trajectory is too far posterior, tenting of the dura may occur, with failure to puncture the CSF space, even though anterior-posterior (AP) screening may show that the needle tip has crossed the midline. Repositioning may be needed in such cases. Severe acute neck or radicular pain indicates that the needle has been directed too far anteriorly and has come into contact with an exiting nerve root. Clumsy technique is known to have caused cord puncture, but permanent neurological damage as a result is unlikely.

5. Following removal of the stilette, CSF will drip from the end of the needle, and a sample may be collected if required.

6. Under fluoroscopy a small amount of contrast medium is injected to verify correct needle-tip placement. This will flow away from the needle tip and gravitate anteriorly to layer behind the vertebral bodies. Transient visualization of the dentate ligaments is obtained.

7. Injection is continued slowly until the required amount has been delivered. The cervical canal should be opacified anteriorly from the foramen magnum to C7/T1. If contrast tends to flow into the

head before filling the lower cervical canal, tilt the table feet down slightly, and vice versa if contrast is flowing into the thoracic region without filling the upper cervical canal.

Radiographic views

After needle withdrawal, two AP radiographs are obtained with the tube angulated cranially and caudally, in turn, along with both oblique views once again with cranial and caudal tube tilt. Soft and penetrated lateral views are needed to ensure full assessment of the cervico-thoracic junction. Lastly, a further lateral view of the craniocervical junction is taken with mild neck flexion because all too often the extended neck position prevents full visualization of the upper cervical cord up to the foramen magnum.

Aftercare

Although many centres request the patient to remain sitting or semi-recumbent for about 6 h, allowing the patient to remain ambulant does not increase the incidence of side effects. A high fluid intake is generally encouraged; though evidence for its usefulness is lacking.

LUMBAR RADICULOGRAPHY

This may be performed by injection of contrast medium into the lumbar thecal sac. If for any reason lumbar puncture is not possible, e.g. because of lumbar spine deformity or arachnoiditis, it is possible to introduce the contrast medium from above by cervical injection. Dilution of the contrast as it passes downwards is a major disadvantage.

Indications

Suspected lumbar root or cauda equina compression, spinal stenosis and conus medullaris lesions in patients who are unable or unwilling to undergo MRI.

Contraindications

Lumbar puncture is potentially hazardous in the presence of raised intracranial pressure. It may be difficult to achieve satisfactory intrathecal injection in patients who have had a recent lumbar puncture, since subdural CSF accumulates temporarily, and this space may be entered rather than the subarachnoid space. Accordingly an interval of 1 week or so is advisable.

14

Contrast medium

The contrast medium is the same as that used for cervical myelography. The maximum dose is again the equivalent of 3 g of iodine, and may be given as 10 ml of contrast medium of 300 mg ml^{-1} concentration, or 12.5 ml of 240 mg ml^{-1}.

Equipment

Tilting fluoroscopic table.

Patient preparation

As for cervical myelography.

Preliminary images

AP and lateral projections of the region under study are taken. Preliminary examination of radiographs is helpful to assess the anatomy of the spine, in order to facilitate the lumbar puncture, and to assist in interpretation of the images. It is important to draw the surgeon's attention to any question of ambiguous segmentation, either lumbarization or sacralization. There is a potential danger of operating at the wrong level if this is not made absolutely clear in the report. A clear description of any anomaly is required, together with a statement of how the vertebrae have been numbered in the report.

Technique

1. The lumbar thecal sac is punctured at L2/3, L3/4 or L4/5. The higher levels tend to be away from the most common sites of disc herniation and stenosis, and puncture may, therefore, be easier.
2. Lumbar puncture can technically be performed in the lateral decubitus position, in the sitting position, or even in the prone position. In the prone position the needle is guided under fluoroscopy, usually at the L2/L3 interspinous space with the patient lying on a folded pillow. This is important, because in the prone position the spinous processes are approximated due to lordosis, rendering puncture more difficult. In addition, spinal extension produces a relatively narrow thecal sac. The sitting position allows easy lumbar puncture, but is unsatisfactory for two reasons. First, the injected contrast medium drops through a large volume of CSF to accumulate in the sacral sac and becomes diluted as it descends. Second, patients may faint in this position, a complication that can be very dangerous, since the radiologist is on the wrong side of the table to help in preventing the patient from coming to any harm.

3. If lumbar puncture is carried out in the lateral decubitus position (described below) moderate spinal flexion is desirable, but there is no need for the extreme flexion sometimes demanded of the patient. A small pillow is placed under the dependent lumbar angle to keep the spine straight. The relevant interspace is one or two spinous processes above the plane of the iliac crest (L4/L5). If the spinous process cannot be felt, lateral fluoroscopy may help.

4. In obese patients the apparent soft-tissue midline gravitates below the spinal midline. The midline position may be verified while introducing local anaesthetic (1% lidocaine) into the skin and subcutaneous tissue, though there is no need to infiltrate the interspinous ligament. A 22G spinal needle should be used. It should be introduced with only a 10–15° cranial angulation. The passage of the needle through the interspinous ligament has a very characteristic sensation of moderate smooth resistance. Lack of resistance implies passage in the fatty tissues lateral to the midline, and a gritty sensation means impingement on the bone of the spinous process.

5. There is a tendency in inexperienced operators to introduce the needle at too steep a cranial angle, which a casual inspection of the spinous process anatomy can show to be incorrect. While traversing the interspinous ligament, the bevel should be in the coronal plane to avoid deflection to one side or the other, but once well established in the ligament may be turned to penetrate the thecal sac parallel to its long axis.

6. There is a characteristic sudden loss of resistance as the needle enters the thecal sac, and at this time the stilette should be withdrawn to verify CSF flow out of the needle. In the prone position suction using a 2-ml syringe may be necessary to obtain CSF. It should then be reintroduced and the needle advanced about 2 mm to ensure that the whole of the bevel has entered the thecal sac. A flexible connector is attached, taking care not to disturb the needle position.

7. Most difficulties are technical, arising from non-midline positioning of the needle, but in the presence of canal stenosis it may be difficult to find a position among the crowded roots where good CSF flow will take place. In most cases, radiologists will prefer to observe the entry of contrast medium into the thecal sac on the fluoroscopic screen, and this is especially important if there has been any difficulty in achieving a good needle position.

8. After the contrast medium has been injected, the patient turns to lie prone, and a series of films is obtained. Before taking films ensure that the relevant segment of the spinal canal is adequately filled with contrast medium. This usually requires some degree of feet-down tilt of the table, and a footrest should be in place to support the patient.

14

Radiographic views

1. AP and oblique views are obtained. (About 25° of obliquity is usual, but tailored in the individual case to profile the exit sleeves of the nerve roots of the cauda equina.)
2. A lateral view with a horizontal beam is useful, but further laterals in the erect or semi-erect position on flexion and extension add a dynamic dimension to the study.
3. Some radiologists advocate lateral decubitus frontal oblique views, to allow full entry of contrast medium into the dependent root sleeves of the whole lumbar and lower thoracic thecal sac. When turning patients from one side to the other ensure that they turn through the prone position, as turning supine will produce irretrievable contrast medium dilution.

At this stage the study will be complete as far as the question of root compression is concerned. The films should be carefully reviewed at this stage to ensure that all areas are fully covered, as the next manoeuvre will make any return to this area impossible. If the study is good, the patient should be screened in the lateral decubitus position, and tilted level or slightly head down until the contrast medium flows up to lie across the thoraco-lumbar junction. The patient may then be turned to lie supine and films of the conus and lower thoracic area obtained in the AP projection.

Additional technique

Post-myelographic MDCT is helpful for good visualization of the conus and cause of root compression and should routinely be done after myelography.

THORACIC MYELOGRAPHY

If the thoracic spine is the primary region of interest the lumbar puncture injection is made with the patient lying on one side, with the head of the table lowered and the patient's head supported on a bolster or pad to prevent contrast medium from running up into the head. If an obstruction to flow is anticipated, about half the volume of contrast medium may be injected and observed as it flows upwards. If an obstruction is encountered, the contrast medium is allowed to accumulate against it, and the remainder of the contrast medium is then injected slowly (this may cause some discomfort or pain and patience must be used). This manoeuvre will, in some cases, cause a little of the contrast medium to flow past the obstructing lesion and demonstrate its superior extent. If there is no obstruction, the full volume is injected. When the injection is complete, lateral radiographs may be taken and the patient then turned to lie supine. Further AP views are then taken.

CERVICAL MYELOGRAPHY BY LUMBAR INJECTION

The technique proceeds as for thoracic myelography, but the patient remains in the lateral decubitus position until the contrast medium has entered the neck. With the head raised on a pad or bolster, contrast will not flow past the foramen magnum. When all the contrast has reached the neck the patient is turned to lie prone, and the study then completed as for a cervical injection study.

CT MYELOGRAPHY

CT myelography (CTM) should be delayed for up to 4 h after injection to allow dilution of the contrast medium. A very high concentration may cause difficulty in resolving the cervical nerve roots. Turning the patient a few times prior to CT ensures even distribution and reduces layering effects. In studying the spinal cord a delay is not required though, again, good mixing of the CSF with contrast medium is essential. The superior contrast resolution of CT allows the definition of very dilute contrast medium, e.g. beyond a spinal block, thus avoiding the need for a cervical puncture. Nerve root exit foramina may be studied by CTM in both the lumbar and cervical region, and it has been shown to be a sensitive technique, though it fails to demonstrate far lateral disc lesions. Delayed CTM is needed in suspected syringomyelia.

PAEDIATRIC MYELOGRAPHY

A few points need to be borne in mind when carrying out myelography in the paediatric age group:

1. General anaesthetic is essential for all children aged 6 years or younger, and for many children up to the age of 12 years.
2. Lumbar puncture in cases of spinal dysraphism carries the risk of damaging a low-lying cord due to tethering. The thecal sac is usually wide in these conditions and the needle should be placed laterally in the thecal sac. In addition, as low a puncture as possible will minimize the risk, though in practice spinal cord injury is very uncommon or masked by the neurologic deficit already present.
3. In dysraphism, the frequent association of cerebellar tonsillar herniation precludes lateral C1/2 puncture.

14

Aftercare

Most patients may be discharged home after being allowed to rest for a few hours after the study. The practice of automatic hospitalization for myelography can no longer be justified in the light of improved contrast media with very low rates of serious morbidity. The patient may remain ambulant. A good fluid intake is generally advised though its value is unproven.

Complications

1. Headache occurs in about 25% of cases, slightly more frequent in females.
2. Nausea and vomiting occur in about 5%.
3. Subdural injection of contrast medium. This occurs when only part of the needle bevel is within the subarachnoid space. Contrast medium initially remains loculated near the end of the needle, but can track freely in the subdural space to simulate intrathecal flow. When in doubt, the injection should be stopped, and AP and lateral views obtained with the needle in situ. The temptation of interpreting such an examination should be resisted and the patient re-booked.
4. Extradural injection of contrast medium outlines the nerve roots well beyond the exit foramina.
5. Intramedullary injection of contrast medium. This is a complication of lateral cervical puncture or in a low-lying spinal cord, and is recognized as a slit-like collection of contrast medium in the spinal canal. Small collections are without clinical significance.

LUMBAR DISCOGRAPHY

Aims

There is strong evidence to support the role of discography in identifying patients with lumbar discogenic pain, but only moderate and limited supportive evidence in cervical and thoracic discogenic pain:

1. To opacify the disc with contrast medium injected into the nucleus pulposus in order to demonstrate degeneration and herniation
2. To provoke and reproduce the pain for which the patient is being investigated and to assess its response to anaesthetic injection.

Indications

Given the present status of MRI, any request for discography must be considered with great care, as it is a painful procedure and not without risk. If infection occurs the disc will be permanently damaged. The indications are:

1. Suspected discogenic pain without radicular signs
2. Confirmation of normal discs above or below a proposed surgical fusion.

Contraindications

1. None absolute (except allergy to iodine)
2. Any local or distant sepsis will add to the risk of infective discitis
3. Patient not a surgical candidate due to comorbidity.

Contrast medium

Non-ionic contrast media such as iopamidol or iohexol. A normal disc will usually allow up to 1.0 ml to be injected.

Equipment

1. Radiographic equipment as for myelography. Biplane screening is essential to ensure correct needle positioning
2. Discography needles – a set of two needles are used for each level:
   (a) Outer needle, 21G, 12.5 cm
   (b) Inner needle, 26G, 15.8 cm.

Patient preparation

The procedure and its aim are explained to the patient. It is important (1) that patients are asked to describe what pain they experience and (2) that patients should not be told that they may get symptomatic pain. This precaution reduces the chance of obtaining a programmed response from the patient. No other preparation is needed. The procedure is done under local anaesthesia. Pre-medication and analgesia may alter the patient's subjective response to discography, diminishing its efficacy and usefulness. Diazepam may, however, be required in very anxious patients. Some authors recommend broad-spectrum antibiotic cover (e.g. cephalosporins) given immediately before the examination to minimize the risk of infection.

Preliminary radiographs

AP and lateral films should be available or obtained.

Technique

1. There are two possible needle approaches:
   (a) The posterior approach, which traverses the spinal canal
   (b) The lateral oblique extradural approach, which avoids puncture of the dura and the vulnerable part of the posterior annulus. This is the preferred approach and can be carried

14

out with the patient in the prone or left lateral decubitus position. The left lateral decubitus position is preferred, with the patient's head resting on a pillow and a pad placed in the lumbar angle to maintain a straight spine. Moderate spinal flexion is useful, especially at L5/S1.

2. Full aseptic technique is mandatory; there should be no compromise on this point. The operator and any assistant should be gowned, masked, capped and gloved, and the patient should be draped. The level to be examined is determined by fluoroscopy, and the skin is anaesthetized, usually a hand's breadth from the spinous processes.

3. The outer 21G needle is then directed towards the posterior aspect of the disc under intermittent fluoroscopic control, at an angle of 45–60° to the vertical. An additional caudal tilt may be necessary for the L5/S1 level. This needle should reach but not traverse the annulus fibrosus. This point is recognized by a distinct feeling of resistance when the outer fibres are encountered. The 26G needle is then introduced through the 21G needle and the entry of its tip into the nucleus pulposus confirmed in two planes with the aid of the image intensifier prior to contrast medium injection.

4. Contrast medium is injected slowly using a 1-ml syringe. This is done under intermittent fluoroscopic control, while the pain response, the disc volume and its radiographic morphology are monitored. The resistance to flow will gradually increase in a normal disc during the 0.5–1.0-ml stage.

Radiographic views

1. AP and lateral films are obtained at each level examined.
2. At the end of the procedure after needle removal, AP and lateral films are taken in the standing position.
3. Films in flexion and extension may be useful.

Computed tomography post discogram

Thin-section CT slices aid in optimizing morphological grading of disc abnormalities, with particular reference to the status of the annulus and the degree and extent of annular tears.

Patient interrogation

Normal discs and some abnormal discs are asymptomatic. In the symptomatic abnormal discs, the pattern and distribution of pain are noted, together with any similarity to the usual symptomatology. At each symptomatic level local anaesthetic (bupivacaine hydrochloride 0.5%) may be injected to test its efficacy in producing symptomatic relief.

Aftercare

Simple analgesia may be required and overnight admission is usually advised to ensure adequate pain control.

Complications

1. Discitis is the most important complication. Pain with or without pyrexia after a few days indicates this development. Narrowing of the disc space with a variable degree of end-plate sclerosis is seen after a few weeks. Most cases are due to low-grade infection and require treatment with antibiotics.
2. With the transdural approach, post-lumbar puncture headache and/or vomiting may occur.

Further Reading

Buenaventura RM, Shah RV, Patel V, et al. Systematic review of discography as a diagnostic test for spinal pain: an update. Pain Physician 2007;10(1): 147–64.

Colhoun E, McCall IW, Williams L, et al. Provocation discography as a guide to planning operations on the spine. J Bone Joint Surg Br 1988;70(2):267–71.

McCulloch JA, Waddell G. Lateral lumbar discography. Br J Radiol 1978;51(607):498–502.

Tehranzadeh J. Discography 2000. Radiol Clin North Am 1998;36(3):463–95.

INTRADISCAL THERAPY

The ability to carry out successful discography will enable the radiologist, with the cooperation of interested clinicians, to carry out therapeutic procedures such as mechanical percutaneous disc removal, laser therapy and intradiscal electrothermal therapy (IDET). While each has advocates, none is widely utilized, and the practice of such methods should be subject to very strict selection criteria and rigorous audit of the outcomes.

FACET JOINT ARTHROGRAPHY

Indications

This is performed for diagnostic and therapeutic purposes, primarily at the lumbar level. Intra-articular injection is the only effective means for assessing the facet joints as a source of back pain. The only indication, therefore, is suspected pain of facet joint origin. Such pain may strongly resemble radicular pain, and patients have often been managed on this basis over a long period of time without success.

Affected facets are usually degenerate as visualized on plain radiographs, CT or MRI. The facet joint capsule is richly innervated by the dorsal ramus of the lumbar spinal nerves.

14

The procedure is valid in that many patients with degenerate facets do not have facet joint pain, and the role of the facet joint in the back pain of the individual patient cannot, therefore, be determined without facet joint injection. The arthrogram is not, therefore, a study of pathological anatomy; the visualization of the joint is important only to verify the needle position. Having visualized the joint, local anaesthetic can be injected to judge the patient's response. In cases obtaining good relief of symptoms, further management will then consist either of a programme of regular steroid injection therapy, cryolysis, radiofrequency or spinal fusion to prevent facet movement.

Equipment

1. As for myelography
2. A 22G spinal needle is appropriate for the study.

Contrast medium

Non-ionic contrast medium 0.1–0.2 ml should be used.

Technique

1. This is an outpatient procedure which involves the simultaneous injection of both joints at each level to be studied. More than one level should not be examined in each session to avoid diagnostic confusion. Needle placement can be done using fluoroscopy or CT guidance.
2. Using fluoroscopy the joint space is profiled by slowly rotating the patient from a prone position into a prone oblique orientation with the relevant side raised.
3. Sterile procedures are required.
4. The spinal needle is inserted and advanced perpendicularly to the facet joint, under fluoroscopic control. Caudal needle angulation is sometimes needed if the iliac crest overlies the L5/S1 facet joints. Alternatively the needles can be placed by simultaneous advancement into the joints using CT guidance.
5. In the majority of cases a noticeable 'give' indicates that the capsule is penetrated.
6. Contrast medium injection confirms correct needle placement by demonstrating immediate opacification of a superior and inferior recess.
7. Correct needle placement is documented showing intra-articular injection. The arthrographic appearances are not of any diagnostic consequence.
8. For diagnostic purposes up to 1 ml of 0.5% bupivacaine hydrochloride (Marcaine) is injected in the facet joint and the response over the ensuing 24-h period documented. For therapeutic injection, 0.5 ml of 0.5% Marcaine mixed with 0.5 ml

of Depo-Medrone (methylprednisolone 40 mg ml^{-1}) is injected
after arthrography.

Further Reading

Fairbank JC, Park WM, McCall IW, et al. Apophyseal injection of local
anaesthetic as a diagnostic aid in primary low back syndromes. Spine
1981;6:598–605.

McCall IW, Park WM, O'Brien JP. Induced pain referral from posterior lumbar
elements in normal subjects. Spine 1979;4(5):441–6.

Maldague B, Mathurin P, Malghem J. Facet joint arthrography in lumbar
spondylolysis. Radiology 1981;140(1):29–36.

Mooney V, Robertson J. The facet syndrome. Clin Orthop Relat Res
1976;115:149–56.

PERCUTANEOUS VERTEBRAL BIOPSY

The percutaneous approach to obtaining a representative sample
of tissue for diagnosis prior to therapy is both easy and safe,
avoiding the morbidity associated with open surgery. It has a
success rate of around 90%. Accurate lesion localization prior to
and during the procedure is required. Vertebral body lesions may
be biopsied under either CT or fluoroscopic control. Small lesions,
especially those located in the posterior neural arch, are best
biopsied under CT control. A preliminary CT scan is helpful,
whatever method is finally chosen to control the procedure.

Indications

Suspected vertebral or disc infection and vertebral neoplasia. Note
that the presence of a more accessible lesion in the appendicular
skeleton should be sought by radionuclide bone scanning, before
vertebral biopsy is undertaken.

Contraindications

1. Biopsy should not be attempted under any circumstances in the
presence of abnormal and uncorrected bleeding or clotting time or
if there is a low platelet count.
2. Lesions suspected of being highly vascular, e.g. aneurysmal bone
cyst or renal tumour metastasis are relatively dangerous, and a
fine-needle aspiration should be used instead of a trephine needle
for these cases.

Equipment

Numerous types of biopsy needle are available. The commonest type
used is the Jamshidi set. A trephine needle with an internal diameter
of 2 mm or more is required, minimizing histological distortion and
reducing sampling error without increasing the complication rate.
Specimen quality is higher with the Jamshidi type.

14

Patient preparation

Sedation/analgesia and, where necessary, general anaesthesia are required, preferably administered and monitored by an anaesthetist.

Technique

1. For a fluoroscopy-guided procedure the lateral decubitus position is used. For CT control the prone position is preferable.
2. The skin entry point distance from the mid-line is about 8 cm for the lumbar region and 5 cm in the thoracic region.
3. The aim of the procedure is to enter the vertebral body at about 4 o'clock or 8 o'clock (visualizing the body with the spinous process at 6 o'clock). Local anaesthetic may be injected via a 21G spinal needle to allow deep infiltration of the soft tissues into close proximity to the periosteum.
4. The biopsy needle is advanced at between 30 and 45° to the sagittal plane in the thoracic and lumbar spine, respectively.
5. When the biopsy needle impinges on the cortex of the vertebral body its position is confirmed fluoroscopically in both AP and lateral planes, or on a single CT section. The trocar and cannula are then advanced through the cortex and the trocar is then withdrawn.
6. Using alternate clockwise and anticlockwise rotation the biopsy cannula is advanced approximately 1 cm.
7. By twisting the needle firmly several times in the same direction the specimen is severed.
8. At least two cores of bone may be obtained by withdrawing the needle back to the cortex, angulating and re-entering the vertebral body.
9. The needle is then withdrawn while simultaneous suction is applied by a syringe attached to the hub.
10. To remove the specimen, the plunger is inserted at the sharp end of the needle and the tissue is pushed out. Any blood clot should be included as part of the specimen.
11. In suspected infection the end-plate rather than the disc is biopsied. Most cases are due to osteomyelitis extending to the disc space. If there is a paravertebral abscess, aspiration and culture of its contents is preferable to vertebral biopsy.

Aftercare

1. Overnight stay with routine nursing observation and analgesia if needed
2. The approach to a thoracic lesion should be extrapleural, but if any doubt exists, a chest X-ray should be obtained after the procedure, as there is a small risk of pneumothorax or haemothorax.

Complications

These are rare, but there are potential risks to nearby structures in poorly controlled procedures, including the lung and pleura, aorta, nerve roots and spinal cord. Local bleeding is an occasional problem.

Further Reading
Babu NV, Titus VT, Chittaranjan S, et al. Computed tomographically guided biopsy of the spine. Spine 1994;19(21):2436–42.
Shaltot A, Michell PA, Betts JA, et al. Jamshidi needle biopsy of bone lesions. Clin Radiol 1982;33:193–6.
Stoker DJ, Kissin CM. Percutaneous vertebral biopsy: a review of 135 cases. Clin Radiol 1985;36:569–77.
Tehranzadeh J, Tao C, Browning CA. Percutaneous needle biopsy of the spine. Acta Radiol 2007;48(8):860–8.

BONE AUGMENTATION TECHNIQUES

The vertebral bodies can collapse in osteoporosis and metastatic disease. The injection of small amounts of bone cement directly into the vertebral body (vertebroplasty) strengthens the vertebral body and is successful in control of spinal pain. Pre-procedure radiographs and an MRI scan are obtained, while a spinal surgeon is on standby should any complications require surgical intervention. Multiple levels can be treated in this manner with placement of the needle in the vertebral body using either a transpedicular approach or a posterolateral approach. Careful aseptic technique and fluoroscopic/CT guidance during cement injection is essential to avoid cement migration into the canal and/or veins. An allied technique (kyphoplasty) in addition partially restores vertebral body height in osteoporotic vertebral fractures.

Further Reading
Burton AW, Rhines LD, Mendel E. Vertebroplasty and kyphoplasty: a comprehensive review. Neurosurg Focus 2005;18(3):e1.
Hide IG, Gangi A. Percutaneous vertebroplasty: history, technique and current perspectives. Clin Radiol 2004;59(6):461–7.

NERVE ROOT BLOCKS

LUMBAR SPINE

14

This is undertaken in difficult diagnostic cases, usually in the presence of multilevel pathology, especially in postoperative situations. If the injected local anaesthetic in the perineural space abolishes the patient's symptoms, it is concluded that pain is originating from the injected nerve root. Therapeutic instillation of local anaesthetic with steroid (e.g. triamcinolone, betamethasone [Celestone Soluspan]) has proved successful as a means of treating sciatica in patients with disc prolapse, especially in a foraminal location. It is crucial that a review of the MRI images takes place before the procedure is carried out to ensure that the correct level and side are in accordance with the patient's symptoms. The objective is to place the needle *outside* the nerve root sleeve so that the injected substances diffuse between the disc prolapse and the compressed nerve. Reduction of the inflammatory response induced by the herniated disc can be slow and improvement of symptoms can take up to 8–12 weeks.

The accurate placement of the tip of a spinal needle is confirmed by the injection of a small amount of contrast medium. This is important to avoid injection in one of the lumbar vessels as, rarely, paraplegia presumed to be due to inadvertent intra-arterial injection has been reported. This risk needs to be communicated in the informed consent with the patient prior to the procedure.

Under local anaesthetic control, the needle is advanced using fluoroscopic or CT guidance, to a point inferior and lateral to the ipsilateral pedicle. The extra-foraminal nerve roots are outlined by contrast medium and for diagnostic purposes a small amount of 0.5% bupivacaine is instilled as a means of assessing the correct level responsible for the patient's sciatica.

CERVICAL SPINE

Perineural root sleeve therapy can also be used in cervical radiculopathy. Correct needle placement using CT and fluoroscopy is very important, utilizing contrast medium injection for confirmation prior to the therapeutic injection of lidocaine (bupivacaine is not used in the cervical spine) and steroid. There is a real risk of inadvertent vascular injection, particularly in the vertebral artery. CT fluoroscopic guidance at the required foraminal level is used to ensure the needle traverses in a horizontal or slightly downward course posterior to the carotid and jugular vessels. The needle tip is aimed towards the outer rim of the posterior bone outline of the foramen so as to avoid the vertebral vessels and the nerve root.

Further Reading

Blankenbaker DG, De Smet AA, Stanczak JD, et al. Lumbar radiculopathy: treatment with selective lumbar nerve blocks. Comparison of effectiveness of triamcinolone and betamethasone injectable suspensions. Radiology 2005;237(2):738–41.

Herron LD. Selective nerve root block in patient selection for lumbar surgery: surgical results. J Spinal Disord 1989;2(2):75–9.

Schellhas KP, Pollei SR, Johnson BA, et al. Selective cervical nerve root blockade: experience with a safe and reliable technique using an anterolateral approach for needle placement. Am J Neuroradiol 2007;28(10):1909–14.

Wagner AL. Selective lumbar nerve root blocks with CT fluoroscopic guidance: technique, results, procedure time, and radiation dose. Am J Neuroradiol 2004;25(9):1592–4.

Wagner AL. CT fluoroscopic-guided cervical nerve root blocks. Am J Neuroradiol 2005;26(1):43–4.

Weiner BK, Fraser RD. Foraminal injection for lateral lumbar disc herniation. J Bone Joint Surg Br 1997;79(5):804–7.

14

Lacrimal system and salivary glands

Methods of imaging the nasolacrimal drainage apparatus

1. Conventional/digital subtraction dacryocystography
2. CT dacryocystography
3. Magnetic resonance dacryocystography.

Further Reading
Ansari SA, Pak J, Shields M. Pathology and imaging of the lacrimal drainage system. Neuroimaging Clin N Am 2005;15(1):221–37.

DIGITAL SUBTRACTION AND CT DACRYOCYSTOGRAPHY

Dacryocystography allows visualization of the lacrimal system by direct injection of contrast into the canaliculus of the eyelid. It may be combined with CT imaging performed immediately following lacrimal system contrast injection. CT imaging gives additional diagnostic information, particularly about adjacent structures.[1]

Indications

Epiphora – to demonstrate the site and degree of obstruction.

Contraindications

None.

Contrast medium

Low osmolar contrast material (LOCM) 300, 0.5–2.0 ml per side.
The use of Lipiodol is to be discouraged.

Equipment

1. Digital subtraction radiography unit
2. Silver punctum or lachrymal dilator and lacrimal probe set
3. Lacrimal cannula or 18G blunt needle with polythene catheter (the catheter technique has the advantage that the examination can be performed on both sides simultaneously).

Patient preparation

0.5% bupivacaine eye drops.

Technique

1. The lacrimal sac is massaged to express its contents prior to injection of the contrast medium. The lower eyelid is everted to locate the lower canaliculus at the medial end of the lid.
2. The lower punctum normally measures 0.3 mm in diameter and is gently dilated. The lower lid should be drawn laterally to straighten the curve in the canaliculus. To avoid perforation, the cannula is initially positioned perpendicular to the eyelid margin as it enters the punctum. The cannula is then rotated by 90° horizontally along the natural curve of the lower canaliculus.
3. Care is taken not to advance the cannula too far into the canaliculus as proximal stenosis can be missed.
4. The upper canaliculus may also be cannulated if there is difficulty with the lower canaliculus.
5. The contrast medium is injected and a digital subtraction run at one image per second is obtained. This allows for a dynamic study in real time.

Images

Appropriate images are filmed/digitally stored.

Aftercare

A protective eye patch for 30–60 min may be necessary in view of the local anaesthetic used.

Complications

Perforation of the canaliculus.

Reference

1. Freitag SK, Woog JJ, Kousoubris PD, et al. Helical computed tomographic dacryocystography with three dimensional reconstruction: a new view of the lacrimal drainage system. Ophthal Plast Reconstr Surg 2002;18(2): 121–32.

MRI OF LACRIMAL SYSTEM

15

The lacrimal system can be assessed with MRI (MR dacryocystography) either following topical administration of eye drops containing a dilute gadolinium solution (sterile 0.9% NaCl solution containing 1:100 diluted gadolinium chelate) or by direct injection of a dilute gadolinium solution into the lacrimal canaliculus. The less-invasive, topical administration technique is more widely used. MR is useful in the diagnosis of obstruction level in the lacrimal system for patients with epiphora and in assessment of surrounding soft tissues.

Methods of imaging the salivary glands

1. **Plain films**: for calculus disease (sialithiasis)
2. **Conventional sialography**: less commonly performed than in the past; many indications replaced by non-invasive cross-sectional imaging
3. **CT**: thin-section unenhanced CT for diagnosis of sialithiasis ± intravenous (i.v.) contrast medium, e.g. in suspected tumour or abscess
4. **Ultrasound (US)**: ideal investigation for superficial salivary gland disease and a sensitive test for sialithiasis
5. **MRI**: ± i.v. contrast medium for assessment of inflammatory or malignant disease, may include MR spectroscopy for characterization of focal mass and MR sialography
6. **Radionuclide imaging (sialoscintigraphy)**.

Further Reading

MRI of Lacrimal System

Coskun B, Ilgit E, Onal B, et al. MR dacryocystography in the evaluation of patients with obstructive epiphora treated by means of interventional radiologic procedures. Am J Neuroradiol 2012;33(1):141–7.

Methods of Imaging the Salivary Glands

Bialek EJ, Jakubowski W, Zajkowski P, et al. US of the major salivary glands: anatomy and spatial relationships, pathological conditions and pitfalls. RadioGraphics 2006;26(3):745–63.

Freling NJ. Imaging of salivary gland disease. Semin Roentgenol 2000;35(1):12–20.

Rabinov JD. Imaging of salivary gland pathology. Radiol Clin North Am 2000;38(5):1047–57.

Yousem DM, Kraut MA, Chalian AA. Major salivary gland imaging. Radiology 2000;216(1):19–29.

CONVENTIONAL AND DIGITAL SUBTRACTION SIALOGRAPHY

Indications

1. Recurrent pain or swelling
2. Identify sequelae of previous infections and radiotherapy
3. Sicca syndrome
4. Dilatation mild strictures.

Contraindications

Clinically active infection or inflammation.

Contrast medium

1. LOCM 240–370 mg I ml^{-1}
2. Lipiodol Ultra Fluid.

Neither contrast medium has a clear advantage over the other. Higher iodine concentration in Lipiodol provides excellent ductal delineation. However, foreign body reactions have been reported with lipid-soluble contrast agents. Newer, water-soluble contrast agents have similar iodine concentration to Lipiodol and are now used routinely.

Equipment

Equipment varies widely depending on the operator's preference:

1. Skull unit (using macroradiography technique) or fluoroscopic unit
2. Silver lacrimal dilator and probe set (size OO to 2)
3. Silver cannula or blunt needle (18G to 24G) with polythene catheter
4. Focused light and magnifying glasses.

Patient preparation

Any radio-opaque artifacts are removed (e.g. false teeth).

Preliminary images

Parotid gland

1. Antero-posterior (AP) with the head rotated 5° away from the side under investigation. Centre to the mid-line of the lower lip
2. Lateral, centred to the angle of the mandible
3. Lateral oblique, centred to the angle of the mandible, and with the tube angled 20° cephalad.

Submandibular gland

1. Inferosuperior using an occlusal film. This is a useful view to show calculi
2. Lateral, with the floor of the mouth depressed by a wooden spatula
3. Lateral oblique, centred 1 cm anterior to the angle of the mandible, and with the tube angled 20° cephalad.

Technique

1. The orifice of the parotid duct is adjacent to the crown of the second upper molar, and may be obscured by a mucosal bite ridge. Gentle abduction of the cheek using the thumb and index finger assists identification and cannulation of the parotid duct.
2. The orifice of the submandibular duct is on, or near, the sublingual papilla, lying next to the lingual frenulum. It is smaller than the parotid duct orifice and is more difficult to identify and cannulate. Raising the tip of the tongue, to touch the hard palate, puts tension on the papilla.
3. If the orifice is not visible, a sialogogue (e.g. citric acid) is placed in the mouth to promote secretion from the gland, and so render the orifice visible. The orifice is gently dilated using the silver probe and the cannula or polythene catheter is introduced into the duct. Care must be taken when advancing the cannula into the submandibular duct, due to the risk of painless perforation into the floor of the mouth.
4. Alternatively, modified Seldinger technique can be used, where a 0.018 inch guide wire is placed within the duct and a 22 gauge polythene catheter is advanced over the wire.
5. The catheter can be held in place by the patient gently biting on it. Up to 2 ml of contrast medium are injected. The injection is terminated immediately if any pain is experienced. The duct and acini should not be overfilled, as this may obscure ductal pathology.

Images

1. Dynamic images can be acquired during the injection at one frame a second. The advantage of the catheter technique is that both sides can be examined simultaneously
2. The occlusal film for the submandibular gland may be omitted, as this is only to demonstrate calculi
3. Post-secretory – the same views are repeated 5 min after the administration of a sialogogue. The purpose of this is to demonstrate sialectasis.

Aftercare

None.

Complications

1. Local pain
2. Damage to the duct orifice or ductal perforation
3. Infection should be suspected if local pain persists 24 h after the procedure – the patient should be evaluated for antibiotic therapy.

MRI of sialography

MR sialography is a non-invasive technique which exploits inherent tissue contrast on highly T2-weighted sequences. Good ductal delineation is therefore achieved without cannulation of the ducts. MR sialography can be used safely in both acute and sub-acute sialadenitis, which are contraindications for conventional sialography. This also eliminates the risk of ductal injury, post-procedure strictures and the ionizing radiation associated with conventional sialography:

1. Patients are fasted for 4 hours before examination.
2. Heavily T2-weighted, fast spin-echo (HASTE and 3d T2 TSE) sequences with frequency-selective fat suppression are used for ductal evaluation.
3. Non-contrast studies can be useful in differentiating benign or low-grade malignant from high-grade malignant tumours.
4. Contrast enhancement is useful in the differential diagnosis of cystic from solid lesions, and when determining the degree of perineural spread of malignant disease.[1]
5. Diffusion-weighted imaging and MR spectroscopy are increasingly used for the characterization of salivary gland masses.[2]
6. Gadolinium-enhanced scans with T1 weighting and fat suppression are obtained in the axial plane; sagittal and coronal images may be obtained at the radiologist's discretion.

References
1. Yousem DM, Kraut MA, Chalian AA. Major salivary gland imaging. Radiology 2000;216(1):19–29.
2. Lee YY, Wong KT, King AD, et al. Imaging of salivary gland tumours. Eur J Radiol 2008;66(3):419–36.

Further Reading
Shah GV. MR imaging of salivary glands. Neuroimaging Clin N Am 2004;14(4):777–808.

Thyroid and parathyroids

Methods of imaging the thyroid and parathyroid glands

1. Plain film (limited to crude assessment of superior mediastinal extension of thyroid goitre and any secondary tracheal displacement and narrowing)
2. Ultrasound (US)
3. Computed tomography (CT)
4. Magnetic resonance imaging (MRI)
5. Radionuclide imaging, including positron emission tomography (PET).

ULTRASOUND OF THYROID

Indications

1. Palpable thyroid mass
2. Screening high-risk patients
3. Suspected thyroid tumour
4. 'Cold spot' on scintigraphy or increased avidity on PET
5. Suspected retrosternal extension of thyroid
6. Guided aspiration or biopsy.

Contraindications

None.

Patient preparation

None.

Equipment

High-frequency transducer – minimum 10 MHz (though in larger patients and assessment of larger goitres lower-frequency probe may be needed). Linear array for optimum imaging.

Technique

The patient is supine with the neck extended. Longitudinal and transverse scans are taken of both lobes of the thyroid and the isthmus. Nodules are assessed for echogenicity, margins and architecture. If there is retrosternal extension, angling downwards and scanning during swallowing may enable the lowest extent of the thyroid to be visualized. Cervical lymph nodes should be routinely assessed at the same time.

Fine-needle aspiration (FNA) is a frequent adjunct to ultrasound examination; US characterization of nodules is limited and ideally US should be undertaken with the facility to proceed to FNA where there is concern about the US appearance.

ULTRASOUND OF PARATHYROID

Normal parathyroid glands cannot be visualized by US because of their small size and similar texture to surrounding adipose tissue. US is performed using a similar technique to thyroid for the detection of parathyroid enlargement by adenomas, hyperplasia and carcinoma. Scanning whilst the patient's head is turned can reveal deeper glands. Scanning for ectopic glands should include the neck below the thyroid down to the superior mediastinum, superiorly to the hyoid region and laterally to the carotid sheaths.

Further Reading

Gharib H, Papini E, Paschke R, et al. American Association of Clinical Endocrinologists, Associazione Medici Endocrinologi, and European Thyroid Association medical guidelines for clinical practice for the diagnosis and management of thyroid nodules. Endocrine Practice 2010;16(Suppl 1): 1–43.

Johnson NA, Tublin ME, Ogilvie JB. Parathyroid imaging: technique and role in the preoperative evaluation of primary hyperparathyroidism. Am J Roentgenol 2007;188(6):1706–15.

CT AND MRI OF THYROID AND PARATHYROID

Indications

1. In staging of known thyroid malignancy
2. To assess extension of substernal goitre and tracheal compromise.

As a result of its iodine content, normal thyroid is hyperdense relative to adjacent soft-tissues on non-contrast-enhanced CT. Other than for staging medullary thyroid cancer, CT of the thyroid is routinely performed without intravenous (i.v.) contrast which interferes with subsequent radionuclide thyroid imaging or treatment. Particular care must be taken if iodinated i.v. contrast is administered to hyperthyroid patients (see Chapter 2). For MRI, gadolinium-based i.v. contrast agents can be used without compromise.

In parathyroid disease, contrast-enhanced CT and MRI are used:

16

1. To detect ectopic or otherwise occult parathyroid adenomas in primary hyperparathyroidism
2. In patients with persistent or recurrent hyperparathyroidism following neck exploration.

Further Reading

Gharib H, Papini E, Paschke R, et al. American Association of Clinical Endocrinologists, Associazione Medici Endocrinologi, and European Thyroid Association medical guidelines for clinical practice for the diagnosis and management of thyroid nodules. Endocrine Practice 2010;16(Suppl 1):1–43.

Johnson NA, Tublin ME, Ogilvie JB. Parathyroid imaging: technique and role in the preoperative evaluation of primary hyperparathyroidism. Am J Roentgenol 2007;188(6):1706–15.

RADIONUCLIDE THYROID IMAGING

Indications

1. Assessment of thyroid uptake prior to radio-iodine therapy for benign conditions
2. Follow-up assessment of treated thyroid malignancy
3. Assessment of neonatal hypothyroidism[1]
4. To locate ectopic thyroid tissue, e.g. lingual or in a thyroglossal duct cyst
5. Evaluation of toxic nodular goitre and thyroiditis.

Contraindications

Pregnancy.

Radiopharmaceuticals

1. *^{99m}Tc-pertechnetate*, 80 MBq max (1 mSv ED). Pertechnetate ions are trapped in the thyroid by an active transport mechanism, but are not organified. Cheap and readily available, it is an acceptable alternative to ^{123}I.
2. *^{123}I-sodium iodide*, 20 MBq max (4 mSv ED). Iodide ions are trapped by the thyroid in the same way as pertechnetate, but are also organified, allowing overall assessment of thyroid function. ^{123}I is the agent of choice, but as a cyclotron product is therefore relatively expensive with limited availability. (*^{131}I-sodium iodide* can also be used for imaging but is associated with a significantly higher radiation dose, so is generally used in the context of whole-body imaging post ^{131}I ablation.)

Equipment

1. Gamma-camera
2. Pinhole, converging or high-resolution parallel hole collimator.

Patient preparation

None, but uptake may be reduced by antithyroid drugs, iodine-based preparations and radiographic iodinated contrast media.

Technique

^{99m}Tc-pertechnetate

1. I.v. injection of pertechnetate
2. After 15 min, immediately before imaging, the patient is given a drink of water to wash away pertechnetate secreted into saliva
3. Start imaging 20 min post injection when the target-to-background ratio is maximum
4. The patient lies supine with the neck slightly extended and the camera anterior. For a pinhole collimator, the pinhole should be positioned to give the maximum magnification for the camera field of view (usually 7–10 cm from the neck)
5. The patient should be asked not to swallow or talk during imaging. An image is acquired with markers on the suprasternal notch, clavicles, edges of neck and any palpable nodules.

^{123}I-sodium iodide

The technique is similar to that for pertechnetate except:

1. Sodium iodide may be given i.v. or orally
2. Imaging is performed 3–4 h after i.v. administration or 24 h after an oral dose
3. A drink of water is not necessary, since ^{123}I is not secreted into saliva in any significant quantity.

Images

200 kilocounts or 15 min maximum:

1. Anterior
2. LAO and RAO views as required, especially for assessment of multinodular disease
3. Large field of view image if retrosternal extension or ectopic thyroid tissue is suspected.

Analysis

The percentage thyroid uptake may be estimated by comparing the background-subtracted attenuation-corrected organ counts with the full syringe counts measured under standard conditions before injection.

Additional techniques

1. Whole-body ^{131}I imaging is often performed after thyroidectomy and ^{131}I ablation for thyroid cancer to locate sites of metastasis.
2. Perchlorate discharge tests can be performed to assess possible organification defects, particularly in congenital hypothyroidism.[1]

16

Aftercare

None.

Complications

None.

Other techniques

Metastatic thyroid cancer can be evaluated using diagnostic ^{123}I or therapeutic ^{131}I whole-body scans as above. When these scans are negative, but serum thyroglobulin is raised, FDG PET-CT is often positive.

Metastatic medullary carcinoma of the thyroid can be imaged with either pentavalent DMSA, indium-labelled octreotide, MIBG or, more recently, FDG PET-CT. These techniques are discussed in Chapter 11.

Reference

1. El-Desouki M, Al-Jurayyan N, Al-Nuaim A, et al. Thyroid scintigraphy and perchlorate discharge test in the diagnosis of congenital hypothyroidism. Euro J Nucl Med 1995;22:1005–8.

Further Reading

Martin WH, Sandler MP, Gross MD. Thyroid, parathyroid, and adrenal gland imaging. In: Sharp PF, Gemmell HG, Murray AD, editors. Practical Nuclear Medicine. 3rd ed. London: Springer-Verlag; 2005. p. 247–72.

Richards PS, Avril N, Grossman AB, et al. Thyroid cancer. In: Husband J, Reznek R, editors. Imaging in Oncology. 3rd ed. London: Informa; 2009. p. 642–79.

Sarkar SD. Benign thyroid disease: what is the role of nuclear medicine? Semin Nucl Med 2006;36(3):185–93.

RADIONUCLIDE PARATHYROID IMAGING

Indications

Pre-operative localization of parathyroid adenomas and hyperplastic glands.

Contraindications

Pregnancy.

Radiopharmaceuticals

1. ^{99m}Tc-*methoxyisobutylisonitrile (MIBI or sestamibi)*, 500 MBq typical, 900 MBq max (11 mSv ED) and ^{99m}Tc-*pertechnetate*, 80 MBq max (1 mSv ED). Both MIBI and pertechnetate are trapped by the thyroid, but only MIBI accumulates in hyperactive parathyroid tissue. With computer subtraction of pertechnetate from MIBI images, abnormal accumulation of MIBI may be seen. MIBI also washes out of normal thyroid tissue faster than parathyroid, so delayed images (1–4 h) can highlight abnormal parathyroid activity.
2. ^{99m}Tc-*tetrofosmin (Myoview)* can be used as an alternative to MIBI, and is as effective if the subtraction technique is used, but not as good for delayed imaging since differential washout is not as great as for MIBI.
3. ^{201}Tl-*thallous chloride* (80 MBq max, 18 mSv ED) was previously used in conjunction with ^{99m}Tc-pertechnetate, but is increasingly being replaced by the technetium agents due to their superior imaging quality and lower radiation dose.

Equipment

1. Gamma-camera (small field of view preferable for thyroid images, large field of view for chest images)
2. High-resolution parallel hole collimator. A pinhole collimator can also be used, but may result in repositioning magnification errors that compromise subtraction techniques
3. Imaging computer capable of image registration and subtraction.

Patient preparation

None, but uptake may be modified by antithyroid drugs and iodine-based medications, skin preparations and recent iodinated contrast media.

Technique

A variety of imaging protocols have been used, with either pertechnetate or MIBI administered first, with subtraction and possibly additional delayed imaging, and using MIBI alone with early and delayed imaging. Subtraction techniques are most sensitive, but additional delayed imaging may increase sensitivity slightly and improve confidence in the result. The advantage of administering pertechnetate first is that MIBI injection can follow within 30 min with the patient still in position to minimize movement, and if subtraction shows a clearly positive result, the patient does not need to stay for delayed imaging. With MIBI injected first, pertechnetate can only be administered after several hours when washout has occurred:

1. 80 MBq ^{99m}Tc-pertechnetate is administered i.v. through a cannula which is left in place for the second injection.

2. After 15 min the patient is given a drink of water immediately before imaging, to wash away pertechnetate secreted into saliva.
3. The patient lies supine with the neck slightly extended and the camera is positioned anteriorly over the thyroid.
4. The patient should be asked not to move during imaging. Head-immobilizing devices may be useful, and marker sources may aid repositioning.
5. 20 min post injection, a 10-min 128×128 image is acquired.
6. Without moving the patient, 500 MBq ^{99m}Tc-MIBI is injected i.v. through the previously positioned cannula (to avoid a second venepuncture which might cause patient movement).
7. 10 min post injection, a further 10-min 128×128 image is acquired.
8. A chest and neck image should then be acquired on a large field of view camera to detect ectopic parathyroid tissue.
9. Computer image registration and normalization is performed and the pertechnetate image subtracted from the 10-min MIBI image.
10. If a lesion is clearly visible in the subtracted image, the patient can leave.
11. If the lesion is not obvious, late MIBI imaging can be performed at hourly intervals up to 4 h if necessary to look for differential washout.

Additional techniques

1. In patients in whom pertechnetate thyroid uptake is suppressed, e.g. with use of iodine-containing contrast media or skin preparations, oral ^{123}I (20 MBq) administered several hours before MIBI may be considered.
2. SPECT and SPECT-CT may be used to improve localization and small lesion detection.
3. Dynamic imaging with motion correction may reduce motion artifact.

Aftercare

None.

Complications

None.

Further Reading

Johnson N, Tublin ME, Ogilvie JB. Parathyroid imaging: technique and role in the preoperative evaluation of primary hyperparathyroidism. Am J Roentgenol 2007;188(6):1706–15.

Kettle AG, O'Doherty MJ. Parathyroid imaging: how good is it and how should it be done. Semin Nucl Med 2006;36(3):206–11.

Palestro CJ, Tomas MB, Tronco GG. Radionuclide imaging of the parathyroid glands. Semin Nucl Med 2005;35(4):266–76.

Breast

Methods of imaging the breast

1. Mammography
2. Ultrasound (US)
3. Magnetic resonance imaging (MRI)
4. Radionuclide imaging
5. Imaging-guided biopsy/pre-operative localization.

MAMMOGRAPHY

Indications

1. Focal signs in women aged >40 years in the context of triple (i.e. clinical, radiological and pathological) assessment at a specialist, multidisciplinary diagnostic breast clinic
2. Following diagnosis of breast cancer, to exclude multifocal/ multicentric/bilateral disease
3. Breast cancer follow-up, no more frequently than annually or less frequently than biennially for at least 10 years
4. Population screening of asymptomatic women with screening interval of 3 years, in accordance with NHS Breast Screening Programme policy:
   (a) By invitation, women aged 47–73 years in England, Northern Ireland and Wales and 50–70 years elsewhere in UK
   (b) Women >73 years, by self-referral (there is no upper age limit)
5. Screening of women with a moderate/high risk of familial breast cancer who have undergone genetic risk assessment in accordance with National Institute for Health and Clinical Excellence (NICE) guidance
6. Screening of a cohort of women who underwent the historical practice of mantle radiotherapy for treatment of Hodgkin's disease when aged <30 years. These women have a breast cancer risk status comparable to the high-risk familial history group[1]
7. Investigation of metastatic malignancy of unknown origin.

Not indicated

1. Asymptomatic women without familial history of breast cancer, aged <40 years
2. Investigation of generalized signs/symptoms, e.g. cyclical mastalgia or non-focal pain/lumpiness
3. Prior to commencement of hormone replacement therapy
4. To assess the integrity of silicone implants
5. Individuals affected by ataxia-telangiectasia mutated (ATM) gene mutation with resultant high sensitivity to radiation exposure, including medical X-rays
6. Routine investigation of gynaecomastia.

Equipment

Conventional film-screen mammographic technology has largely been superseded by full-field digital mammography (FFDM) which has a higher sensitivity in:

1. Women aged <50 years
2. Pre/peri-menopausal women
3. Dense fibroglandular breast tissue.[3]

Ongoing developments of FFDM include:

1. *Tomosynthesis* which creates a single three-dimensional image of the breast by combining data from a series of two-dimensional radiographs acquired during a single sweep of the X-ray tube. Ongoing studies suggest that this technique may improve diagnostic accuracy in screening of the order of 30%, reduce recall by an estimated 40% and has a radiation dose of approximately 50% of that of a single mammographic exposure
2. *Contrast-enhanced digital mammography*, i.e. angiomammography. Two approaches are being developed: temporal sequencing (in which images pre and post contrast are subtracted with a resultant angiomammogram) and dual energy imaging (in which imaging at low and high energies detailing, respectively, parenchyma and fat with and without iodine are obtained. The subsequent views can then be subtracted
3. *Computer-aided detection (CAD)* software can assist film reading by placing prompts over areas of potential mammographic concern. There is evidence that, even in the screening setting, single reading in association with CAD may offer sensitivities and specificities comparable to that of double reading.[4]

If conventional film-screen mammographic imaging is to be carried out, it should be performed on a dedicated unit which includes in its specification:

1. Dual-focus X-ray tube: 0.1/0.3 focal spot size
2. Dual filtration: molybdenum/rhodium

3. Choice of rotating target material: molybdenum/rhodium/tungsten
4. 18 × 24 cm and 24 × 30 cm interchangeable buckys
5. Automatic/semi-automatic and manual exposure control
6. Carbon fibre table top assembly with reciprocating or oscillating grid, average grid ratio 5:1
7. Magnification assembly; magnification factors 1.8/2.0
8. Contact spot compression.

Technique

Standard mammographic examination comprises imaging of both breasts in two views, namely the mediolateral oblique (MLO) and craniocaudal (CC) positions. Screening methodology is bilateral, two-view (MLO and CC) mammography at all screening rounds.

Additional views may be required to provide adequate visualization of specific anatomical sites:

1. Lateral/medial extended CC
2. Axillary tail
3. Mediolateral/lateromedial.

Compression of the breast is an integral part of mammographic imaging resulting in:

1. Reduction in radiation dose
2. Immobilization of the breast, thus reducing blurring
3. Uniformity of breast thickness allowing even penetration
4. Reduction in breast thickness thus reducing scatter/noise achieving higher resolution.

Adaptation of the technique can provide additional information:

1. Spot compression, to remove overlapping composite tissue
2. Magnification (smaller focal spot combined with air-gap), to provide morphological analysis.

In the presence of subpectoral implants, the push back technique of Ecklund[2] can aid visualization of breast tissue.

References
1. Hancock SL, Tucker MA, Hoppe RT. Breast cancer after treatment of Hodgkin's disease. J Natl Cancer Inst 1993;85:25–31.
2. Eklund GW, Busby RC, Miller SH, et al. Improved imaging of the augmented breast. Am J Roentgenol 1988;151:469–73.
3. Pisano ED, Gatsonis C, Hendrick E, et al. Diagnostic performance of digital versus film mammography for breast cancer screening. N Engl J Med 2005;353:1773–83.
4. Gilbert FJ, Astley SM, McGee MA, et al. Single reading with computer-aided detection and double reading of screening mammograms in the United Kingdom National Breast Screening Program. Radiology 2006;241:47–53.

Further Reading

Health Technology Assessment. The clinical effectiveness and cost-effectiveness of different surveillance mammography regimes after the treatment for primary breast cancer: systematic reviews registry database analyses and economic evaluation. Health Technology Assessment 2011;15(34):1–322.

NICE Clinical Guidelines. The Classification and Care of Women at Risk of Familial Breast Cancer in Primary, Secondary and Tertiary Care. (CG 41 October 2006. http://www.nice.org.uk/nicemedia/live/10994/30244/30244.pdf (last accessed 11/2012)

Tucker AK, Ng YY. In: Tucker AK, Ng YY, editors. Textbook of Mammography. 2nd ed. Edinburgh: Churchill Livingstone; 2001. p. 18–64.

Willet AM, Michell MJ, Lee MJR. Association of Breast Surgery: Best Practice Diagnostic Guidelines for Patients Presenting with Breast Symptoms www.associationofbreastsurgery.org.uk. 2010. or http://www.associationofbreastsurgery.org.uk/media/4585/best_practice_diagnostic_guidelines_for_patients_presenting_with_breast_symptoms.pdf (last accessed 11/2012).

ULTRASOUND

Indications

1. Focal signs in women aged <35 years in the context of triple (i.e. clinical, radiological and pathological) assessment at a specialist, multidisciplinary diagnostic breast clinic
2. As an adjunctive method to improve diagnostic sensitivity and specificity in women aged >35 years with a mammographic and/or clinical abnormality
3. Following diagnosis of breast cancer to assess initial tumour size or response to neo-adjuvant therapy
4. Assessment of implant integrity
5. Diagnosis, drainage guidance and follow-up of breast abscess
6. Targeting diagnostic biopsy/pre-operative localization of both palpable and impalpable breast lesions
7. To guide axillary lymph node biopsy, thus informing choice of surgical management.[1]

Not indicated

1. For screening in any age group
2. In the investigation of generalized signs/symptoms, e.g. cyclical mastalgia or non-focal pain/lumpiness
3. In the routine investigation of gynaecomastia.

Equipment

Hand-held, high-frequency (8–18 MHz) contact US is widely used in breast imaging, with concomitant advantages of cost, accessibility and safety. Proprietary stand-off gels can be useful when assessing superficial lesions and the nipple-areolar complex.

Technique

1. The patient's arm on the side to be examined should be placed behind the head.
2. The patient lies supine for examination of the medial aspect of the breast.
3. The patient lies in the lateral, oblique position for examination of the lateral and axillary aspects of the breast and axilla.

Additional technique

Elastography is a non-invasive US technique, which provides a visual representation of the stiffness (elasticity) of both normal and abnormal tissue.[2] US imaging is used to examine tissue, both before and after minimal compression. A colour-coded image is generated with dark tissue representing least compressible tissue, i.e. with a higher index of suspicion of malignancy.

References

1. Damera A, Evans AJ, Cornford EJ, et al. Diagnosis of axillary nodal metastases by ultrasound guided core biopsy in primary operable breast cancer. Br J Cancer 2003;89:1310–13.
2. Zhi H, Ou B, Luo B-M, et al. Comparison of ultrasound elastography, mammography and sonography in the diagnosis of solid breast lesions. J Ultrasound Med 2007;26:807–15.

Further Reading

Stavros AT. Breast Ultrasound. Philadelphia, PA: Lippincott, Williams & Wilkins; 2003.

MAGNETIC RESONANCE IMAGING

Indications

1. Detection/exclusion of recurrent malignant disease in the conserved breast ≥6 months following surgery. Mature scar tissue, which may mimic malignancy morphologically, does not enhance with resultant high negative predictive value
2. Assessment of implant integrity
3. Monitoring response to neo-adjuvant therapy
4. Combined with mammography, as a screening tool[1] in women deemed to be at high risk of developing breast cancer (see above, mammography section)
5. In carefully selected cases, to clarify equivocal or suspicious mammographic and US findings
6. Investigation of occult breast cancer. 0.3% of patients present with malignant axillary lymphadenopathy but normal breast triple assessment.

Indications under evaluation

1. Detection of unsuspected multifocal/multicentric/contralateral disease. This may be of particular value in the pre-operative staging of invasive lobular disease. A high proportion of lesions identified on MRI can be located on second look US and are, therefore, amenable to conventional biopsy. All biopsy techniques can be adapted for use with MRI guidance
2. MRI may have a role in the pre-operative evaluation of the extent of high grade (Grade 3) ductal carcinoma in situ (DCIS).

Technique

1. Contraindications as for standard MRI examinations
2. Lying prone, with breasts placed in a dedicated surface coil, images are obtained pre and post contrast ($0.1–0.2$ mmol kg^{-1} gadolinium chelate contrast, given i.v. via pump injector) in either axial fat suppression or coronal subtraction sequences. The presence, amount, speed and morphology of the pattern of enhancement are analysed
3. For implant integrity non-enhanced scanning is adequate.

Reference

1. Leach MO, Boggis CR, Dixon AK, et al. Screening with magnetic resonance imaging of a UK population at high familial risk of breast cancer: a prospective multi-centre cohort study (MARIBS). Lancet 2005;365:1769–78.

Further Reading

Mann RM, Kuhl CK, Kinkel K, et al. Breast MRI: guidelines from the European Society of Breast Imaging. European Radiology 2008;18(7):1307–18.

Morris EA. Diagnostic breast MR imaging: current status and future directions. Radiol Clin North Am 2007;45(5):863–80.

RADIONUCLIDE IMAGING

Intra-operative sentinel node identification

A sentinel lymph node is the first node to which malignant cells are likely to spread from the primary tumour. The lower axillary sentinel lymph node(s) can be identified at operation following injection of a combination of radioisotope (^{99m}Tc colloidal albumin, particle size 3–80 nm) and blue dye. The subareolar route allows rapid (i.e. within minutes) uptake to lymph nodes via the plexus of Sappey.

Positron emission tomography scanning
(see Chapter 11)

Hybrid positron emission tomography (PET)-CT scanning with ^{18}F-fluorodeoxyglucose (FDG) may provide additional information in carefully selected cases where re-staging of disease, monitoring response to treatment or the detection of distant metastases is required.

17

Further Reading

Clarke D, Khonji NI, Mansel RE. Sentinel node biopsy in breast cancer: ALMANAC trial. World J Surg 2001;25:819–22.

Lim HS, Yoon W, Chung TW, et al. FDG PET/CT for the detection and evaluation of breast diseases: usefulness and limitations. Radiographics 2007;27(Suppl. 1):S197–213.

IMAGE-GUIDED BREAST BIOPSY

Indications

1. Diagnostic biopsy: to obtain specimen of tissue for histological analysis. Comprise the majority of biopsy procedures
2. Therapeutic biopsy: US-guided, large-volume (up to 7G needle), vacuum-assisted techniques can be used to excise:
   (a) small (<2 cm) fibroadenomata
   (b) parenchymal distortion (with no evidence of atypia on diagnostic core)
   (c) impalpable papillary lesions
   (d) complex cysts.

Equipment

1. Require either:
   (a) US guidance; using hand-held, high-frequency (8–18-MHz) probe. The avoidance of radiation combined with accessibility of the technique results in this approach being used wherever possible

   OR

   (b) X-ray guidance; applying the principle of stereotaxis whereby imaging a static object from two known angles from a known zero point can provide data from which the x, y and z co-ordinates can be calculated. Small-field digital stereotactic equipment can be purchased as an add-on to conventional mammography machines, thus providing the most common approach to X-ray-guided biopsy, namely with the patient in the seated, upright position. Less commonly, the small-field digital stereotactic system is attached to a prone table (dedicated to biopsy use) with resultant increased accessibility for posteriorly sited lesions and reduction in syncopal episodes; advantages which can be reproduced by the use of an appropriate biopsy chair allowing the adoption of the lateral decubitus position in conjunction with an upright imaging system

2. Automated biopsy gun. Choice of needle depends on the nature of the mammographic abnormality. For US-guided biopsy of masses, 14G biopsy needle is adequate. For biopsy of clustered microcalcifications and parenchymal distortions, large-volume needles (up to 7G) in conjunction with vacuum-assisted techniques increase diagnostic accuracy.

Patient preparation

1. Consent
2. For patients receiving anticoagulant treatment. A benefit/risk discussion should underpin decisions for each patient prior to proceeding to biopsy but in general:
   (a) aspirin – no contraindication
   (b) warfarin – if decision taken to proceed to biopsy the INR must be <1.5
   (c) clopidogrel – cessation for no less than 7 days prior to biopsy.

Technique

1. Standard skin cleansing and local anaesthetic infiltration
2. Biopsy needle introduced via automated biopsy gun
3. At the time of biopsy, when the mammographic target *may* be completely removed by diagnostic biopsy or to confirm concordance of the target site with other imaging modalities, a titanium marker can be deployed either via an introducer or the large-volume biopsy needle. Some tissue markers comprise not only a radio-opaque clip but a series of collagen pellets rendering the marker ultrasonically visible for up to 6 weeks
4. Confirmatory imaging should accompany all cases:
   (a) Non-calcified lesion – US (orthogonal views) of needle position during procedure
   (b) Calcified lesion – X-ray of microcalcification in cores obtained by US or X-ray guidance.

Complications

1. Bleeding
2. Infection
3. Milk fistula (in the lactating breast)
4. Damage to adjacent tissue, e.g. pneumothorax. Careful technique, with needle alignment parallel to chest wall should avoid this.

PRE-OPERATIVE LOCALIZATION

Pivotal to the success of this technique is close multidisciplinary team working at pre-operative discussion/planning, accurate communication between the imaging department and theatre, and postoperative confirmation of adequacy of surgery at the multidisciplinary team (MDT) meeting.

The technique involves the insertion of a thin metal wire (or several wires) through the skin with the wire tip positioned within the lesion itself. The position of the wire is secured and the wire is then used by the surgeon to guide excision of the lesion.

17

Equipment

1. Localizing wire
2. Non-allergenic adhesive to fix the wire to adjacent skin
3. Swabs – coloured to be easily identifiable as separate from those used in theatre
4. Image guidance:
   (a) The avoidance of radiation and accessibility of the technique results in US being the method of image guidance of choice, particularly if the original pre-operative biopsy was achieved via US guidance. Lesions which on US are visible <4 cm from skin can be amenable to the technique of skin marking, avoiding the requirement of a localizing wire. Following discussion with the surgeon, the operative position of the patient should be reproduced. With the US probe immediately overlying the lesion, the skin is marked and the depth to target is measured. At operation, the site of the skin mark is incised and dissection through the relevant distance is undertaken
   (b) X-ray guidance using fenestrated grid or stereotactic devices can be used for the placement of the localizing wire.

Patient preparation

As for image-guided biopsy.

Technique

1. Standard skin cleansing and local anaesthetic infiltration
2. In cases of extensive (i.e. >2 cm) microcalcification, the placement of multiple wires may aid adequacy of excision
3. After wire placement, mammograms (orthogonal views) indicating the precise position of the tip of the localizing wire are taken. These must be available to the surgeon at the time of operation

4. Using magnification technique (see Mammography section), X-ray of the surgical specimen is undertaken to confirm excision of the mammographic lesion both at the time of operation (allowing further sampling) and at the postoperative MDT.

Further Reading

Liberman L. Percutaneous image-guided core breast biopsy. Radiol Clin North Am 2002;40:483–500.

NHSBSP Publication No 20. Quality Assurance Guidelines for Surgeons in Breast Cancer Screening 3rd edn NHSBSP: Sheffield. 2003. http://www.cancerscreening.nhs.uk/breastscreen/publications/nhsbsp20-3rd.pdf (last accessed 11/2012).

Sedation and monitoring

SEDATION

Sedation is the use of a drug or drugs to produce a state of depression of the central nervous system that enables interventional procedures or treatment to be carried out. Sedative drugs may be combined with drugs used for pain relief (analgesia). Sedation is only part of a 'package' of care comprising pre-assessment, properly informed consent, adequate facilities, good techniques and risk avoidance.[1]

Over recent years the number and complexity of diagnostic imaging and image-guided interventional procedures in radiology departments has increased; often these patients are frail, medically unfit, unable to cooperate or lie still. The relief of anxiety, discomfort and pain allows patients to tolerate these procedures. Some drugs, such as benzodiazepines, have purely sedative effects but others, such as opioids, have combined sedative and analgesic effects. Although sedative and analgesic agents are generally safe, catastrophic complications related to their use can occur, often as a result of incorrect drug administration or inadequate patient monitoring.[2] The incidence of adverse outcomes is reduced by improved understanding of the pharmacology of drugs used, appropriate monitoring of sedated patients and by recognizing those at increased risk of adverse event.

There is a continuum between the main types of sedation (Fig. 18.1) defined as:

1. **Anxiolysis**: the patient is alert and calm
2. **Conscious sedation**: a state of depression of the central nervous system that enables diagnostic and therapeutic procedures to be carried out, but during which the patient remains conscious, retains protective reflexes and is able to understand and respond to verbal commands

Figure 18.1 The continuum of patient conscious level from mild sedation to general anaesthesia.

3. **Deep sedation**: in which these criteria are not fulfilled and airway or ventilation intervention may be required. Deep sedation requires the presence of an anaesthetist
4. **General anaesthesia**.

The joint Royal College of Radiologists/Royal College of Anaesthetists Working Party on Sedation and Anaesthesia in Radiology recommended establishment of local guidelines for sedation in radiology.[3] These should include:

1. Each patient must have a pre-procedure evaluation to assess their suitability for sedation
2. The operator must not supervise the sedation
3. Nurses and technicians should not administer drugs without medical supervision
4. All staff carrying out sedation should have undertaken training in sedation and resuscitation, and should have knowledge and experience of the sedative drugs, monitoring and resuscitation equipment
5. There should be periodic retraining and assessment of staff
6. There should be an appropriate recovery area
7. Resuscitation equipment and appropriate reversal drugs must be immediately available.

Preparation

Sympathetic patient management with an explanation of the procedure may reduce anxiety and remove the need for any medication. Sedation should be explained and consent obtained. Patients who are to be given intravenous (i.v.) sedation should undergo a period of fasting before the procedure; 6 h fasting for solid food and 2 h for clear liquids.

Resuscitation and monitoring equipment and oxygen delivery devices should be checked and venous access established.

Equipment

1. Appropriate drugs, including reversal agents
2. Monitoring equipment – see page 361
3. Resuscitation equipment – see page 365.

Pre-assessment

It is essential to anticipate and reduce the risk of potential problems before the procedure. Pre-assessment must include:

1. Evaluation of the patient's airway
2. Full assessment of the patient's medical, drug and allergy history
3. Cardio-respiratory reserve assessment.

18

DRUGS

As part of a sedation protocol the following may be used:

1. Combination of a sedative drug and an analgesic drug (e.g. i.v. midazolam and i.v. opiate). Intravenous analgesic and sedative drugs have a synergistic sedative effect and the dose of each drug must be reduced by up to 70% when administered together. It is best to give the i.v. analgesic first and then titrate the dose of i.v. sedative
2. Analgesic drug alone (e.g. i.v. opiate)
3. Sedative drug alone (e.g. i.v. midazolam).

Analgesic drugs

Analgesic drugs are used for pain control and improve patient comfort. For some procedures local anaesthesia or oral analgesia (using paracetamol 1 g or ibuprofen 400 mg taken 1–2 h before the procedure) will be appropriate. For more invasive interventional radiology procedures the use of intravenous analgesia may be required.

LOCAL ANAESTHESIA

For recommended doses see Table 18.1.

Commonly used local anaesthetics for subcutaneous infiltration are:

1. *Lidocaine 1%.* Lidocaine may be used in combination with adrenaline (epinephrine) and is supplied in pre-mixed ampoules for this purpose. Adrenaline causes local vasoconstriction, decreases drug absorption and will increase the intensity and duration of action of lidocaine. Lidocaine is also available as a 2% solution.

Table 18.1 Recommended doses of local anaesthetic drugs

Drug	Onset of effect	Duration of effect	Maximum total recommended dose	Route of administration
Lidocaine 1% (1% = 10 mg ml^{-1})	10–15 min	1–2 h	*without adrenaline*: 3 mg kg^{-1} (max 200 mg) *with adrenaline*: 7 mg kg^{-1} (max 500 mg)	Subcutaneous injection
Bupivacaine 0.25% (0.25% = 2.5 mg ml^{-1})	15–30 min	2–3 h	2 mg kg^{-1} (max 150 mg)	Subcutaneous injection

2. *Bupivacaine 0.25%.* Has slower onset but longer duration of action than lidocaine. The effect of adrenaline is much less pronounced in combination with bupivacaine. Bupivacaine is also available as a 0.5% solution.

INHALATIONAL ANALGESIA

A mixture of 50% nitrous oxide and 50% oxygen (Entonox®) may be used. This has both analgesic and sedative properties.

INTRAVENOUS ANALGESIA

These drugs are used for pain control but also have a dose-dependent sedative effect. Most commonly used are the opioid drugs morphine, pethidine and fentanyl. These drugs must be given in small, divided doses and dose-titrated to the patient's need. It is extremely important to titrate the dosage to effect rather than assume a fixed dose based on body weight. The maximum recommended dose must not be exceeded because of the risk of adverse events, particularly respiratory depression. For recommended dosage see Table 18.2.

The opioid drugs can cause:

1. Nausea and vomiting
2. Hypotension
3. Respiratory depression
4. Bradycardia.

Effects of opioids can be reversed by the competitive antagonist naloxone (dose 0.4–2 mg). Naloxone should be administered

Table 18.2 Recommended doses of intravenous analgesic drugs

Drug	Maximum total recommended dose	Onset of effect	Duration of effect	Route of administration
Morphine	100 µg kg^{-1} body weight	5–10 min	4–5 h	Intravenous injection
Pethidine	1 mg kg^{-1} body weight	5 min	1–2 h	Intravenous injection
Fentanyl	1 µg kg^{-1} body weight	1 min	0.5–1 h	Intravenous injection

These drugs should be used in divided doses and the maximum total dose must not be exceeded. It is always important to titrate the dosage of medication to effect rather than assume a fixed dose based on body weight.

18

intravenously in a solution containing 0.4 mg in 10 ml and given in 1 ml increments. It has peak effect at 1–2 min with duration of 20–60 min. As a result of the relatively short duration of action, repeated doses of naloxone may be necessary.

SEDATIVE DRUGS

For conscious sedation in the radiology department, the water-soluble benzodiazepine midazolam is the drug of choice. Midazolam has superseded diazepam because the latter has active metabolites and longer duration of effect. Midazolam produces:

1. Dose-dependent anxiolysis
2. Intense amnesia (for 20–30 min)
3. Sedation
4. Muscle relaxation.

Midazolam is given i.v. It has a rapid onset of effect, within 1–5 min, and a variable duration of effect of 1–4 h. The sedative dose is 70 µg kg^{-1} body weight (for average adult approx. 4–5 mg) and the sleep dose is 100–200 µg kg^{-1} (>7 mg). Typically, 2–2.5 mg is administered i.v. over 30–120 s with further 0.5-mg doses titrated as required. Rarely are total doses of more than 5 mg required. Smaller doses of 1–3 mg must be used in the elderly.

The effects of midazolam can be reversed by the competitive antagonist **flumazenil**; onset of flumazenil is within 1–3 min with a half-life of 7–15 min. The dose of flumazenil should be titrated every 1–2 min starting with 200 µg up to a maximum of 1 mg. The clinical effect depends on the dose of flumazenil and sedative given. Note: the half-life of flumazenil is shorter than that of midazolam, therefore re-sedation effects can occur.

Remifentanil is a potent ultra-short-acting synthetic opioid analgesic drug, the sedative dose range by intravenous infusion is 0.025–0.1 µg kg^{-1} min^{-1}, at higher doses it can cause marked respiratory depression. Dexmedetomidine is an agonist of α_2-adrenergic receptors; it can provide sedation, analgesia and anxiolysis without respiratory depression when given as an intravenous infusion at 0.2–1 µg kg^{-1} h^{-1}. The use of i.v. anaesthetic agents, such as ketamine and propofol, can result in the patient moving quickly from a state of sedation to anaesthesia with concomitant risks. These drugs should only be used by those who have undergone appropriate specialist training.

Sedation of children

Each child should be individually assessed. In most circumstances parents should stay with the child, and with patience and encouragement the need for sedation may be avoided in some cases. Short procedures such as CT can often be achieved in neonates by keeping them awake and then feeding the child and swaddling just prior to the procedure. Often, children over the age of 4–5 years will not need sedation and will cooperate. If venous access is required, local anaesthetic cream, e.g. Ametop, can be applied to a suitable vein prior to insertion of a cannula. Oral sedation does not work well in children over the age of 4 and older children who are unable to co-operate will usually require general anaesthetic.

It is important to ensure that all monitoring and resuscitation equipment is suitable for paediatric use. A nurse, experienced in the care of sedated children, should be present throughout. When drugs are given which are likely to result in loss of consciousness, the primary care of the patient should be under the direct supervision of an anaesthetist.

For many years chloral hydrate has been the mainstay for sedation of young children for a variety of procedures. Triclofos, which is an active metabolite of chloral hydrate, causes less gastric irritation and vomiting. Alimemazine (Vallergan) is a sedating antihistamine, with anticholinergic effects and can be used in combination with triclofos. The recommendations in Table 18.3 are made as being suitable for the majority of patients, in respect of both safety and efficacy. It is recognized that, for certain patients, deviation from these guidelines will be appropriate on clinical or weight grounds (Table 18.3).

Vomiting is not uncommon after oral sedation is given. If the child vomits within 10 min of administration the dose can be repeated. After 10 min a reduced dose of 50–70% of the Triclofos + Alimemazine dose can be repeated. The dose should not be repeated after 20 min as significant absorption may have occurred.

Table 18.3 Sedation recommendations made as being suitable for the majority of child patients. These doses are used to achieve deep sedation: a nurse should be present throughout

Age/weight	Sedation	Dose
<1 month old	Feed only or Triclofos	30 mg kg^{-1}
>1 month old but <5 kg	Triclofos	50–70 mg kg^{-1}
5–10 kg	Triclofos	100 mg kg^{-1}
>10 kg up to 4 years	Triclofos + Alimemazine	100 mg kg^{-1} (maximum 2 g) 1 mg kg^{-1} (maximum 30 mg)
Over 4 years	Consider oral sedation (as above) or general anaesthetic	

On the night before the procedure or scan parents should be asked to try to keep the child awake for as long as possible. The child should be woken early on the relevant day and no 'naps' allowed on the journey to the hospital. This will ensure that the child is already tired prior to administration of the sedation. The sedative medication usually takes about 45 min to take effect.

Children should have nothing to eat or drink prior to sedation as follows:

1. *Breast fed only*: Last feed 2 hours before sedation
2. *Under 1 year or on formula, or weaning onto a soft diet*: Last feed/milk 4 h before sedation, but can have clear fluids up to 2 h before
3. *Over 1 year*: Light meal, such as fruit juice, milk, toast or cereal 4 h before sedation, clear fluids up to 2 h before sedation.

Complications of sedation

Early recognition and treatment of complications is essential to reduce morbidity and mortality from sedation in all patients.

Minor complications include:

1. Syncope
2. Phlebitis
3. Emesis
4. Agitation
5. Rash.

Major complications are rare, but include:

1. Bradycardia
2. Hypotension

3. Hypoxia

4. Death.

Sedation causes a reduction in muscle tone of the oropharynx and at deeper levels of sedation the glottic reflexes may fail. Major complications of sedation are most often due to airway obstruction and respiratory depression. The following patient groups are at high risk:

1. *Elderly patients.* Old age is an independent risk factor for sedation. The effects of sedative drugs are more pronounced and prolonged in the elderly. Small incremental doses of sedatives are required.
2. *Chronic obstructive pulmonary disease.* These patients have a blunted ventilator drive. Supine position impairs chest wall function and oxygenation. Patients may need supplemental oxygen and bronchodilators. Local anaesthesia should be used for pain whenever possible and sedative drugs should be used sparingly.
3. *Coronary artery disease.* Under-sedation will increase cardiac oxygen demand but over-sedation can cause hypotension, hypoxaemia and decrease myocardial oxygen delivery leading to myocardial ischaemia. Patients should be given supplemental oxygen.
4. *Hepatic dysfunction or renal failure.* Altered drug metabolism in renal and liver disease increases the risk of overdose when using opioids and benzodiazepines. These drugs should be used in reduced doses. In children, similarly, Triclofos should be avoided in those with end-stage liver failure and used with caution in cholestasis. In renal impairment dose reduction should be considered.
5. *Drug addicts.* These patients may exhibit unpredictable requirements and drug-seeking behaviour. Local anaesthetics and short-acting benzodiazepines are preferred; reversal agents should be avoided.

References

1. Royal College of Radiologists. Safe Sedation, Analgesia and Anaesthesia within the Radiology Department. London: The Royal College of Radiologists; 2003. http://www.rcr.ac.uk/publications.aspx?PageID=310& PublicationID=186 (last accessed 11/2012).
2. Martin ML, Lennox PH. Sedation and analgesia in the interventional radiology department. J Vasc Interv Radiol 2003;14(9 Pt 1):1119–28.
3. Royal Radiologists/Royal College of College of Anaesthetists joint publication. Sedation and Anaesthesia in Radiology. London: The Royal College of Radiologists; 1992.

Further Reading

American College of Radiology. ACR-SIR Practice guideline for sedation/ analgesia. 2010. www.acr.org

Patatas K, Koukkoulli A. The use of sedation in the radiology department. Clin Radiol 2009;64:655–63.

NICE clinical guideline 112. Sedation for diagnostic and therapeutic procedures in children and young people. 2010. www.nice.org.uk/guidance/CG112 (last accessed 11/2012).

MONITORING

18

Monitoring should be used:

1. In all patients receiving any form of sedation
2. For those at risk of haemorrhage
3. In any prolonged or complicated procedure.

The purpose is to observe and assess response of the patient to any psychological or physiological stress imposed by the procedure or sedative agents administered and allow appropriate therapeutic action to be taken.

Equipment

1. *Pulse oximetry.* Pulse oximetry is the most sensitive monitoring method to detect hypoxaemia. It is the minimum requirement for safe monitoring and may suffice as the sole monitoring device in the young and fit. It accurately measures the oxygen saturation of blood and provides information on pulse rate and adequacy of the circulation. The oxygen saturation should be maintained at or above 95%. Most pulse oximeters have a short lag time in demonstrating desaturation. Due to the nature of the oxygen dissociation curve, patients may rapidly desaturate from 90% to 70%. Oxygen saturation of 90% is an emergency and corrective action should be taken immediately. The pulse oximeter signal may be affected by interference from nail polish, light, movement and cold extremities.

2. *Electrocardiograph.* A continuous electrocardiography monitor will provide information on pulse rate and rhythm, presence of arrhythmia and signs of ischaemia, but does not monitor circulation or cardiac output.

3. *Automated blood pressure monitor.* Minimum acceptable mean arterial pressure is 60 mmHg, but patients with cardiac disease or hypertension require higher pressures. Falsely high arterial pressure readings are obtained with cuffs which are too small. Manual blood pressure measurements are inconvenient and inconsistent. The blood pressure monitor may impede function of the pulse oximeter so should not be on the same arm. The monitor should be set to 5-min recording intervals; nerve damage has been reported with prolonged use.

Monitor alarms may be the first signal of an adverse event and should not be silenced. If there is any doubt repeat measurement should be performed.

Technique

Monitoring should include assessment of:

1. The patient's level of consciousness
2. Ability to maintain airway
3. Adequacy of respiratory function – respiratory rate and pattern
4. Adequacy of cardiac function – pulse and skin colour
5. Pain level
6. Side effects or complications of any drugs administered
7. Hydration and urine output during prolonged procedures.

The patient should be monitored by a trained professional who should have no other role at the time of the procedure than to continuously monitor these parameters. The radiologist performing the procedure should not monitor the patient.

Vital signs (pulse, blood pressure and respiratory rate) should be regularly measured. Any adverse events must be fully recorded in the patient's notes. Monitoring should continue into the recovery period.

SEDATION AND MONITORING FOR MAGNETIC RESONANCE IMAGING

Sedation should be given in a quiet area close to the scanner and there should be an appropriate recovery area available.

The MRI scan room is a challenging environment in which to monitor the patient. The scanner is noisy, potentially claustrophobic and any patient inside the scanner is relatively inaccessible.

All equipment used for monitoring and all anaesthetic equipment must be MR-compatible, e.g. MR-compatible pulse oximeters with fibre-optic cabling. Potential problems include effects from the gradient field and radiofrequency fields. Heat induction in conducting loops formed by ECG leads can cause superficial burns and induced current in monitoring equipment may produce unreliable readings or malfunction of syringe drivers resulting in incorrect drug-dose delivery (see Chapter 1). Responsibility for safe use of MRI monitoring equipment should be allocated to a small number of experienced and appropriately trained staff.

RECOVERY AND DISCHARGE CRITERIA

The effects of most agents used for sedation and analgesia last longer than the duration of the procedure; therefore, monitoring of the patient must continue into the recovery period. Once the patient is alert and orientated and vital signs have returned to their baseline values or acceptable levels, the patient can be considered fit to be moved from the radiology department. The overall responsibility for the patient's care until discharge is with the consultant radiologist or main operator and every unit should have written guidelines for discharge criteria.

18

Further Reading

Sedation and Monitoring for Magnetic Resonance Imaging

American Society of Anesthesiologists Task force on anesthetic care for magnetic resonance imaging. Practice advisory on anesthetic care for magnetic resonance imaging: A report by the American Society of Anesthesiologists Task force on anesthetic care for magnetic resonance imaging. Anesthesiology 2009;110:459–79.

Medical emergencies

Medical emergencies occurring in the radiology department may be due to:

1. Medication or radiographic contrast given
2. Procedure-related complications
3. Deterioration of pre-existing morbidities.

Patients may develop cardiac arrhythmias, hypotension, inadequate ventilation or adverse drug/radiographic contrast reactions. Complications arise from sedative drug administration, invasive procedures and human error; poor monitoring and organizational failings may contribute.

If a complication occurs, rapid recognition of the problem and effective management are essential. A call must be made to summon the hospital medical emergency or cardiac arrest team for any medical emergency event that is not immediately reversed or if ongoing care will be required.

The basic principles are summarized in the ABC of resuscitating the acutely ill patient:

1. Airway – ensuring a patent airway
2. Breathing – providing supplemental oxygen and adequate ventilation
3. Circulation – restoration of circulating volume.

These early interventions should proceed in parallel with diagnosis and definitive treatment of the underlying cause. If cardiac arrest is suspected, the adult advanced life support algorithm in Figure 19.1 should be followed.

EQUIPMENT

A regularly checked and stocked resuscitation trolley should be kept in the radiology department and contain:

1. A defibrillator
2. A positive pressure breathing device (Ambu bag) and mask

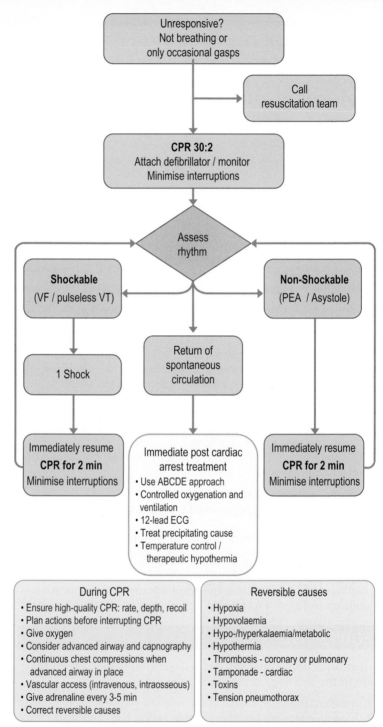

Figure 19.1 Adult advanced life support algorithm. Reproduced with the kind permission of the Resuscitation Council (UK).

3. Supplemental oxygen and oxygen delivery devices
4. Suction equipment
5. An intubation tray with airways, laryngoscopes and endotracheal tubes
6. Intravenous (i.v.) cannulas and i.v. fluids
7. Drugs:
   (a) Sedative reversal drugs including naloxone and flumazenil
   (b) Resuscitation drugs including adrenaline (epinephrine), atropine and hydrocortisone
8. Pulse oximeter
9. Non-invasive blood pressure device and appropriately sized brachial cuffs
10. An electrocardiograph.

19

RESPIRATORY EMERGENCIES

In all cases it is essential to call for urgent anaesthetic assistance if the medical emergency event is not immediately reversed.

RESPIRATORY DEPRESSION

Sedative and analgesic drugs can cause depression of respiratory drive and compromise of the airway leading to hypoxia and hypercapnia. The clinical signs are:

1. Decreased, shallow, laboured breathing
2. Decreased oxygen saturations
3. In partial airway obstruction; snoring and paradoxical chest wall movement.

The patient should immediately be placed in the supine position. If the airway is compromised it can be maintained by opening the mouth, tilting and extending the head, and lifting the chin. Supplemental oxygen must be provided. If respiratory depression is due to sedative drugs then reversal agents should be considered.

LARYNGOSPASM

This is airway obstruction due to tonic contractions of laryngeal and pharyngeal muscles. Risk factors include excessive secretions and mechanical irritation:

1. In partial obstruction stridor will be present. Partial airway obstruction can be treated with oxygen, coughing and calming measures.
2. In complete obstruction there will be chest wall movement but no air movement. Immediate anaesthetic assistance is required.

BRONCHOSPASM

This is constriction of bronchial airways by increased smooth muscle tone leading to small-airway obstruction. Risk factors are pre-existing asthma, airway irritation, histamine release and smoking. The signs include:

1. Wheeze
2. Tachypnoea and dyspnoea
3. Decreased oxygen saturations
4. Use of accessory respiratory muscles
5. Tachycardia
6. Silent chest.

Treatment includes high-flow oxygen, nebulized salbutamol 2.5–5 mg, nebulized ipratropium bromide 0.25–0.5 mg and i.v. hydrocortisone 100–200 mg.

ASPIRATION

Aspiration of blood or gastric contents into the lungs occurs when protective reflexes are lost and, if severe, can cause hypoxia, requiring mechanical ventilation. Risk factors are:

1. Post-procedure nausea and vomiting
2. Obesity
3. Hiatus hernia
4. Non-adherence to fasting guidelines.

The patient should be placed on their side in the head-down position, high-flow oxygen should be administered, airway adjuncts should be removed and the airway suctioned.

PNEUMOTHORAX

This is likely to be related to a procedure such as lung biopsy (see also Chapter 7). Presentation is with unilateral pleuritic chest pain and dyspnoea:

1. For asymptomatic small pneumothorax the patient should be observed.
2. For symptomatic small pneumothorax simple aspiration should be performed and the patient subsequently observed.
3. If the pneumothorax is >2 cm in depth (which is equivalent to 49% of the volume of the hemithorax) an intercostal chest drain should be inserted.
4. If the dyspnoea increases rapidly and the patient becomes cyanosed, tension pneumothorax should be suspected and air

should be aspirated immediately by insertion of a 16G cannula through the second intercostal space in the mid-clavicular line.

CARDIOVASCULAR EMERGENCIES

In all cases it is essential to call for urgent anaesthetic assistance if the medical emergency event is not immediately reversed.

HYPOTENSION

This is defined as a fall of greater than 25% from the patient's pre-procedure systolic blood pressure. Hypotension may be a manifestation of shock, which is a state of circulatory failure resulting in inadequate tissue perfusion to vital organs. The signs of hypotension are pallor, faints, tachycardia, and reduction in capillary refill and oliguria. The common causes are:

1. Pharmacological vasodilatation
2. Myocardial depression
3. Hypovolaemia due to procedure-related haemorrhage or haematoma
4. Sepsis
5. Vasovagal event.

The treatment depends on cause; pressure should be applied to any developing haematoma, the patient placed in the Trendelenburg position and oxygen administered. In the case of haemorrhage or haematoma, normalization of blood pressure is not the initial priority until bleeding is controlled. Hypotension is treated at first by the administration of an i.v. fluid bolus such as Hartmann's solution 10 ml kg^{-1} and the patient immediately re-assessed.

TACHYCARDIA

This is classified as a heart rate greater than 100 beats min^{-1} and is associated with stimulation of the sympathetic nervous system due to:

1. Under-sedation
2. Pain
3. Hypotension
4. Hypoxia.

Heart rates of up to 160 beats min^{-1} are generally well tolerated, but tachycardia-induced hypotension or myocardial ischaemia require urgent treatment.

BRADYCARDIA

This is classified as a heart rate less than 60 beats min^{-1} and may be due to sedative depressant effect, vasovagal or secondary to hypoxia or pain. Management is as follows:

1. If the patient is non-symptomatic, monitor closely.
2. If hypotension or bradycardia <40 beats min^{-1} is present an anticholinergic drug such as atropine 0.3–0.6 mg may be given i.v.
3. If the patient develops asystole, pulseless electric activity or ventricular fibrillation then confirm diagnosis – unconscious, apnoeic, absent carotid pulse. Call for help, defibrillator and cardiac arrest team, and follow the advanced life support algorithm outlined in Figure 19.1.

ADVERSE DRUG REACTIONS

CONTRAST MEDIA REACTION

This is also discussed in detail in Chapter 2. Suggested management is as follows:

1. Nausea/vomiting – patient reassurance. Retain i.v. access and observe
2. Urticaria – retain i.v. access and observe. If troublesome give an antihistamine by slow i.v. injection, e.g. chlorphenamine maleate 10–20 mg. If severe urticaria add i.v. hydrocortisone 100 mg
3. Hypotension with bradycardia (vasovagal reaction)
4. Mild wheeze (see above)
5. Anaphylaxis – rare, most often mild, but may be life-threatening. Iodinated i.v. contrast media are the commonest cause of anaphylaxis in the radiology department; however, other possible causes include gadolinium agents, opioid drugs, antibiotics, aspirin, latex and local anaesthetics. Anaphylaxis is a hypersensitivity reaction which causes a range of symptoms and signs including: oedema of face and airway, wheeze, cyanosis, tachycardia, hypotension, erythema and urticaria. Anaphylaxis is likely when all of the following three criteria are met:
   (a) Sudden onset and rapid progression of symptoms
   (b) Life-threatening Airway ± Breathing ± Circulation problems
   (c) Skin or mucosal changes (flushing, urticaria, angio-oedema)
      It should be noted however, that skin or mucosal changes alone do not indicate anaphylactic reaction and that these changes are subtle or absent in up to 20% of anaphylactic reactions.
      The recommended management plan for anaphylaxis is the UK Resuscitation Council algorithm in Figure 19.2
6. Unconscious/unresponsive/pulseless/collapse – see Figure 19.1.

Figure 19.2 Anaphylaxis algorithm. Reproduced with the kind permission of the Resuscitation Council (UK).

LOCAL ANAESTHETIC TOXICITY

Accidental i.v. injection of local anaesthetic or systemic absorption can result in toxicity due to membrane effects on the heart and central nervous system:

1. Early signs of toxicity are tingling around mouth and tongue, light-headedness, agitation and tremor.
2. More severe reactions include sudden loss of consciousness, with or without tonic-clonic convulsions and cardiovascular collapse.

The immediate management includes stopping injection, calling for help, maintaining airway (including securing the airway with intubation if required), 100% oxygen, ensuring adequate i.v. access, ventilator and cardiovascular support, and control of seizures. In the event of a cardiac arrest, resuscitation should be prolonged.

Patient consent

INTRODUCTION

It is a legal requirement that consent be obtained from a patient before any medical care can be provided, with the exception of emergencies where consent cannot be obtained.

Consent can take two forms: implied or express. When patients attend for low-risk procedures consent is often implied and has been taken by the referring clinician prior to the patient arriving in the radiology department on behalf of the reporting clinician, for example a chest radiograph.

Express consent is required for more complex procedures. It may be appropriate for this to take the form of verbal consent; as long as the discussion and granting of consent are documented in the patient notes, for example a nephrostogram.

The General Medical Council (GMC) requires written consent to be obtained in the following circumstances (GMC 2008):[1]

- The investigation or treatment is complex or involves significant risks
- There may be significant consequences for the patient's employment, or social or personal life
- Providing clinical care is not the primary purpose of the investigation or treatment
- The treatment is part of a research programme or is an innovative treatment designed specifically for their benefit.

The three components of consent are: voluntariness, information and capacity. For consent to be valid consent must be voluntarily given, the patient must have information regarding the treatment concerned and must be competent to do so.

VOLUNTARINESS

Consent should be given freely without undue influence to either accept or refuse treatment. It is the responsible clinician's duty to ensure that the patient is not under pressure from relatives or carers to consent to medical treatment. Doctors should also guard against exerting pressure on patients, especially if the patient's wishes do not agree with their own.

It is useful to create a suitable environment to facilitate voluntary consent taking. It is good practice to take consent prior to the patient entering the operating room, as this environment places the patient under pressure and may invalidate consent.[2] Suitable environments, which allow privacy and sufficient time for the patient to understand the information provided and to ask questions, include outpatient clinic and ward quiet rooms.

After taking consent the patient may change their mind and decline to confirm consent at the time of the procedure. The doctor should explore the patient's decision without being coercive and provide any support or additional information that the patient requests. The withdrawal of consent and subsequent discussion should be clearly documented in the patient's notes.

Patients may occasionally withdraw consent during a procedure. Should this occur, the doctor should immediately stop the procedure (even temporarily) and explore the patient's concerns. Medication or pain may affect the patient's capacity at this time. However, if the patient wishes the procedure to end and there is no possibility of immediate harm, the patient's wishes should be accepted as a withdrawal of consent and the procedure halted.[2]

Patients who are detained by the Police, Criminal Justice systems and Immigration Authorities and those detained under Mental Health legislation may be particularly vulnerable to coercion. Doctors should ensure that patients understand their rights to refuse or withdraw consent. Patients who are detained under Mental Health legislation can be treated for their mental illness and not physical illness. Where mentally ill people also lack capacity to consent to interventions, the advice below should be followed.

INFORMATION

Who?

The person providing care should take consent for the procedure. If this responsibility is delegated, the individual taking consent should have sufficient knowledge of the procedure.[3] Confirmation of consent, done at the time of the procedure, remains the responsibility of the doctor performing the procedure.[2]

When?

For non-urgent procedures consent should be taken at least 24 hours prior to the procedure to allow the patient to consider the options available to them and change their mind if they wish to.[4] There is no specific time limit on consent as long as the information provided to the patient has not changed with the passage of time.

What?

The GMC recommends the following information be provided to the patients prior to any procedure (GMC 2008):[1]

- The diagnosis and its prognosis
- Treatment or management options for the condition, including the option not to treat
- The purpose of any proposed investigation or treatment and what it will involve
- The potential benefits, risks and burdens, and the likelihood of success, for each option; this should include information, if available, about whether the benefits or risks are affected by which organization or doctor has chosen to provide care
- Whether a proposed investigation or treatment is part of a research programme or is an innovative treatment designed specifically for their benefit
- The people who will be mainly responsible for and involved in their care, what their roles are, and to what extent students may be involved
- Their right to refuse to take part in teaching or research
- Their right to seek a second opinion
- Any bills they will have to pay
- Any conflicts of interest that you, or your organization, may have
- Any treatments that you believe have greater potential benefit for the patient than those you or your organization can offer.

The GMC advises that doctors discuss these matters with patients, encourage them to ask questions, listen to their concerns and ask for and respect their views.

Importantly, when providing information about risks, doctors should include all significant risks, however unlikely. Furthermore, material information that the individual is likely to attach meaning to because of their unique circumstances should also be provided. For example, the risk of losing kidney function following renal artery stenting is of particular risk in a patient with a single kidney, however small that risk may be. Doctors who omit this information leave themselves vulnerable to 'Failure to warn' litigation charges.

20

Visual aids depicting risk are helpful in clarifying numerical data. These may be produced within departments or doctors may use smartphone applications.

Information literature should be clear and concise and designed for patients.[2] Many radiologists make use of patient information booklets compiled by professional societies such as the RCR, CIRSE and BSIR, which go some way to providing standardized complication rates for common procedures.

- http://www.cirse.org/index.php?pid=612,
- http://www.rcr.ac.uk/content.aspx?PageID=323
- http://www.bsir.org/content/PatientsHome.aspx

CAPACITY

The Mental Capacity Act 2005 of England is underpinned by five statutory principles:

- All persons are assumed to have capacity unless the contrary is demonstrated
- All practicable steps must be taken to assist the person in making a decision
- The person should not be considered to lack capacity if they choose to make an unwise decision
- Any decision made or act done under this Act on behalf of a person lacking capacity should be in that person's best interests
- Any act done or decision made should be the least restrictive possible that would ensure a good outcome.

The Adults with Incapacity (Scotland) Act has similar requirements and includes an expectation that interested parties should be consulted and that incapacitated people are encouraged to use existing skills.

The legislation together with the GMC guidelines require doctors to assume that patients have the capacity to accept or decline a treatment or intervention, unless the doctor has demonstrated and documented that the person lacks capacity.

ASSESSMENT OF CAPACITY

It is important to remember that capacity is not generalized. Capacity assessments aim to establish whether the person in question has capacity to make a specific decision at a specific time. Someone may have the capacity to consent to have their nightclothes changed on the ward, but not to the siting of a PICC line, as the process of the latter is more complex and requires greater mental processing abilities to evaluate risks and benefits.

In order to undertake a capacity assessment, a two-stage test of capacity should occur.

1. Does the person have an impairment (of mind or brain) or is there a disturbance affecting the way their mind or brain works?
2. If so, does the impairment mean that the person is unable to make the decision at the time needed?

An assessment of capacity need only be undertaken if there is a doubt about the person's mental functioning at the time.

In order to assess capacity, the following need to be evaluated (Mental Capacity Act 2005: Code of Practice):[5]

- Does the person have a general understanding of what decision they need to make and why they need to make it?
- Does the person have a general understanding of the likely consequences of making or not making this decision?
- Is the person able to understand, retain, use and weigh up the information relevant to this decision?
- Can the person communicate their decision (by talking, using sign language or other means)? Would the services of a professional (such as a speech and language therapist) be helpful?
- And in more complex or serious decisions: Is there a need for a more thorough assessment (perhaps by involving another professional expert)?

Patients are deemed to lack capacity if they cannot:

- Understand information about the decision to be made (the Act calls this 'relevant information')
- Retain that information in their mind
- Use or weigh that information as part of the decision-making process, or
- Communicate their decision (by talking, using sign language or any other means).

Only one of the above needs to be absent for the person to lack capacity, although more than one is often present.

Capacity to consent is best established by the clinician offering the proposed intervention, as they will have sufficient knowledge of the risks and benefits involved. For more complex procedures or where there is an underlying illness contributing to difficulties in reasoning (e.g. dementia) it may be of benefit to work in collaboration with expert colleagues (e.g. psychiatrists).

20

SUPPORTING PATIENTS TO MAKE DECISIONS

Before a patient can be deemed to lack capacity to consent to a procedure, all practicable steps should be taken to support the person to make the decision. Making use of images or visual aids, involving family members, interpreters or other professionals may be beneficial. Where a treatment can safely be delayed to allow the person to regain capacity, this should be done.

Doctors may encounter patients who choose not to undergo treatments or procedures offered to them even though this may result in significant morbidity or death. Patients have the right to make unwise decisions and doctors should guard against coercion.[6]

In these cases all discussions with the patient, a comprehensive and contemporaneous documentation of the capacity assessment and consent procedure should be entered into the patient's medical notes. The RCR recommends that in these cases the notes are witnessed by a third party.[2] If this patient later loses the capacity to consent to a procedure, clinicians must not then perform the intervention in the patient's best interests: under the Mental Capacity Act this would be considered a criminal offence of ill-treatment.

ACTING FOR PATIENTS WHO LACK CAPACITY

When a person has been established to lack capacity to decide on treatment offered, the treating clinician may lawfully treat the patient in their best interests. Prior to proceeding, the clinician should take into consideration any previously expressed wishes. These may be formalized in Advance Statements or may be ascertained from other sources: family, carers or other professionals involved in providing care to the person previously.

Clinicians should establish if any proxy decision-makers have been appointed. Under English law a person may have designated a Lasting Power of Attorney (LPA) to make health and welfare decisions on their behalf once they no longer have mental capacity.

Note however:

- Within the health and welfare LPA agreement there is an explicit declaration made determining whether the attorney is empowered to give or refuse consent for treatments specifically deemed to be life-sustaining so clarification should be sought.
- Separate Lasting Power of Attorney arrangements can also be made for property and financial decisions but these alone do not confer any power for the attorney to make health-related decisions on behalf of the patient.

- Similarly, any older Enduring Power of Attorney arrangements still in force (made pre 2007) allow only proxy financial, not health or welfare, decisions to be made.
- Scottish law makes no distinction between differing powers of attorney.

When acting in a person's best interests, clinicians should do so in the least restrictive manner possible. If less invasive alternatives exist to the preferred intervention, then these should be attempted first.

20

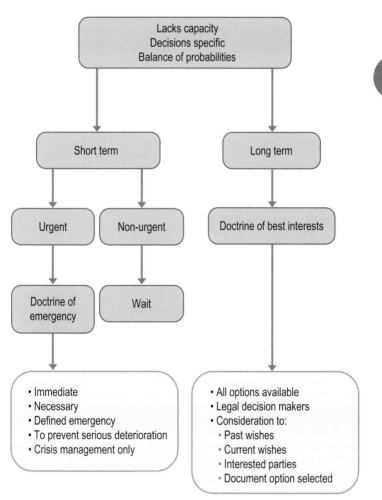

Figure 20.1 Decision-making flow chart.

In an emergency situation where consent cannot be obtained, clinicians can act in the patient's best interest to administer emergency treatment. Treatment should be immediate and necessary to prevent further deterioration. No further treatment may be given until a capacity and if necessary a best interest's assessment has been undertaken.

Clinicians are directed to the MCA 2005 and Adults with Incapacity (Scotland) Act 2000 Codes of Practice for details on the roles of powers of attorney. These can be stored as PDF documents on computers or smart phones. Seeking legal advice from employment lawyers or protection societies is recommended if clinicians are unclear of how to proceed.

DOCUMENTING ASSESSMENT OF CAPACITY

Most hospitals have standardized pre-printed consent forms for patients who lack capacity. In addition to completion of these forms, the authors recommend contemporaneous documentation of assessment of capacity in the patient's notes or the relevant radiology report. Documentation should include the following information:

- Full patient details
- The details of the intended intervention
- The specific reason the patient has been deemed to lack capacity and how this judgement was reached (as above)
- Attempts that have been made to assist the patient to make his/her own decision and why these were unsuccessful
- The likelihood that the patient may regain capacity and the reason the intervention needs to be performed before this can occur
- The steps taken to establish the patient's previously expressed wishes including the names of the family members consulted
- The names and designation of clinical colleagues consulted in deciding on the proposed intervention
- The name of the clinician responsible for performing the procedure
- The name and designation of any clinician who has provided a second opinion.

SHARED DECISION-MAKING

As part of the Liberating the NHS White paper published in May 2011, there is an increasing requirement of clinicians to involve patients in decisions about their care. 'No decision about me without me' requires clinicians to agree on treatment plans in partnership with their patients. There is a growing expectation from the public for doctors to provide sufficient information for patients to allow them to make their own decisions. This is particularly important in procedures where there is lack of consensus and there is a perceived variance of risk between the clinician and the patient (Fig. 20.1).

In these cases, clear documentation of all information given and the decision arrived at should be made. It may be advisable to include the patient in the correspondence to other clinicians, so that they have a written copy available to them.

References

1. General Medical Council. Consent: Patients and Doctors making decisions together. http://www.gmc-uk.org/guidance/ethical_guidance/consent_guidance_index.asp 2008 (last accessed 11/2012).
2. The Royal College of Radiologists. Standards for patient consent particular to radiology. 2nd ed. London: The Royal College of Radiologists; 2012. http://www.rcr.ac.uk/publications.aspx?PageID=310&PublicationID=372 (last accessed 11/2012).
3. The Medical Protection Society. Consent to Medical Treatment in the UK. MPS 2011; http://www.medicalprotection.org/mps-guide-to-consent.pdf (last accessed 11/2012).
4. O'Dwyer HM, Lyon SM, Fotheringham T, et al. Informed consent for interventional radiology procedures: a survey detailing current European practice. Cardiovasc Interv Radiol 2003;26:428–33.
5. Mental Capacity Act. Code of practice. 2005. www.publicguardian.gov.uk/mca/code-of-practice.htm (last accessed 11/2012).
6. Ms B v An NHS Hospital Trust 2002 2 All ER 449.

20

Appendix

Average effective dose equivalents for some common examinations

Examination	Effective dose equivalent (mSv)	Miles travelled by car*	Equivalent period of natural background radiation	Probability of radiation effect occurring ($\times 10^{-6}$) (fatal somatic)	
				Male	Female
Chest (PA)	0.02	50	3 days	0.27	0.47
Skull	0.1	250	2 weeks	1.7	1.7
Cervical spine	0.1	250	2 weeks		
Thoracic spine	1.0	2500	6 months	7.0	11
Lumbar spine	2.4	5000	14 months	25	26
Hip (1 only)	0.3	750	2 months		
Pelvis	1.0	2500	6 months	3.9	3.9
Abdomen	1.5	3750	9 months	9.4	9.5
Extremity (e.g. hand, foot)	<0.01	<25	<1.5 days		
Barium Meal	5.0	12500	2.5 years	26	31
Small bowel	6.0	15000	3 years		
Large bowel	9.0	22500	4.5 years	37	38
i.v. urography	4.6	11500	2.5 years	26	37

Continued

Examination	Effective dose equivalent (mSv)	Miles travelled by car*	Equivalent period of natural background radiation	Probability of radiation effect occurring ($\times 10^{-6}$) (fatal somatic)	
				Male	*Female*
Computed tomography					
Head	2.0	5000	1 year	62	69
Chest	8.0	20000	4 years	330	370
Abdomen	8.0	20000	4 years	330	370

*ICRP 60.

Appendix ● II

Dose limits – the Ionising Radiation Regulations 1999[1]

Body part etc.	Dose limit (mSv)			
	Employees 18 years or over	Special circumstances[#]	Trainees aged under 18 years	Other persons (including any person below 16 years)
Effective dose in any calendar year	20	50 (not more than 100 mSv averaged over 5 years)	6	1 (5*)
Equivalent dose for the skin in a calendar year as applied to the dose averaged over any area of 1 cm², regardless of the area exposed. Equivalent dose for hands, forearms, feet and ankles in a calendar year	500	500	150	50
Equivalent dose for the lens of the eye in a calendar year	150	150	50	15

Continued

	Dose limit (mSv)			
Body part etc.	Employees 18 years or over	Special circumstances#	Trainees aged under 18 years	Other persons (including any person below 16 years)
Equivalent dose for the abdomen of a woman of reproductive capacity at work, being the equivalent dose from exposure to ionizing radiation averaged throughout the abdomen in any consecutive 3-monthly period	13	13	n/a	n/a

#If an employer demonstrates to the Health and Safety Executive (HSE) that it cannot meet the 20 mSv/calendar year limit. It may apply this limit after notifying HSE, the employees concerned and the approved dosimetry service.

*The dose limit for persons who are exposed to ionizing radiation from a medical exposure of another person but are not 'comforters or carers'[2] is 5 mSv in any period of 5 consecutive calendar years.

References

1. Crown copyright 1999 with the permission of the Controller of Her Majesty's Stationery Office.
2. A 'comforter and carer' is defined in IRR 99 as an individual who (other than as part of his occupation) knowingly and willingly incurs an exposure to ionizing radiation resulting from the support and comfort of another person who is undergoing or who has undergone any medical exposure.

Appendix III

The Ionising Radiation (Medical Exposure) Regulations 2000 with the Ionising Radiation (Medical Exposure) (Amendment) Regulations 2006 and the Ionising Radiation (Medical Exposure) (Amendment) Regulations 2011[1]

These Regulations, together with the Ionising Radiations Regulations 1999 (S.I. 1999/3232) partially implement, as respects Great Britain, Council Directive 97/43/Euratom (OJ No. L180, 9.7.97, p. 22) laying down basic measures for the health protection of individuals against dangers of ionizing radiation in relation to medical exposure. The regulations impose duties on those responsible for administering ionizing radiation to protect persons undergoing medical exposure whether as part of their own medical diagnosis or treatment or as part of occupational health surveillance, health screening, voluntary participation in research or medico-legal procedures.

They replaced The Ionising Radiation (Protection of Persons Undergoing Medical Examination or Treatment) Regulations 1988.

1. Commencement

These regulations came into force:

1. Except for regulation 4(1) and 4(2) on 13 May 2000
2. As regards regulation 4(1) and 4(2) on 1 January 2001
3. As regards Ionising Radiation (Medical Exposure) (Amendment) Regulations 2006 on 1 November 2006
4. As regards Ionising Radiation (Medical Exposure) (Amendment) Regulations 2011 on 25th July 2011.

2. Glossary of [some of the] terms

Adequate training means training which satisfies the requirements of Schedule 2; and the expression *adequately trained* shall be similarly construed.

Appropriate authority means the Commission for Healthcare, Audit and Inspection established under section 41 of the Health and social Care (Community Health and Standards) Act 2003 as regards England, the National Assembly for Wales as regards Wales, or the Scottish Ministers as regards Scotland.

Child means a person under the age of 18 in England and Wales or a person under the age of 16 in Scotland.

Clinical audit means a systematic examination or review of medical radiological procedures which seeks to improve the quality and the outcome of patient care through structured review whereby radiological practices, procedures and results are examined against agreed standards for good medical radiological procedures, intended to lead to modification of practices where indicated and the application of new standards if necessary.

Diagnostic reference levels means dose levels in medical radiodiagnostic practices or, in the case of radioactive medicinal products, levels of activity, for typical examinations for groups of standard-sized patients or standard phantoms for broadly defined types of equipment.

Dose constraint means a restriction on the prospective doses to individuals which may result from a defined source.

The Directive means Council Directive 97/43/Euratom laying down measures on health protection of individuals against the dangers of ionizing radiation in relation to medical exposure.

Employer means any natural or legal person who, in the course of a trade, business or other undertaking, carries out (other than as an employee), or engages others to carry out, medical exposures or practical aspects, at a given radiological installation.

Employer's procedures means the procedures established by an employer pursuant to regulation 4(1).

Equipment means equipment which delivers ionizing radiation to a person undergoing a medical exposure and equipment which directly controls or influences the extent of such exposure.

Ethics committee means:

   (a) An ethics committee established or recognized in accordance with Part 2 of the Medicines for Human Use (Clinical Trials) Regulations 2004, or

   (b) The Ethics Committee constituted by regulations made by the Scottish Ministers under section 51(6) of the Adults with Incapacity (Scotland) Act 2000, or

   (c) Any other committee established to advise on the ethics of research investigations in human beings, and recognized for that purpose by or on behalf of the Secretary of State, the National Assembly for Wales of Scottish Ministers.

Individual detriment means clinically observable deleterious effects that are expressed in individuals or their descendants the appearance of which is either immediate or delayed and, in the latter case, implies a probability rather than a certainty of appearance.

Ionizing radiation means the transfer of energy in the form of particles or electromagnetic waves of a wavelength of 100 nanometres or less or a frequency of 3×10^{15} hertz or more capable of producing ions directly or indirectly.

Medical exposure means any exposure to which regulation 3 applies and which involves an individual being exposed to ionizing radiation.

Medical physics expert means a person who holds a science degree or its equivalent and who is experienced in the application of physics to the diagnostic and therapeutic uses of ionizing radiation.

Medico-legal procedure means a procedure performed for insurance or legal purposes without a medical indication.

Operator means any person who is entitled, in accordance with the employer's procedures, to carry out practical aspects including those to whom practical aspects have been allocated pursuant to regulation 5(3), medical physics experts as referred to in regulation 9 and, except where they do so under the direct supervision of a person who is adequately trained, persons participating in practical aspects as part of practical training as referred to in regulation 11(3).

Patient dose means the dose concerning patients or other individuals undergoing medical exposure.

Practical aspect means the physical conduct of any of the exposures referred to in regulation 3 and any supporting aspects including handling and use of radiological equipment, and the assessment of technical and physical parameters including radiation doses, calibration and maintenance of equipment, preparation and administration of radioactive medicinal products and the development of films.

Practitioner means a registered healthcare professional who is entitled in accordance with the employer's procedures to take responsibility for an individual medical exposure.

Quality assurance means any planned and systematic action necessary to provide adequate confidence that a structure, system, component or procedure will perform satisfactorily and safely complying with agreed standards and includes quality control.

Quality control means the set of operations (programming, coordinating, implementing) intended to maintain or to improve quality and includes monitoring, evaluation and maintenance at required levels of performance.

Radioactive medicinal product has the meaning given in the Medicines (Administration of Radioactive Substances) Regulations 1978.

Referrer means a registered healthcare professional who is entitled in accordance with the employer's procedures to refer individuals for medical exposure to a practitioner.

Registered healthcare professional means a person who is a member of a profession regulated by a body mentioned in section 25(3) of the National Health Service Reform and Health Care Professions Act 2002.

3. These Regulations apply to the following medical exposures

1. The exposure of patients as part of their own medical diagnosis or treatment including any exposure of an asymptomatic individual
2. The exposure of individuals as part of occupational health surveillance
3. The exposure of individuals as part of health screening programmes
4. The exposure of patients or other persons voluntarily participating in medical or biomedical, diagnostic or therapeutic, research programmes
5. The exposure of individuals as part of medico-legal procedures.

4. Duties of the employer

1. The employer shall ensure that written procedures for medical exposures including the procedures set out in Schedule 1 are in place and:
    (a) shall take steps to ensure that they are complied with by the practitioner and operator; or
    (b) where the employer is concurrently practitioner or operator, he shall comply with these procedures himself.
2. The employer shall ensure that written protocols are in place for every type of standard radiological practice for each equipment.
3. The employer shall establish:
    (a) recommendations concerning referral criteria for medical exposures, including radiation doses, and shall ensure that these are available to the referrer
    (b) quality assurance programmes for standard operating procedures
    (c) diagnostic reference levels for radiodiagnostic examinations falling within regulation 3(a), (b), (c) and (e) having regard to European diagnostic reference levels where available
    (d) dose constraints for biomedical and medical research programmes falling within regulation 3(d) where no direct medical benefit for the individual is expected from the exposure.

4. The employer shall take steps to ensure that every practitioner or operator engaged by the employer to carry out medical exposures or any practical aspect of such exposures:

   (a) complies with the provisions of regulation 11(1); and

   (b) undertakes continuing education and training after qualification including, in the case of clinical use of new techniques, training related to these techniques and the relevant radiation protection requirements; or

   (c) where the employer is concurrently practitioner or operator, he shall himself ensure that he undertakes such continuing education and training as may be appropriate.

5. Where the employer knows or has reason to believe that an incident has or may have occurred in which a person, while undergoing a medical exposure was, otherwise than as a result of a malfunction or defect in equipment, exposed to ionizing radiation to an extent much greater than intended, he shall make an immediate preliminary investigation of the incident and, unless that investigation shows beyond a reasonable doubt that no such overexposure has occurred, he shall forthwith notify the appropriate authority and make or arrange for a detailed investigation of the circumstances of the exposure and an assessment of the dose received.

6. The employer shall undertake appropriate reviews whenever diagnostic reference levels are consistently exceeded and ensure that corrective action is taken where appropriate.

5. Duties of the practitioner, operator and referrer

1. The practitioner and the operator shall comply with the employer's procedures.

2. The practitioner shall be responsible for the justification of a medical exposure and such other aspects of a medical exposure as is provided for in these Regulations.

3. Practical aspects of a medical exposure or part of it may be allocated in accordance with the employer's procedures by the employer or the practitioner, as appropriate, to one or more individuals entitled to act in this respect in a recognized field of specialization.

4. The operator shall be responsible for each and every practical aspect which he carries out as well as for any authorization given pursuant to regulation 6(5) where such authorization is not made in accordance with the guidelines referred to in regulation 6(5).

5. The referrer shall supply the practitioner with sufficient medical data (such as previous diagnostic information or medical records) relevant to the medical exposure requested by the referrer to enable the practitioner to decide on whether there is a sufficient net benefit as required by regulation 6(1)(a).

6. The practitioner and the operator shall cooperate, regarding practical aspects, with other specialists and staff involved in a medical exposure, as appropriate.

7. For the avoidance of doubt, where a person acts as employer, referrer, practitioner and operator concurrently (or in any combination of these roles) he shall comply with all the duties placed on employers, referrers, practitioners or operators under these Regulations accordingly.

6. Justification of Individual Medical Exposures

1. No person shall carry out a medical exposure unless:
   - (a) it has been justified by the practitioner as showing a sufficient net benefit giving appropriate weight to the matters set out in paragraph (2); and
   - (b) it has been authorized by the practitioner or, where paragraph (5) applies, the operator; and
   - (c) in the case of a medical or biomedical exposure as referred to in regulation 3(d), it has been approved by an ethics committee; and
   - (d) in the case of an exposure falling within regulation 3(e), it complies with the employer's procedures for such exposures; and
   - (e) in the case of a female of child-bearing age, he has enquired whether she is pregnant or breast feeding, if relevant.

2. The matters referred to in paragraph (1)(a) are:
   - (a) the specific objectives of the exposure and the characteristics of the individual involved
   - (b) the total potential diagnostic or therapeutic benefits, including the direct health benefits to the individual and the benefits to society, of the exposure
   - (c) the individual detriment that the exposure may cause and
   - (d) the efficacy, benefits and risk of available alternative techniques having the same objective but involving no or less exposure to ionizing radiation.

3. In considering the weight to be given to the matters referred to in paragraph (2), the practitioner justifying an exposure pursuant to paragraph (1)(a) shall pay special attention to:
   - (a) exposures on medico-legal grounds
   - (b) exposures that have no direct health benefit for the individuals undergoing the exposure and
   - (c) the urgency of the exposure, where appropriate, in cases involving:
     - (i) a female where pregnancy cannot be excluded, in particular if abdominal and pelvic regions are involved, taking into account the exposure of both the expectant mother and the unborn child and

      (ii) a female who is breast feeding and who undergoes a nuclear medicine exposure, taking into account the exposure of both the female and the child.

4. In deciding whether to justify an exposure under paragraph (1)(a) the practitioner shall take account of any data supplied by the referrer pursuant to regulation 5(5) and shall consider such data in order to avoid unnecessary exposure.

5. Where it is not practicable for the practitioner to authorize an exposure as required by paragraph (1)(b), the operator shall do so in accordance with guidelines issued by the practitioner.

7. Optimization

1. In relation to all medical exposures to which these Regulations apply except radiotherapeutic procedures, the practitioner and the operator, to the extent of their respective involvement in a medical exposure, shall ensure that doses arising from the exposure are kept as low as reasonably practicable consistent with the intended purpose.

2. In relation to all medical exposures for radiotherapeutic purposes the practitioner shall ensure that exposures of target volumes are individually planned, taking into account that doses of non-target volumes and tissues shall be as low as reasonably practicable and consistent with the intended radiotherapeutic purpose of the exposure.

3. Without prejudice to paragraphs (1) and (2), the operator shall select equipment and methods to ensure that for each medical exposure the dose of ionizing radiation to the individual undergoing the exposure is as low as reasonably practicable and consistent with the intended diagnostic or therapeutic purpose and in doing so shall pay special attention to:

    (a) quality assurance

    (b) assessment of patient dose or administered activity and

    (c) adherence to diagnostic reference levels for radiodiagnostic examinations falling within regulation 3(a), (b), (c) and (e) as set out in the employer's procedures.

4. For each medical or biomedical research programme falling within regulation 3(d), the employer's procedures shall provide that:

    (a) the individuals concerned participate voluntarily in the research programme

    (b) the individuals concerned are informed in advance about the risks of the exposure

    (c) the dose constraint set down in the employer's procedures for individuals for whom no direct medical benefit is expected from the exposure is adhered to and

    (d) individual target levels of doses are planned by the practitioner for patients who voluntarily undergo an experimental diagnostic or therapeutic practice from which the patients are expected to receive a diagnostic or therapeutic benefit.

5. In the case of patients undergoing treatment or diagnosis with radioactive medicinal products, the employer's procedures shall provide that, where appropriate, written instructions and information are provided to:
   (a) the patient, where he has capacity to consent to the treatment or diagnostic procedure or
   (b) where the patient is a child who lacks capacity so to consent, the person with parental responsibility for the child or
   (c) where the patient is an adult who lacks capacity so to consent, the person who appears to the practitioner to be the most appropriate person.

6. The instructions and information referred to in paragraph (5) shall:
   (a) specify how doses resulting from the patient's exposure can be restricted as far as reasonably possible so as to protect persons in contact with the patient
   (b) set out the risks associated with ionizing radiation and
   (c) be provided to the patient or other person specified in paragraph (5) as appropriate prior to the patient leaving the hospital or other place where the medical exposure was carried out.

7. In complying with the obligations under this regulation, the practitioner and the operator shall pay special attention to:
   (a) the need to keep doses arising from medico-legal exposures as low as reasonably practicable
   (b) medical exposures of children
   (c) medical exposures as part of a health screening programme
   (d) medical exposures involving high doses to the patient
   (e) where appropriate, females in whom pregnancy cannot be excluded and who are undergoing a medical exposure, in particular if abdominal and pelvic regions are involved, taking into account the exposure of both the expectant mother and the unborn child and
   (f) where appropriate, females who are breast feeding and who are undergoing exposures in nuclear medicine, taking into account the exposure of both the female and the child.

8. The employer shall take steps to ensure that a clinical evaluation of the outcome of each medical exposure, is recorded in accordance with the employer's procedures or, where the employer is concurrently practitioner or operator, shall so record a clinical evaluation, including, where appropriate, factors relevant to patient dose.

9. In the case of fluoroscopy:

   (a) the operator shall ensure that examinations without devices to control the dose rate are limited to justified circumstances and

   (b) no person shall carry out an examination without an image intensification or equivalent technique.

8. Clinical audit

The employer's procedures shall include provision for the carrying out of clinical audit as appropriate.

9. Expert advice

1. The employer shall ensure that a medical physics expert shall be involved in every medical exposure to which these Regulations apply in accordance with paragraph (2).

2. A medical physics expert shall be:

   (a) closely involved in every radiotherapeutic practice other than standardized therapeutic nuclear medicine practices

   (b) available in standardized therapeutic nuclear medicine practices and in diagnostic nuclear medicine practices

   (c) involved as appropriate for consultation on optimization, including patient dosimetry and quality assurance, and to give advice on matters relating to radiation protection concerning medical exposure, as required, in all other radiological practices.

10. Equipment

1. The employer shall draw up, keep up-to-date and preserve at each radiological installation an inventory of equipment at that installation and, when so requested, shall furnish it to the appropriate authority.

2. The inventory referred to in paragraph (1) shall contain the following information:

   (a) name of manufacturer

   (b) model number

   (c) serial number or other unique identifier

   (d) year of manufacture and

   (e) year of installation.

3. The employer shall ensure that equipment at each radiological installation is limited to the amount necessary for the proper carrying out of medical exposures at that installation.

11. Training

1. Subject to the following provisions of this regulation no practitioner or operator shall carry out a medical exposure or any practical aspect without having been adequately trained.

2. A certificate issued by an institute or person competent to award degrees or diplomas or to provide other evidence of training shall, if such certificate so attests, be sufficient proof that the person to whom it has been issued has been adequately trained.

3. Nothing in paragraph (1) above shall prevent a person from participating in practical aspects of the procedure as part of practical training if this is done under the supervision of a person who himself is adequately trained.

4. The employer shall keep and have available for inspection by the appropriate authority an up-to-date record of all training undertaken by all practitioners and operators engaged by him to carry out medical exposures or any practical aspect of such exposures or, where the employer is concurrently practitioner or operator, of his own training, showing the date or dates on which training qualifying as adequate training was completed and the nature of the training.

5. Where the employer enters into a contract with another to engage a practitioner or operator otherwise employed by that other, the latter shall be responsible for keeping the records required by paragraph (4) and shall supply such records to the employer forthwith upon request.

12. Enforcement

1. The provisions of these Regulations shall be enforced as if they were health and safety regulations made under section 15 of the Health and Safety at Work etc. Act 1974 and, except as provided in paragraph (2), the provisions of that Act, as regards enforcement and offences, shall apply for the purposes of these Regulations.

2. The enforcing authority for the purposes of these Regulations shall be the appropriate authority.

13. Defence of due diligence

In any proceedings against any person for an offence consisting of the contravention of these Regulations it shall be a defence for that person to show that he took all reasonable steps and exercised all due diligence to avoid committing the offence.

SCHEDULE 1

Regulation 4(1)

Employer's procedures
The written procedures for medical exposures shall include:

1. procedures to identify correctly the individual to be exposed to ionizing radiation

2. procedures to identify individuals entitled to act as referrer or practitioner or operator

3. procedures to be observed in the case of medico-legal exposures

4. procedures for making enquiries of females of child-bearing age to establish whether the individual is or may be pregnant or breast feeding

5. procedures to ensure that quality assurance programmes are followed

6. procedures for the assessment of patient dose and administered activity

7. procedures for the use of diagnostic reference levels established by the employer for radiodiagnostic examinations falling within regulation 3(a), (b), (c) and (e), specifying that these are expected not to be exceeded for standard procedures when good and normal practice regarding diagnostic and technical performance is applied

8. procedures for determining whether the practitioner or operator is required to effect one or more of the matters set out in regulation 7(4) including criteria on how to effect those matters and in particular procedures for the use of dose constraints established by the employer for biomedical and medical research programmes falling within regulation 3(d) where no direct medical benefit for the individual is expected from the exposure

9. procedures for the giving of information and written instructions as referred to in regulation 7(5)

10. procedures for the carrying out and recording of an evaluation for each medical exposure including, where appropriate, factors relevant to patient dose

11. procedures to ensure that the probability and magnitude of accidental or unintended doses to patients from radiological practices are reduced so far as reasonably practicable.

SCHEDULE 2

Regulation 2(1)

Adequate training

Practitioners and operators shall have successfully completed training, including theoretical knowledge and practical experience, in:

1. such of the subjects detailed in section A as are relevant to their functions as practitioner or operator and

2. such of the subjects detailed in section B as are relevant to their specific area of practice.

A. Radiation production, radiation protection and statutory obligations relating to ionizing radiations

1. Fundamental physics of radiation
    1.1. Properties of radiation
        Attenuation of ionizing radiation
        Scattering and absorption
    1.2. Radiation hazards and dosimetry
        Biological effects of radiation
        Risks/benefits of radiation
        Dose optimization
        Absorbed dose, dose equivalent, effective dose and their
            units
    1.3. Special attention areas
        Pregnancy and potential pregnancy
        Infants and children
        Medical and biomedical research
        Health screening
        High dose techniques
2. Management and radiation protection of the patient
    2.1 Patient selection
        Justification of the individual exposure
        Patient identification and consent
        Use of existing appropriate radiological information
        Alternative techniques
        Clinical evaluation of outcome
        Medico-legal issues
    2.2 Radiation protection
        General radiation protection
        Use of radiation protection devices
        – Patient
        – Personal
        Procedures for untoward incidents involving overexposure to
            ionizing radiation
3. Statutory requirements and advisory aspects
    3.1. Statutory requirements and non-statutory recommendations
        Regulations
        Local rules and procedures
        Individual responsibilities relating to medical exposures
        Responsibility for radiation safety
        Routine inspection and testing of equipment
        Notification of faults and health department hazard
            warnings
        Clinical audit

B. Diagnostic radiology, radiotherapy and nuclear medicine

4. Diagnostic radiology
    4.1. General
        Fundamentals of radiological anatomy
        Fundamentals of radiological techniques
        Production of X-rays
        Equipment selection and use
        Factors affecting radiation dose
        Dosimetry
        Quality assurance and quality control
    4.2. Specialized techniques
        Image intensification/fluoroscopy
        Digital fluoroscopy
        Computed tomography scanning
        Interventional procedures
        Vascular imaging
    4.3. Fundamentals of image acquisition, etc.
        Image quality vs. radiation dose
        Conventional film processing
        Additional image formats, acquisition, storage and display
    4.4. Contrast media
        Non-ionic and ionic
        Use and preparation
        Contraindications to the use of contrast media
        Use of automatic injection devices

5. Radiotherapy
    5.1. General
        Production of ionizing radiations
        Use of radiotherapy
        – Benign disease
        – Malignant disease
        – External beam
        – Brachytherapy
    5.2. Radiobiological aspects for radiotherapy
        Fractionation
        Dose rate
        Radiosensitization
        Target volumes
    5.3. Practical aspects for radiotherapy
        Equipment
        Treatment planning
    5.4. Radiation protection specific to radiotherapy
        Side effects – early and late
        Toxicity
        Assessment of efficacy

6. Nuclear medicine
   6.1. General
      Atomic structure and radioactivity
      Radioactive decay
      The tracer principle
      Fundamentals of diagnostic use
      Fundamentals of therapeutic use
      – Dose rate
      – Fractionation
      – Radiobiology aspects
   6.2. Principles of radiation detection, instrumentation and equipment
      Types of systems
      Image acquisition, storage and display
      Quality assurance and quality control
   6.3. Radiopharmaceuticals
      Calibration
      Working practices in the radiopharmacy
      Preparation of individual doses
      Documentation
   6.4. Radiation protection specific to nuclear medicine
      Conception, pregnancy and breast feeding
      Arrangements for radioactive patients
      Disposal procedures for radioactive waste

Reference

1. Crown copyright 2000. With the permission of the Controller of Her Majesty's Stationery Office.

Index

Page numbers followed by 'f' indicate figures, 't' indicate tables, and 'b' indicate boxes.

C